Inside the AIDS Fight

Inside the AIDS Fight

*Memoir of an Epidemiologist
at the Pandemic Front Lines*

HARRY W. HAVERKOS, M.D.

Foreword by Dale Lawrence, M.D.

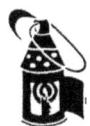

McFarland & Company, Inc., Publishers
Jefferson, North Carolina

The author utilized the artificial intelligence software ChatGPT in editing this work prior to delivering the manuscript to the publisher. The composition of the text is his own.

Portions of this work appeared in Harry W. Haverkos, *On the Front Lines of the AIDS Pandemic*. Saarbrücken: LAP Lambert Academic Publishing, 2012. Copyright Harry W. Haverkos.

ISBN (print) 978-1-4766-9614-0
ISBN (ebook) 978-1-4766-5440-9

LIBRARY OF CONGRESS CATALOGING DATA ARE AVAILABLE

Library of Congress Control Number 2025018267

© 2025 Harry W. Haverkos. All rights reserved

No part of this book may be reproduced or transmitted in any form or by any means, electronic or mechanical, including photocopying or recording, or by any information storage and retrieval system, without permission in writing from the publisher.

Front cover images: Dr. Harry Haverkos with bust of Dr. Moricz Kaposi, University of Vienna, Austria (photograph by Dr. Lynne Haverkos; 1995); *background* © janews/Shutterstock.

Printed in the United States of America

McFarland & Company, Inc., Publishers
Box 611, Jefferson, North Carolina 28640
www.mcfarlandpub.com

In loving memory
of Lynne M. Haverkos, M.D., M.P.H.
(1951–2023)
Medical school classmate, soulmate,
and cherished wife of 45 years

Acknowledgments

I express my gratitude to the following individuals for their invaluable assistance and encouragement: Carolyn Arakaki, Dr. Barry Blinderman, Brandon Brauer, Colleen Brauer, Dr. Dan Burnett, Dr. Zachary Brooks, Dr. Richard Byyny, Bridget Clark, Dr. Kathryn Clark, Paul Clark, Dr. James Curran, Dr. Eric Deussing, Dr. Peter Drotman, Dr. Jay Epstein, Dr. Steven Gitterman, Dr. Michael Gorman, Daniel Haverkos, Dr. Lynne Haverkos, Rebecca Haverkos, Bob Hersh, Mary Hilspertshauser, Don Jaspers, Dr. Tom Jernigan, Dr. Melanie Kerber, Dr. Mark Kortepeter, Dr. Dale Lawrence, Brent Leung, Ralph Lindeman, Sophia Lyons, Dee Martinez, Dr. Heather Miller, Dr. Andrew Moss, Fran Niehaus, Dr. Steve Patterson, Dr. Jim Quinn, Dr. Vern Schinski, Laura Sturza, Mehmet Tamay, Dr. Sten Vermund, Dr. Bryant Webber, and Dr. Hao Zhang.

Special appreciation goes to Dr. Jim Quinn for his prompt and insightful suggestions, diligently reviewing each chapter draft. I extend heartfelt thanks to Bridget Clark for her work on the index; to Colleen Brauer for her expertise in graphic design and compiling the manuscript for the publisher; and to Laura Sturza, my writing instructor.

Table of Contents

Acknowledgments vi
Foreword by Dale Lawrence, M.D. 1
Abbreviations 3
Preface 7
Prologue 10

1. The Emergence of AIDS 11
2. Joining the Epidemic Intelligence Service (EIS) 20
3. Surveillance: Gathering Information for Action 33
4. National Study of Gay Men 47
5. The Search for the AIDS Virus 59
6. HIV Transmission Via Blood 71
7. Workplace Transmission Concerns 84
8. Haitian Connections 97
9. Out of Africa? 108
10. Nitrite Inhalants and Kaposi's Sarcoma 122
11. Early Attempts at Treatment 131
12. A Health Science Administrator at the National Institutes of Health (NIH) 139
13. The Multicenter AIDS Cohort Study (MACS) 146
14. U.S. Army and Heterosexual Transmission 163
15. HIV Therapy: HPA-23 to AZT 173
16. What Causes Kaposi's Sarcoma? 185

17. Paradigm Shift: From Koch's Postulates to Rothman's Sufficient Causal Theory	203
18. Multifactorial Causes of Infectious and Chronic Diseases	222
Epilogue	234
Appendix A: Report Form—AIDS Surveillance	237
Appendix B: Questionnaire—AIDS Case-control Study	240
Appendix C: Leading Causes of Death in the United States Since 1900	253
Chapter Notes	255
Bibliography	271
Index	275

Foreword

by Dale Lawrence, M.D.

This memoir by Dr. Harry Haverkos unveils a series of events that unfolded during a period of national and global bewilderment, as the world grappled with the emergence of a new and universally fatal disease with uncertain transmission routes. Beginning his heroic investigations in 1981 at the CDC and collaborating with shocked physician-epidemiologists, Dr. Haverkos shares his own and others' contributions to controlling a pandemic unparalleled in modern medical history. I had the privilege of participating in the early AIDS investigations alongside him, which not only changed history but garnered retrospective acclaim. Witnessing his career span various agencies of the United States Public Health Service, the U.S. Department of Health and Human Services, and the Walter Reed Army Medical Center in Washington, D.C., was truly remarkable.

The AIDS pandemic persists, still claiming 630,000 lives globally in 2022 (World Health Organization estimate). However, the exponential growth and spread in the first half-decade seemed to foretell that the next four or more decades (1981–2024) might be an unparalleled global catastrophe.

Dr. Haverkos and others conducted investigations that paved the way for the implementation of epidemiologically guided preventive measures to curtail the transmission of HIV, even before the virus was officially identified. Subsequent to the identification of the agent, extensive therapeutic clinical research was undertaken to suppress patients' HIV and reduce its transmissibility.

The legacy of the AIDS pandemic goes beyond medical advancements, encompassing a profound transformation of society. This includes the influential impact on health policy, medical research, legal and judicial perceptions, and patient self-advocacy. The dynamics of patients' fear and isolation prompted the establishment of collaborative partnerships with medical scientists, clinicians, and others, facilitating discoveries and service delivery. This collaborative effort extended globally through initiatives such as the President's Emergency Plan for AIDS Relief (PEPFAR), continuing to shape responses to the present day.

Dr. Haverkos's undergraduate and medical education, combined with his specialty training and research, uniquely positioned him for a "date with destiny." The memoir recounts over 30 years of career experiences, providing an unparalleled perspective on the sweep of history. This history he recounts is composed of individual ideas, investigations, conversations, decisions, actions, and coincidences. In this narrative journey, Dr. Haverkos reveals previously unexplored moments that kept shaping the trajectory of the AIDS pandemic.

Throughout his career, spanning individual and organizational roles, Dr. Haverkos dedicated himself to combating AIDS, leaving an indelible mark on the unfolding history of this global health crisis.

Dale Lawrence, M.D., M.P.H., Captain (ret.), U.S. Public Health Service, Epidemic Intelligence Service, 1973.

Abbreviations

Abbreviation	Explanation
ACE	Angiotensin-converting enzyme
ACTG	AIDS Clinical Trials Group
ACT-UP	AIDS Coalition to Unleash Power
ARC	Addiction Research Center, Baltimore, Maryland
ARC	AIDS-related complex
ARC	American Red Cross
AZT	Azidothymidine
CABG	Coronary Artery Bypass Grafting
CDC	Communicable Disease Center, 1946–1966 (National Communicable Disease Center, 1967–1970 Center for Disease Control, 1970–1992 Centers for Disease Control, 1992–present)
CDER	Center for Drug Evaluation and Research
CHD	Coronary Heart Disease
CMV	Cytomegalovirus
DAVDP	Division of Anti-Viral Drug Products
DDT	Dichlordiphenyltrichloroethene
EIS	Epidemic Intelligence Service
FDA	Food and Drug Administration
FSW	Food-services worker
GRID	Gay-related immunodeficiency
HAV	Hepatitis A virus
HBV	Hepatitis B virus
HCV	Hepatitis C virus

Abbreviation	Explanation
HCW	Health care worker
HHS	Health and Human Services
HHV-8	Human herpes virus, type 8
HIV	Human immunodeficiencey virus
HSV-1	Herpes simplex virus, type 1
HSV-2	Herpes simplex virus, type 2
HTLV-I	Human T-lymphotrophic virus, type 1
HTLV-II	Human T-lymphotrophic virus, type 2
HTLV-III	Human T-lymphotrophic virus, type 3
IARC	International Agency for Research on Cancer
IHA	Indirect hemagglutination assay
IND	Investigational New Drug
JAMA	*Journal of the American Medical Association*
KS	Kaposi's sarcoma
KSOI	Kaposi's sarcoma and opportunistic infections
LAV	Lymphadenopathy-associated virus, 1983 (Lymphadenopathy AIDS virus, 1986)
LBGTQ	Lesbian, Bisexual, Gay, Transgender, Queer
LSD	Lysergic acid diethylamide
MACS	Multicenter AIDS Cohort Study
MAI	*Mycobacterium avium-intracellulare*
MCOT	Medical College of Ohio at Toledo
MMWR	Morbidity and Mortality Weekly Report
MSM	Men who have sex with men
NCI	National Cancer Institute
NDA	New Drug Application
NEJM	*New England Journal of Medicine*
NIAID	National Institute of Allergy and Infectious Diseases
NIDA	National Institute on Drug Abuse
NIH	National Institutes of Health
NIR	No increased risk
PCP	*Pneumocystis carinii* pneumonia
PHS	Public Health Service

Abbreviations

Abbreviation	Explanation
Projet SIDA	AIDS Project
PSW	Personal services worker
SEER	Surveillance, Epidemiology, and End Results
SIVcpz	Simian immunodeficiency virus-chimpanzee
SV40	Simian virus, type 40
TB	Tuberculosis
TSS	Toxic shock syndrome
USPSTF	United States Preventive Services Task Force
USU	Uniformed Services University of the Health Sciences
VZV	Varicella-zoster virus
WHO	World Health Organization

Preface

This volume serves as a memoir, blending science, history, detective storytelling, and coming-of-age narrative. Providing a unique insider's perspective on the AIDS fight, it traces the journey from my initial encounter with an AIDS patient in 1980 to the groundbreaking moment when French virologists received the Nobel Prize in 2008. The narrative unfolds the relentless pursuit of understanding and combating the AIDS pandemic.

Advocating for a paradigm shift in understanding AIDS, this book challenges the notions of HIV as the sole cause, as per Robert Koch's postulates. Instead, it embraces Kenneth Rothman's sufficient-component cause model, asserting that AIDS, like many chronic diseases, has a multifactorial etiology. By presenting this perspective, the book encourages a more nuanced understanding of infectious diseases, moving away from the monolithic view of the 19th century and embracing the complexities of the present day.

I credit my fascination with infectious diseases to Dr. Bruce Ribner, an infectious disease physician at the Medical College of Ohio at Toledo. During a month-long elective as a medical student in the fall of 1975, I worked closely with Dr. Ribner. Each day, we saw patients together, and he encouraged me to read classic articles on infectious diseases like "fever of unknown origin," "subacute bacterial endocarditis," and "streptomycin treatment for tuberculosis," sending me to the library each night.

Upon graduating in June 1976, I began an internal medicine internship at Akron City Hospital in Akron, Ohio. The summer of 1976 presented challenges with Legionnaires' disease, the swine flu epidemic, and Guillain-Barré syndrome. This period heightened my awareness of infectious diseases, and I subscribed to the Center for Disease Control (CDC) publication *Morbidity and Mortality Weekly Report* (*MMWR*), recognizing the CDC's pivotal role in those outbreaks.

Following a three-year residency in internal medicine at Akron, I pursued a two-year research fellowship in infectious diseases at the University of Pittsburgh. My research focused on opportunistic infections among cancer patients and organ transplant recipients, particularly kidney and heart transplant recipients, and interferon therapy for herpesviruses and papillomaviruses.

In October 1980, as I sought infectious disease positions in the Midwest, Dr. Ribner suggested exploring opportunities at the CDC and the Epidemic Intelligence Service, marking a pivotal moment in my career trajectory.

Origins of the CDC

During World War II, the Public Health Service took on the responsibility of malaria control in areas surrounding military camps and training facilities in the United States, mostly concentrated in the South. The Malaria Control in War Areas program, based in Atlanta, was established to oversee this effort. Throughout the war, the program introduced DDT (dichlordiphenyltrichloroethene) for mosquito control and expanded its focus to include other insect-borne diseases like dengue, typhus, and yellow fever. This service continued postwar and was renamed the Communicable Disease Center (CDC) in 1946. Over time, the CDC's mission expanded beyond infectious diseases to cover chronic diseases, nutrition, and environmental and occupational health. In 1970, the name was changed to the Center for Disease Control (CDC) to reflect its broader scope, and in 1992, it became the Centers for Disease Control and Prevention (CDC).[1]

The Epidemic Intelligence Service (EIS), established in 1951 during the Korean War, is a two-year applied epidemiology training program within the CDC. EIS officers, including myself, often enter the U.S. Public Health Service Commissioned Corps, a uniformed service initially associated with the U.S. Navy. EIS officers serve as disease detectives, working alongside subject matter experts on the front lines of public health.[2]

In October 1980, I applied to the CDC's EIS program but was informed that I had missed the September 1 deadline for the class starting in July 1981. However, in November 1980, Ronald Reagan won the presidential election and pledged to cut several government programs, including funding for the CDC. Subsequently, some applicants withdrew their applications for the class of 1981. Taking advantage of this shift, I was invited for an interview in Atlanta on December 8, 1980, and received an offer for an EIS position just two days later.

In July 1981, Dr. James Curran invited me to join a task force on Kaposi's sarcoma and opportunistic infections (KSOI) at the CDC. He informed me that my work would focus on gay men.

Preface

This journey through the AIDS pandemic has undeniably been the most impactful and transformative experience of my life, shaping the trajectory of my entire career. The profound influence of this global health crisis has not only left an indelible mark on my personal journey but has also served as a catalyst for my professional pursuits, motivating me to contribute meaningfully to the field. The challenges and lessons learned from navigating the complexities of the AIDS pandemic have become integral to my professional growth and commitment to making a positive impact in the realm of public health.

Prologue

Back in 1983, the world was just starting to learn about a novel and frightening disease called AIDS. People didn't know much about it, and it was causing a lot of fear and confusion. I was working at the CDC, and my boss, Jim Curran, was too busy to give a talk in Italy about it, so I went instead.

Before I left for Italy, a colleague named Paul Pinsky told me something very important. He had discovered a key difference between two common problems in AIDS patients: Kaposi's sarcoma (a type of cancer) and a lung infection called *Pneumocystis*. The answer lay in a single variable: the enigmatic "poppers." Gay men took these drugs to enhance their sexual experiences.

In Italy, a scientist named Jean-Claude Chermann talked about a new virus called lymphadenopathy-associated virus (LAV), which later became known as HIV. This virus seemed crucial to understanding AIDS.

On my way back to the United States, I started connecting the dots. I became convinced that HIV was the missing piece we were looking for in understanding AIDS. But questions lingered in my thoughts. What role did those volatile nitrites, the "poppers," play in the intricate tapestry of AIDS? Could they be a contributing factor, or cofactor, in the malevolence of AIDS-related Kaposi's sarcoma?

Little did I know that my hypothesis would pave the way for a tumultuous journey, one filled with resistance, skepticism, and the relentless pursuit of knowledge. The stage was set, and I stood on the precipice of discovery, ready to unveil a truth that could reshape the way we thought about infectious diseases.

1

The Emergence of AIDS

June 5, 1981. I read the *Morbidity and Mortality Weekly Report* about case-patients of *Pneumocystis* pneumonia (PCP) in Los Angeles. The report detailed five homosexual men, aged 29 to 36, who had been diagnosed with PCP between October 1980 and May 1981. Tragically, two of them had already passed away. All five men had evidence of cytomegalovirus infection and were known to abuse nitrite inhalants.[1]

I was astonished by the similarities between these patients and a young man I had already treated at the University of Pittsburgh hospital six months earlier. He was the first patient I encountered who would later be diagnosed with AIDS (Acquired Immune Deficiency Syndrome).

December 30, 1980. I was summoned to the microbiology lab to review an open lung biopsy from a 36-year-old man suffering from pneumonia. The biopsy confirmed the presence of *Pneumocystis carinii* (see figure 1). At the time, I was a second-year infectious diseases fellow at University Hospital in Pittsburgh, Pennsylvania, having recently returned from spending the holidays with my family in Ohio.

I visited the patient to assess his condition. E.M. was experiencing shortness of breath and drowsiness following the procedure, so I referred to his medical chart to gather his history. He worked as a manager at a local business and had been unwell for the past 18 months. In the summer of 1979, he weighed over 300 pounds and had developed intermittent fevers and weight loss. He had seen his primary care physician multiple times, but they were unable to provide a diagnosis. When he developed a cough and shortness of breath, he was diagnosed with community-acquired pneumonia. Despite two weeks of antibiotic treatment, his condition did not improve, leading to the open lung biopsy. During the examination, I detected signs of pneumonia while listening to his chest, and I also noticed a few swollen lymph nodes in his neck and armpits during the physical examination. His chest X-ray revealed bilateral amorphous shadows, indicating "whitening" of both lung sides.

At the time, I knew that *Pneumocystis carinii* pneumonia (PCP) was

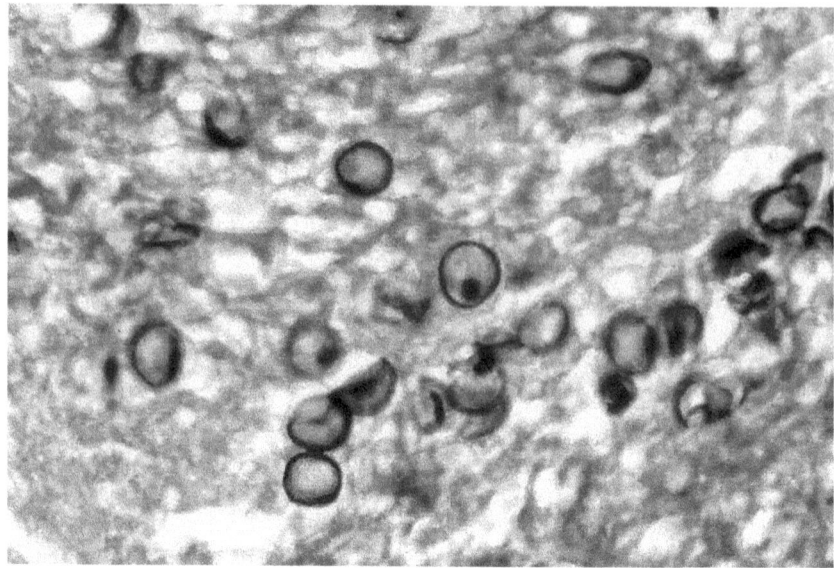

This image shows lung tissue from an AIDS patient with pneumocystosis, stained with methenamine silver. It reveals the distinct cup-shaped forms and dot-like cysts of *Pneumocystis jiroveci* (formerly *Pneumocystis carinii*) (Public Health Images Library [PHIL] ID # 960 CDC/Dr. Edwin Ewing, Jr., 1984).

a rare cause of pneumonia. I had treated another patient—a kidney transplant recipient—for PCP earlier in the year and was in the process of collecting case-patients of pneumonia among immunocompromised patients for a research project. I understood that *Pneumocystis* was an "opportunistic" parasite, meaning it only caused pneumonia in individuals with compromised immune systems. This led me to suspect that E.M. might have a lymphoma, a type of cancer affecting the lymph nodes.

I recommended the first-line therapy for PCP, trimethoprim-sulfamethoxazole, and suggested conducting tests to identify the cause of immunosuppression, such as lymphoma. However, the patient did not respond to the sulfa treatment, and his blood oxygen levels worsened. Despite further testing, we couldn't find any lymphoma or cancer.

During our weekly infectious diseases grand rounds, I presented the patient's medical history to a group of University of Pittsburgh infectious diseases experts, including attending staff, fellows, residents, microbiologists, and other interested individuals. We then visited the patient's bedside where Dr. Monto Ho, our chief, examined him. Dr. Ho made two suggestions: first, he noticed that the open lung biopsy also showed cytomegalovirus, a type of herpesvirus. This raised the question of whether cytomegalovirus infection could cause severe immune suppression.

Second, Dr. Ho recommended contacting the CDC in Atlanta to obtain pentamidine isethionate, a rarely used injectable drug for PCP.

As a public health service, the CDC stored drugs for life-threatening infections, including pentamidine. I called the CDC and spoke with a technician in the parasitology division. Before releasing the pentamidine to us, she inquired about the cause of the patient's immunocompromised state. I mentioned that we were ruling out lymphoma but withheld the fact that we were uncertain about the underlying cause of immunosuppression. I was concerned that she might not release the drug. Fortunately, we obtained the pentamidine, and over the next two weeks of therapy, the patient's breathing improved, leading to his release from the hospital.

Two months later, the patient returned to University Hospital. Following his earlier discharge in January, he experienced intermittent fevers, diarrhea, weight loss, and dehydration. Upon readmission, he was diagnosed with "gay bowel disease," a sexually transmitted perirectal and rectal infection commonly observed in gay men. It was at this point that I learned he was homosexual and the manager of a local gay bathhouse. Regrettably, I had not obtained an adequate sexual history from the patient in December. He was ultimately diagnosed with amebiasis and giardiasis, two protozoan parasitic infections of the gastrointestinal tract. Fortunately, he responded well to antibiotics and intravenous fluids.

Herpes Viruses

During my infectious diseases fellowship at the University of Pittsburgh from July 1979 to June 1981, I had the privilege of training under Dr. Monto Ho, a renowned expert in herpes viruses. Dr. Ho, originally from Taiwan, held several prestigious positions, including chief of infectious diseases, director of the microbiology laboratory, and head of the School of Public Health. His primary focus was on cytomegalovirus (CMV), a type of herpes virus, and he was particularly interested in studying interferon, a derivative of white blood cells, as a potential experimental therapy for viral infections. Notably, Dr. Ho was part of the team that discovered interferon in the 1950s.

At the time, there were five known human herpesviruses:

1. Herpes simplex virus-1 (HSV-1), commonly known as the "cold sore" virus.
2. Herpes simplex virus-2, responsible for genital herpes.
3. Varicella-zoster virus (VZV), which causes chickenpox and shingles.

4. Epstein-Barr virus (EBV), the culprit behind infectious mononucleosis, also known as the "kissing disease."
5. Cytomegalovirus (CMV), a prevalent infection in the United States that is typically harmless. It is estimated that 50–80 percent of Americans become infected by the age of 40. While most individuals with CMV experience no symptoms or only mild illness, it can cause severe complications in newborns and immunocompromised individuals. CMV is also considered an opportunistic infection, capable of causing life-threatening disease in certain populations.

Research on Herpes Viruses

During my fellowship, my research focused on herpes viruses. In the first year, I was assigned a research project while also initiating my own investigations in the field of infectious diseases. Additionally, I had clinical responsibilities overseeing medical students, interns, and residents in an internal medicine clinic. To broaden my knowledge, I spent time in the microbiology laboratory and other relevant sites like venereal disease and dermatology clinics. I also dedicated effort to learning biostatistics through the School of Public Health.

In July 1979, I participated in my initial weekly meeting for our working group focused on HSV-1 and interferon research. The group consisted of Dr. Ho, Dr. George Pazin, an attending physician from the infectious diseases department, and two microbiologists. One topic of great excitement was an upcoming lead article in the August 2, 1979, edition of the *New England Journal of Medicine* (*NEJM*). This article resulted from a series of observations and randomized placebo-controlled clinical trials conducted by our group.

The trials centered around a surgical treatment developed by Dr. Peter Jannetta, a neurosurgeon at Pitt, for a condition called trigeminal neuralgia or *tic douloureux*. The disorder is characterized by intense facial pain that lasts for a few seconds to several hours and can occur numerous times per day, sometimes even up to a hundred times. It can be severely debilitating and is commonly referred to as the "suicide disease." Triggers for the pain episodes include activities such as eating or talking, as well as exposure to wind or loud noises.

Dr. Janetta hypothesized that the disease stemmed from a pulsating artery coming into contact with the trigeminal or fifth cranial nerve in the head, triggering the pain. He developed a surgical procedure known as microvascular decompression, which involved entering the skull through a small hole behind the ear, identifying the problematic artery, and placing a small pad of inert material, such as Teflon, between the artery and the trigeminal ganglion. Successful implementation of the Janetta procedure provided long-lasting pain relief with minimal to no facial numbness.

However, it was observed that nearly 60 percent of patients developed cold sores shortly after the surgery. Dr. Ho saw this as an ideal opportunity to test human leukocyte interferon. He and his colleagues conducted a series of prospective, randomized, placebo-controlled trials to evaluate the effects of interferon administered before and after surgery. In the August 1979 *NEJM*, they reported that out of 18 patients who received a placebo, 10 (56 percent) developed cold sores. On the other hand, out of 19 patients treated with interferon, cold sores developed in five (26 percent). They concluded that interferon, at a well-tolerated dose, reduced the reactivation of HSV-1 after a potent neurosurgical stimulus.[2]

The *NEJM* reviewers raised a question of whether interferon killed the virus (virucidal) or simply blocked one episode of reactivation (virostatic). The research group suggested that my research project was to duplicate the experiment in rabbits. I would infect rabbits with a herpes virus, reenact neurosurgery, give half interferon and half placebo, and then test for herpes virus at autopsy. I was not excited about spending the next two years operating on rabbits, nor about sacrificing the animals.

I went into the next week's meeting with an alternate proposal. I suggested that instead of the animal study, we telephone all of the patients in the randomized trials and ask them about any subsequent episodes of cold sores. If interferon was virucidal, those assigned to interferon should report significantly fewer cold sores following surgery than those receiving placebo. The group was not excited about my proposal. I convincingly argued that they knew who received placebo or interferon and would be biased in the follow-up assessment, but that I was blinded and should conduct the interviews. I drafted my first research proposal and a list of questions and presented it to the group the following week. It was approved.

Labor Day weekend, 1979. I called the 39 patients who had participated in the studies; 37 answered the phone and my questions. Eighteen of the 37 (49 percent) reported one or more cold sores after returning home after surgery; nine treated with interferon and nine with placebo. Clearly, there was no difference. Interferon was virostatic in that setting.

Dr. Ho was disappointed with the results. He could not accept the finding as valid and told me I could not publish the results. He suggested that there must be some bias or confounding variable that we had not taken into account. He recommended that I reconsider conducting the rabbit experiments. I was flabbergasted.

However, in the spring of 1980, Dr. Ho attended a meeting where another group presented preliminary data suggesting that interferon was virostatic and not virucidal. Dr. Ho rushed to me upon his return and suggested that I prepare the paper immediately and submit it to the *NEJM*, so that we might "beat" the other group. He felt more comfortable with our findings now that a second group had confirmed our results. Our findings were published in the September 18, 1980, *NEJM* correspondence section.[3] It was my first scientific publication.

I learned a great deal from this experience, delving deeper into the intricate world of academic medicine than I had initially anticipated. It was my first encounter with conflict among my medical superiors, but certainly not the last. This experience reaffirmed my faith in the scientific method. Valid results should be replicable by other scientists, demonstrating the results' effectiveness. Moreover, I discovered valuable insights about myself. I realized that I possessed the ability to design clinical studies, execute them, analyze the results, and effectively defend my findings. Perhaps there was a promising future for me in medical research.

Opportunistic Infections

During the summer of 1979, I was searching for additional research projects when an opportunity arose while accompanying Dr. John Dowling, an attending physician specializing in infectious diseases, on clinical rounds. We encountered two immunocompromised patients with pneumonia: one was a kidney transplant recipient, and the other had lymphoma. Dowling provided similar recommendations for both patients. First, he advised minimizing the use of immunosuppressive agents, such as reducing the dosage of steroids used to prevent graft-versus-host disease in the transplant patient, and modifying the dosage of cancer chemotherapy for the lymphoma patient. Second, he emphasized the importance of promptly identifying the cause of the pneumonia to initiate appropriate antibiotic treatment.

The surgeons responsible for the transplant patient promptly followed Dowling's advice, performed an open lung biopsy, and identified *Legionella* pneumonia (Legionnaires' disease) as the cause of the pneumonia. They initiated treatment with erythromycin, the preferred agent for *Legionella*, and the patient recovered successfully. However, the oncologists treating the lymphoma patient opted to administer broad-spectrum antibiotics for one week before conducting an open lung biopsy. Ultimately, they diagnosed the patient with chemical pneumonia, a result of lung inflammation induced by chemotherapy, and the patient unfortunately passed away shortly thereafter.

John Dowling noticed a pattern: surgeons working with transplant recipients tended to follow his advice promptly and perform lung biopsies early, while oncologists typically treated initially with broad-spectrum antibiotics and only proceeded to open lung biopsies after a delay if the patients did not show improvement. This led Dowling to pose the research question: what was the appropriate approach for each patient? Did the timing of open lung biopsy during the course of the disease affect the outcome? He invited others to review the medical charts of patients and compare outcomes, and I took on the challenge.

We identified 59 immunocompromised patients with fever and pulmonary infiltrates who underwent open lung biopsy between February 1975 and June 1981. Among them, 31 patients had leukemia or lymphoma diagnosis (Group A) prior to biopsy, 23 were renal or heart transplant recipients (Group B), and four immunocompromised for other reasons. Notably, we excluded E.M., a gay man with PCP, as he did not meet our case definition. Additionally, we were unable to determine the cause of his immune suppression. Among the patients, nine were diagnosed with PCP through open lung biopsy, with six case-patients in cancer patients and three in transplant recipients. We found no significant difference in survival between Group A and Group B. Overall, 53 percent of the patients survived and were medically discharged from the hospital, indicating that nearly half of immunocompromised patients with pneumonia passed away within a month of diagnosis.[4] While we could not definitively prove which approach was superior in managing immunosuppressed patients with pneumonia, this research provided valuable insights into PCP and other infections that occurred in these patients, as well as the potential biases and confounders inherent in retrospective, nonrandomized clinical trials.

The second year of my fellowship was focused on completing research projects and actively participating in the clinical practice of infectious diseases at four hospitals: the University Hospital, the Veterans' Administration Hospital, Magee's Women's Hospital, and Eye and Ear Hospital. During this year, I served as the leader of the infectious diseases team, composed of medical residents and students, providing infectious diseases consultations 24 hours a day, seven days a week. I alternated months with another infectious diseases fellow, ensuring comprehensive coverage of the service. My responsibilities include daily patient examinations, evaluating new consultations, examining diagnostic samples submitted to the microbiology laboratory, and assessing any new "interesting" isolates from other patients in the hospitals.

From Pittsburgh to Atlanta

My training program in Pittsburgh was scheduled to end on June 30, 1981. In the fall of 1980, I began job hunting and reached out to Dr. Bruce Ribner, an infectious diseases physician at my alma mater, the Medical College of Ohio at Toledo. He recommended a fellowship in the Epidemic Intelligence Service (EIS) at the CDC. I flew to Atlanta on December 8, 1980, for an interview and received a job offer just two days later.

As incoming EIS officers, we attended the CDC annual conference in April and interviewed for various assignments. Following the conference, the EIS "match" process took place over the weekend. It was akin to rushing for fraternities in college. In my class, there were 65 officers vying for approximately 95 available positions. While most positions were at the CDC headquarters in Atlanta, there were also opportunities at city and state health departments, as well as the CDC laboratories across the country. We were encouraged to interview with as many groups as possible.

During the weekend, I had the chance to meet department chiefs, former EIS officers, and laboratory personnel, many of whom were renowned scientists. Among the different groups, I was particularly captivated by the Hospital Infections group in Atlanta and their work on antibacterial drug resistance. With the increasing prevalence of antibiotic resistance on the wards in Pittsburgh, I considered this area to be the most compelling.

Additionally, I was impressed by the ongoing research on hepatitis viruses in Phoenix, Arizona. At the time, we were aware of two forms of hepatitis: acute (hepatitis A virus or HAV) and serum (hepatitis B virus or HBV). Acute hepatitis had a relatively short incubation period of two to six weeks and was transmitted through contaminated food or water. Serum hepatitis, on the other hand, was a chronic form transmitted through sexual behavior, blood transfusion, and sharing needles during drug use.

While the weekend was a whirlwind, one interview that stood out was with Dr. Myron Schulz, the chief of the parasitology epidemiology section. He asked me to describe patients with a parasitic infection that I had cared for. I shared stories about an Asian-born woman with obstruction of the stomach caused by anisakiasis, a parasitic roundworm infection from eating raw fish (sushi), as well as a gay man with *Pneumocystis carinii* pneumonia. As a result, I was matched with parasitology.

After the interviews, I returned to Pittsburgh to complete the final two months of my infectious diseases fellowship. In July, my family and I relocated to Atlanta.

Seeing Our Patient a Third Time

In August 1981, I had the opportunity to see E.M. once again at Emory University Hospital in Atlanta. After leaving Pittsburgh in the spring of 1981, he had relocated to live with relatives in the vicinity of Tallahassee, Florida. However, one evening, he found himself apprehended by the police while driving aimlessly, leading to his admission to a local mental hospital. E.M. exhibited troubling symptoms at this point, including disorientation, a persistent fever, and severe emaciation. Subsequently, he was transferred to Atlanta, where a diagnosis revealed that he was suffering from a disseminated *Mycobacterium avium-intracellulare* infection, yet another opportunistic infection.

During this period, I had joined the CDC and made the move to Atlanta as well. Just a few days before his passing, I had the privilege of visiting E.M. Sadly, he passed away alone, with me being the only visitor during his final days.

2

Joining the Epidemic Intelligence Service (EIS)*

> *Since its founding in 1951 by Alexander Langmuir as a service/training program, the Epidemic Intelligence Service, working out of CDC in Atlanta, Georgia, has sent out more than three thousand officers to combat every imaginable human (and sometimes animal) ailment. These young people—doctors, veterinarians, dentists, statisticians, nurses, microbiologists, academic epidemiologists, sociologists, anthropologists, and now even lawyers—call themselves "shoe leather epidemiologists." EIS officers have ventured over the globe in search of diseases, sometimes in airplanes or jeeps, on bicycles, aboard fragile boats, on dogsleds, atop elephants and camels.*
> —Mark Pendergrast, 2010[1]

Monday, July 6, 1981. I reported to the CDC headquarters in Atlanta to attend a mandatory three-week course consisting of a series of lectures, interactive case studies, and a primer on biostatistics, and to participate in a field study. My EIS class consisted of 65 new officers: 55 physicians, four nurses, three academic epidemiologists, two veterinarians, and an anthropologist. Nine of the physicians were international trainees.

Each year, incoming EIS officers conduct a household survey on an assigned topic to get hands-on or "shoe-leather" experience collecting data on a contemporary public health topic. Performing the survey introduced us to field epidemiology and taught us about systemic or probability sampling. Our field study in the second week was a household survey of injuries and violence in Atlanta. Our class designed a questionnaire and assigned groups of two officers to randomly selected house addresses to conduct the survey.

---

*Chapter 2 adapted from H.W. Haverkos, "A recruit enters the Epidemic Intelligence Service," *The Pharos* 79 (1) (Winter 2016): 36–43.

2. Joining the Epidemic Intelligence Service (EIS)

In the classroom, we studied the well-known 1940 Oswego, New York, church picnic outbreak of gastroenteritis. Out of 80 people attending the picnic, 75 were interviewed, and 46 had developed significant diarrheal disease within 24 hours. The source of the outbreak was identified as vanilla ice cream contaminated by one of its preparers. The exercise introduced us to the steps in the investigation of an outbreak, all of which remain applicable today:

- Identify the potential investigation team and resources, and prepare for field work (e.g., administration, clearance, travel, contacts, designation of lead investigator).
- Establish the existence of an epidemic.
- Verify the diagnosis.
- Construct a working case definition.
- Find case-patients systematically, and develop a line listing of case-patients.
- Perform descriptive epidemiology (i.e., orient the data by time, place and person).
- Develop hypotheses that explain the specific exposures that may cause disease.
- Evaluate these hypotheses by appropriate statistical methods using data collected.
- As necessary, reconsider/refine hypotheses and execute additional studies.
- Implement control and prevention measures as early as possible.
- Communicate findings.
- Maintain surveillance to monitor trends and evaluate control/prevention measures.

Before the first class on Monday, I checked into the epidemiology component of parasitology, my assignment as an EIS officer. My supervisor, Dennis Juranek (EIS 1970), a veterinarian and staff parasitologist, asked me to meet with a Dr. James Curran of the venereal diseases division on Tuesday to discuss a new project.

James "Jim" Curran graduated from the University of Notre Dame in 1966 and the University of Michigan Medical School in 1970. After serving a one-year internship (six months in obstetrics and gynecology and six months in internal medicine), he entered the U.S. Public Health Service to fulfill his military commitment. He was assigned to the Venereal Disease Branch at the CDC, and served in Memphis, Tennessee, and Columbus, Ohio, before returning to Atlanta in 1978 to head the Venereal Diseases Research Branch, CDC.

When I met with Curran, he told me that he and others had been working on a number of new diseases rapidly spreading among gay men in New York and California. The CDC pathologists had already confirmed the diagnosis of Kaposi's sarcoma (KS) and *Pneumocystis carinii* pneumonia (PCP) in several patients from biopsy materials (step 3). They had confirmed that those few case-patients represented an epidemic (step 2). Curran asked me if I had heard anything about it. I told him I knew nothing about KS, but I had seen a few patients with PCP (including one gay male) in Pittsburgh during my infectious diseases fellowship. I told him about my work on open lung biopsies among organ transplant recipients and cancer patients and mentioned that I had read the *MMWR* detailing five case-patients of PCP among gay men in Los Angeles.[2] Curran informed me that he intended to conduct interviews with some of my classmates before reaching a final decision on the new team's staffing. For those selected to join the task force, a willingness to collaborate with gay men and a commitment of at least six months were required. I agreed to these conditions.

As I rose to return to class, Jim, upon reviewing my resume, pointed out our shared alma mater, the University of Notre Dame. He mentioned that we had both narrowly missed witnessing national football championships at Notre Dame by just one semester. Intrigued, I thought he might be an enjoyable colleague.

The next day, Jim contacted me and extended an offer to join the task force on Kaposi's sarcoma and opportunistic infections (KSOI). Without hesitation, I accepted the position. My responsibilities would involve establishing a surveillance system for the emerging diseases, encompassing steps 4, 5, and 6.

Early in the second week of class, he called again to ask how I was coming along with my project; I was unprepared and he was unhappy with me. He told me I had to develop and present a case definition and plan to share with my EIS classmates by the end of the third week of class, when we would all disperse on our field assignments. Later that day he called yet again, this time with welcome news: he had arranged for me to skip classes so I would have the necessary time to complete the assignment.

Step 4—Construct a Working Case Definition

I reported to Jim Curran's office first thing on Monday of the third week. He told me to develop a case definition, suggesting that I review the case reports collected in the spring, read about the diseases being reported, review files on requests for the drug pentamidine isethionate, and talk with Kathy Shands (EIS 1979), who had developed a surveillance system for toxic shock syndrome two years earlier.

2. Joining the Epidemic Intelligence Service (EIS)

From my class notes, I knew that surveillance was "information for action," the ongoing systematic collection, analysis, and interpretation of outcome-specific data essential to the planning, implementation, and evaluation of public health practice. Before counting case-patients, one must decide what to count. A case definition is a set of standard criteria for classifying whether a person has a particular disease, syndrome, or other health condition. I spent Monday and Tuesday in the CDC library, reading about KS and the other diseases considered "opportunistic" infections (OIs), including PCP, toxoplasmosis, disseminated herpes virus infections, tuberculosis, and cryptococcosis.

By the end of the week I proposed the following three-part definition:

- Biopsy-proven Kaposi's sarcoma and/or culture or biopsy-confirmed life-threatening "opportunistic" infections at least moderately predictive of immunosuppression;
- Persons between the ages of 15 and 60 years; and
- No prior evidence of underlying immunosuppression, i.e., cancer diagnosis, organ transplant recipients, or use of steroids or other immunosuppressant agents.

I defined "moderately predictive" of an opportunistic infection as those in which at least 50 percent of case-patients reported in the medical literature had occurred in immunocompromised patients. For PCP, essentially every adult case occurred in an immunosuppressed person. A former EIS officer assigned to parasitology, Peter Walzer (EIS 1970), had reviewed all case-patients of PCP reported to the CDC between 1967 and 1970, and 191 of the 194 case-patients he reviewed were clearly linked to immunosuppression. The three outliers were infants.[3]

Other OIs were not as clear cut. By my calculations, cryptococcal meningitis (a fungal infection of the membranes surrounding the brain and spinal cord) occurred in immunocompromised patients in 50 percent of the reports, and in healthy hosts less than 50 percent of the time, so it barely met the criterion for inclusion. Tuberculosis, on the other hand, occurred predominantly in otherwise healthy individuals and less so (15 to 20 percent) in immunocompromised patients, so it was excluded.

The initial list of OIs included PCP, esophageal candidiasis, cryptococcal meningitis, extensive mucocutaneous herpes simplex virus infections, disseminated infection with Mycobacteria species other than *Mycobacterium* tuberculosis, disseminated strongyloidiasis (roundworm infection), and central nervous system toxoplasmosis (protozoan infection of the brain).

I had never heard of Kaposi's sarcoma, much less seen a case during my clinical training, so I had to do more digging. I learned that dermatologists from NYC and California reported 26 case-patients of KS among young gay men between January 1979 and June 1981, including five fatalities. Prior to 1980, approximately 300 new case-patients of biopsy-proven KS occurred annually in the United States, predominantly among men aged 60 or older and renal transplant recipients. In elderly patients, KS appeared as persistent skin lesions and rarely proved fatal. Those 26 gay men had skin lesions of KS by biopsy, but their disease followed a more fulminant course, with spread to the lungs, stomach and intestines. Seven gay men with KS also had PCP—especially striking since both KS and PCP had never been reported in the same patient before.[4]

In 1872, Moritz Kaposi, a Hungarian-born dermatologist at the University of Vienna, described three fatal case-patients of hemangiosarcoma (blood vessel cancer) in elderly men. Since then the disease has borne his name.

In the early 1900s, KS was described in sub–Saharan Africa in adults, mainly young men, and in children; the male-to-female ratio of case-patients in Africa was five to one. Benign, nodular lesions, limited to the extremities, formed one end of the spectrum; florid, disseminated lesions were at the other end; survival ranged from three to 10 years following presentation. There was a lymphadenopathic subvariant of the African form that affected children at a mean age of three years and the male-to-female ratio was three to one. Italian oncologist Gaetano Giraldo, studying KS in Uganda, linked the sarcoma to a herpes virus using electron microscopy and to cytomegalovirus (CMV) infection using blood tests.

In the 1960s and 1970s, oncologists noticed a third form of KS appearing among immunocompromised patients, such as renal transplant recipients, patients on long-term corticosteroids, and patients who were immunocompromised as a result of some other therapeutic regimens or malignancy. The male-to-female ratio of an iatrogenic form of KS was 2.3 to one; some lesions resolved when immunosuppressants were stopped.[5]

Step 5—Find Case-patients Systematically, and Develop a Line Listing of Case-patients

I met with Kathy Shands to discuss the "passive" surveillance system she developed for toxic shock syndrome. In retrospect, she regretted that she had not conducted "active" surveillance. She developed a case definition for TSS, published a series of case-patients occurring in menstruating women in *MMWR*, and asked individuals to call her if they knew of any additional case-patients matching her definition. She received calls, as anticipated, from physicians and nurses, but also from patients, their relatives, and their neighbors. After TSS was linked to a specific brand of tampons (Rely®) and the link was widely reported in the press, physicians stopped reporting case-patients. It appeared that TSS had disappeared.

Fortunately, "active" surveillance for TSS was conducted in the Midwest. Epidemiologists at the Wisconsin and Minnesota State Health Departments identified chiefs of medicine at selected large hospitals and called them regularly to solicit information on potential new case-patients. These chiefs continued to report new TSS case-patients, even after Rely® tampons were taken off the market. Indeed, it was subsequently determined that TSS was caused by streptococcal and staphylococcal exotoxins (toxins released by bacteria into its surroundings) and that risk factors included not only superabsorbent tampons, such as the Rely® tampon, but also surgery and open wounds infected with specific bacterial agents.

Passive surveillance refers to data supplied to the health department by the source of the data, often based on a known set of rules or regulations stipulating reportable conditions. A review of death certificates, for example, constitutes passive surveillance. Given these criteria, undercounting of case-patients occurs often with passive surveillance systems.

Active surveillance, on the other hand, is initiated by the data collector and involves proactive solicitation of reports, typically from selected healthcare providers, generally in addition to requests for passive reporting. Active surveillance systems are more costly, both economically and in terms of time and effort expended. The data generated, however, are usually more reliable.

My conversation with Dr. Shands convinced me that we needed an active system to supplement passive reporting. I proposed that each EIS officer assigned to a field position identify the largest hospitals in their cities and call on chiefs of infectious diseases, oncology, medicine, and dermatology to tell them about our case-patients of PCP and KS, and find out if they had heard of any similar case-patients at their institutions. They would be contacted at regular intervals, and any case-patients reported to me. Jim Curran approved this plan.

We selected six EIS officers from my class and six cities in which to conduct active surveillance: two cities considered by reputation to have a high percentage of gay men—New York City (Polly Thomas) and Los Angeles (David Auerbach); two cities with a moderate percentage of gay men—Albany and Rochester, New York (John Hanrahan and Alain Roisin, respectively); and two cities with a low percentage of gay men—Tallahassee, Florida (Mike Malison) and Oklahoma City (Diane Dwyer).

Curran contacted another 12 EIS officers, assigned to other cities, and encouraged them to look for new case-patients. He also sent a letter to all state health departments asking them to report any potential case-patients to the CDC and giving them my telephone number as the point of contact (passive surveillance).

I developed a two-page case report form that included the patient's name, age, self-reported sexual orientation, diagnosis, how the diagnosis was made (biopsy or culture), and contact information for the reporting physician (Appendix A). EIS officers completed the forms when referring physicians reported case-patients. We avoided collecting information from patients or family members, partly because that approach had created problems (multiple reports of the same patient) during the TSS investigation and partly because our case definition required a more advanced understanding of immunology, microbiology, and pathology. The report form was easy to complete—mainly a series of check boxes—to keep the phone calls with clinicians as short as possible.

Step 6—Perform Descriptive Epidemiology (More in Chapter 3)

I continued reviewing the case reports that others had collected at the CDC, including the five case-patients reported by Michael Gottlieb in the June 5 *MMWR*. One of Gottlieb's patients had a prior lymphoma and was excluded. The four other men were previously healthy gay men who had PCP, extensive mucosal candidiasis, and multiple viral infections, including CMV; one had KS. Three of the four patients had prolonged and unexplained febrile episodes.

The immune system is a complex network of cells, tissues, organs, and substances they make that fight infectious and other diseases. As an immunologist at UCLA, Gottlieb had conducted extensive immunologic studies on his patients. The underlying defect, he suggested, was a decrease in or depletion of one form of white cells, the T-helper lymphocyte, resulting in a change in the ratio of T-helper lymphocytes to T-suppressor lymphocytes.[6]

Step 7—Develop Hypotheses That Explain the Specific Exposures That May Cause Disease

While I was setting up surveillance, Jim Curran charged Dr. Harold Jaffe (EIS 1981) with listing hypotheses of causation and designing a study to test them (Steps 7 and 8). Jaffe listed his leading hypotheses:

2. Joining the Epidemic Intelligence Service (EIS)

- Cytomegalovirus (CMV)
- An environmental toxin, most likely nitrite inhalants
- Immune overload caused by exposure to multiple infectious agents
- A "new" infectious agent, most likely related to herpes or hepatitis viruses

Cytomegalovirus was at the top of everyone's list. Michael Gottlieb had found evidence of CMV infection in his initial five case-patients. Gaetano Giraldo, working with KS patients in Africa, had found evidence of herpes virus infection in KS tissues, and suggested CMV as the causative agent. But why would CMV be causing an epidemic now? Could it be a new or mutated strain now circulating among gay men? And what was its relationship to immunosuppression: was it causing immunosuppression or taking advantage of another immunosuppressive cause—was CMV the chicken or the egg?

Inhalants containing alkyl nitrites, commonly known as "poppers," were discussed as a possible toxic cause of immunosuppression. Michael Gottlieb noted that all five of his patients had used them. The CDC had conducted a survey of 420 men attending venereal disease clinics in New York, San Francisco, and Atlanta, and found that 85 percent of gay men interviewed reported using poppers at least once in the last five years, compared to just 15 percent of heterosexual men. Jim Curran hoped that poppers or some contaminant of those drugs would be implicated as the causative agent because the solution would then be straightforward.

Nitrite inhalants are commonly abused substances in the United States and Europe—used primarily by gay men, adolescents, and young adults to enhance sexual activity by prolonging penile erection. Alkyl nitrites (e.g., amyl, butyl nitrite) are colorless or yellow liquids at room temperature and are highly volatile. They have a fruity odor (often described as unpleasant) and have been nicknamed "poppers" because of the sound made when glass capsules containing amyl nitrite are crushed. The vasodilatory effect following inhalation of amyl nitrite vapor was identified in 1859 and led to the first report of its clinical application to provide relief for angina pectoris in 1867 by a Scottish medical student, T. Lauder Brunton. Amyl nitrite works by relaxing blood vessels and increasing blood flow to the heart while decreasing its workload. It was the preferred treatment for angina pectoris universally from about 1890 until about 1960, when the nitrates (e.g., nitroglycerin, sublingual tablets, dermally applied ointments, and later, transdermal nitrate patches) replaced amyl nitrite as the preferred treatment for angina pectoris. In the late 1960s, pharmacists and drug manufacturers noted widespread purchases

Left: Chemical structure of amyl nitrite (C5H11NO2). *Right:* Chemical structure of butyl nitrite (C4H9NO2).

Chemical structure of nitroglycerin (C3H5N3O9), also known as glyceryl trinitrate.

of amyl nitrite by apparently healthy young men. Those over-the-counter purchases became the impetus for the FDA (Food and Drug Administration) to reinstate the prescription requirement in 1968.[7] Soon thereafter, an underground market for amyl nitrite and other nitrite congeners, such as butyl and isopropyl nitrites, emerged. Those products were initially sold as "room odorizers," and are still being sold, now illegally in the United States, under that guise.

Finally, a novel infectious agent or some hybrid or mutation of a known organism was considered as the possible immunosuppressive agent. A new herpesvirus, particularly a new CMV, generated much discussion, although other viruses also deserved consideration. The

2. Joining the Epidemic Intelligence Service (EIS)

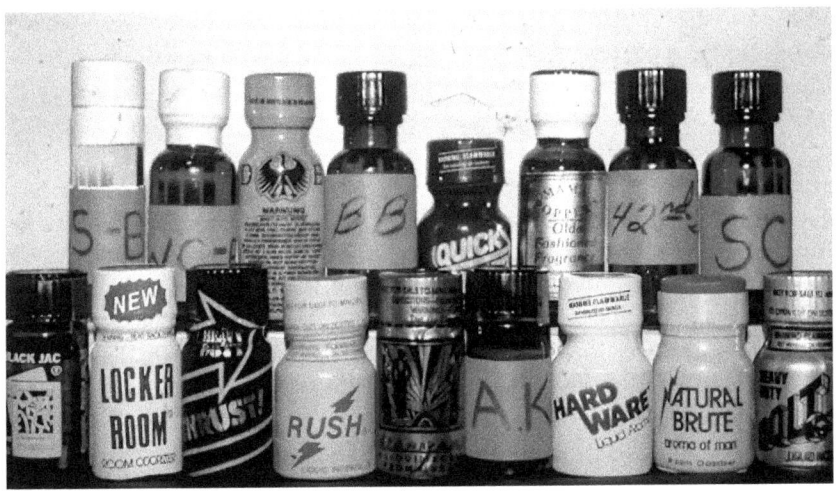

"Poppers," or volatile nitrite inhalants, have been marketed in numerous countries. They come in small glass vials, typically around 30 ml in size, featuring appealing names, as shown. Additionally, they can be found in unlabeled vials. While these vials contain a mix of nitrite congeners, including amyl, butyl, and isopropyl, butyl nitrite held the position of the primary ingredient in the 1980s. Users inhale the vapors released from the vials, emphasizing that they are not meant to be consumed as liquids (courtesy Dr. Alvin Friedman-Kien, with verbal permission 40 years ago).

prevalence of OI clusters among gay men and drug addicts suggested that hepatitis B-like viruses should be considered and sought.

Step 8—Evaluate These Hypotheses by Appropriate Statistical Methods Using Data Collected

For most outbreaks, the investigator must decide between a case-control and a cohort study. In a case-control study the participants are selected on the basis of whether or not they have the disease. Case-patients are those with the disease, controls are those without the disease. A cohort study takes a group of non-diseased persons, characterizes them by suspect exposure levels, follows them over time, and measures the occurrence of disease. The case-control study is generally considered more efficient when the disease is rare, which is usually defined as occurring in less than 20 percent of the population studied. By October 1981, fewer than 100 case-patients were recognized and still alive in the United States. In addition to the condition's rarity, the vast number of exposures requiring investigation, and the difficulty obtaining such personal exposure data favored a case-control design. If a cohort study were chosen, who would be selected as a participant? How long would they be followed? How many would be lost to follow-up? In addition, case-control studies are generally much less costly to implement than a prospective cohort study.

Case-control studies, however, have their own drawbacks. They are often beset by selection, interviewer, and recall biases. How does one determine an appropriate control group? The investigator must always be concerned about information bias and the obscuring effect of confounding variables. Having weighed the pros and cons of each study design, Harold Jaffe chose to conduct a case-control study.

As a starting point, he defined a case as a homosexual male with KS and/or PCP, 18 to 60 years of age, and with no prior evidence of immune suppression. He decided to recruit all patients meeting his case definition in New York City, San Francisco, Los Angeles, and Atlanta.

Defining the ideal control group presented a greater challenge. The use of controls who were very similar to the case-patients could result in overmatching and obscure important risk factors. On the other hand, the use of controls that were very different from case-patients could make comparison difficult, so that differences between case-patients and controls could not be interpreted. Harold Jaffe decided to recruit multiple controls for each case, ranging from persons relatively similar to the case (friend controls) to persons relatively different from the case (heterosexual male controls).

Since obtaining a true random sample of gay men to serve as controls did not appear feasible, he asked health departments, private clinics, private physicians, and case-patients themselves to help recruit controls. Each control was a man of the same race/ethnicity, age, and metropolitan residence as the case to whom he was matched.

Jaffe sought five matched controls per case:

- A friend control—a gay male identified by the case as a friend who had never been a sexual partner;
- Two venereal disease clinic controls—homosexual men who were patients of the venereal disease clinic;
- A private practice gay control—a homosexual patient of a local private practice physician seen for an acute illness and selected randomly from the referring physician's Rolodex or log book;
- A private practice heterosexual control—an exclusively heterosexual patient of a local private physician selected randomly from the physician's Rolodex or log book.

Harold Jaffe and Dr. William Darrow, a sociologist, collaborated on the development of a questionnaire and trained the interviewers

2. Joining the Epidemic Intelligence Service (EIS)

responsible for conducting the interviews (see Appendix B). One of the standout strengths of Jaffe's study was the extensive groundwork he laid in crafting the questionnaire. This meticulous effort ensured that the data collected on the back end was less susceptible to contamination from information bias.

The initial inquiry on the questionnaire aimed to establish the date when the disease symptoms first appeared in the case-patients. Patients were asked to pinpoint the first indication that they were unwell. These indications encompassed various signs and symptoms such as fever, weight loss, skin abnormalities, lymph node enlargement, diarrhea, cough, or shortness of breath. This onset date of illness served as the reference point for all subsequent inquiries, both for case-patients and for their matched controls.

For instance, taking the example of my patient from Pittsburgh, this individual received a PCP diagnosis in December 1980. However, the presence of fevers and weight loss had been noted 18 months prior. It will become evident that several subsequent studies failed to recognize that drug usage and sexual activity declined during the early phase of disease symptoms, which could potentially skew the results.

Task force members and other EIS officers—all physicians—conducted the interviews. The same officer who interviewed a case interviewed all the controls matched to that case.

All of us were trained to conduct the interviews in a consistent, nonjudgmental fashion. At the training, during which Bill Darrow mock-interviewed another CDC employee, I asked if we should be concerned about participants misrepresenting their sexual activity—exaggerating exploits, perhaps, or minimizing certain behaviors. Jim Curran acknowledged the difficulty in collecting such private information, but was emphatic as to the importance of the interview data. He pointed out that we were not looking for the truth *per se*, but for differences between case-patients and controls. Importantly, we would also collect blood samples and mouth and anal swabs from all participants for a more objective investigation of immunologic and infectious markers at our Atlanta lab. Training now complete, we were prepared to enter the field in October.

On Sunday, October 4, Jim Curran, Martha Rogers (EIS 1981), and I flew to New York City. On Monday morning we met others at the New York City Health Department to get our marching orders. Local health officers cleared Harold Jaffe's protocol (Appendix B) through the health department's sanctioning process and arranged for us to begin our study. We conducted interviews of case-patients in hospital rooms, physician offices, or at patients' homes. We interviewed controls at the venereal disease clinics, physician offices, and even in our hotel room. After an interview of about 45 minutes, we drew blood and collected the swabs. Following standard practice of that era, we did not wear gloves to draw blood.

I conducted about 60 interviews that month. The participants seemed impressed that the CDC physicians from Atlanta had traveled to New York to engage face-to-face with them in several settings, including their homes. By attempting to answer all of their questions, we seemed to gain rapport with the subjects and the gay community, demonstrating that the CDC was serious about this outbreak. In turn, I was impressed with how open and apparently honest they were in describing the most intimate details of their lives.

Step 9—As Necessary, Reconsider/Refine Hypothesis and Execute Additional Studies

David Auerbach (EIS 1981) was assigned to the Los Angeles County Health Department, initiated surveillance in Los Angeles area hospitals, and conducted the Los Angeles interviews in the case-control study. He noted that four of the case-patients interviewed were sexual partners of each other and wondered if the CDC could connect patients on the West Coast with each other and with those elsewhere. Bill Darrow, who had trained us to conduct the interviews, joined Auerbach in the effort. They collected the names of sexual partners of case-patients, either directly from the patient, or from close companions of patients who had died, and then compared the names of sexual contacts listed with case-patients of KSOI in the national surveillance line listing (Step 5). Darrow would then crisscross the country to interview those from outside the Los Angeles area.[8] Several patients could not name their sexual partners, but thought they might be able to recognize them in photographs. Auerbach and Darrow sought permission to photograph interviewees and share their photos with other patients. The CDC denied the request because it challenged the promise of confidentiality given to all study participants.

3

Surveillance
Gathering Information for Action

Different scientists were using different acronyms in an alphabet soup that further confused the already befuddled story of a strange new disease of unknown origin. The staffers at the CDC despised the GRID acronym and refused to use it. With the advent of the hemophiliac case-patients, Jim Curran argued that any references to "gay" or "community" should be dropped and something more neutral should be adopted.... Somebody finally suggested the name that stuck: Acquired Immune Deficiency Syndrome. That gave the epidemic a snappy acronym, AIDS, and was sexually neutral. The word "acquired" separated the immune deficiency syndrome from congenital defects or chemically induced immune problems, indicating the syndrome was acquired from somewhere even though nobody knew from where.
—Randy Shilts, 1987[1]

Step 6—Perform Descriptive Epidemiology (i.e., Orient the Data by Time, Place and Person)

During the initial phase of the investigation, on Friday July 24, 1981, Dr. James Curran presented our active surveillance plan to EIS officers assigned to various city and state health departments, including Albany, New York; Atlanta, Georgia; Los Angeles, California; New York City; Oklahoma City; Rochester, New York; and Tallahassee, Florida. The officers were tasked with contacting lead physicians in dermatology, infectious diseases, internal medicine, and oncology at major hospitals in their respective areas to gather information on case-patients of Kaposi's sarcoma and opportunistic infections (KSOI) in previously healthy men.

Curran personally reached out to second-year EIS officers in other cities and sent letters to directors of all state health departments, informing them of the outbreak and instructing them to report any such case-patients to us. He designated my telephone number as the point of contact for passive surveillance.

Prior to my arrival at the CDC, the task force had already documented 41 case-patients of KS and/or PCP. This included five PCP patients from Los Angeles,[2] 26 KS case-patients reported by dermatologists attending a national conference in California,[3] and 10 additional patient reports collected by Jim Curran and Dennis Juranek during their visit to NYC. All but one of these case-patients were white homosexual men.

However, we soon discovered that KSOI was not exclusive to gay men. In late August, we reported a total of 108 previously healthy patients with KS and/or PCP. Among them, 96 were gay men, six had an unknown sexual orientation, five were heterosexual men, and one was a heterosexual woman who engaged in heroin use and prostitution.[4]

In October, I spent a month in New York City participating in our national case-control study. During this period, we temporarily paused our surveillance activities, causing a backlog of telephone calls. Upon returning to Atlanta, my role shifted from field work to primarily conducting phone interviews. I spent several hours each day on the phone, conversing with physicians, the press, patients, and anyone else who called the designated number. For each patient, I filled out a case report form, which can be found in Appendix A.

First Clusters of Heterosexual Men and Women

Dr. Henry Masur from Cornell University identified the first clusters of heterosexual men and women with *Pneumocystis carinii* pneumonia (PCP) in New York City. These case-patients were primarily linked to injection drug abuse. In an article published in the *New England Journal of Medicine* on December 10, 1981, Masur described seven PCP case-patients among drug users, including two homosexual and three heterosexual heroin users, one heterosexual alcoholic, and one heterosexual cocaine addict/alcoholic. Among them, three men were Black, two were white, and two were Hispanic.[5]

Later, Masur reported five women (four heterosexual and one bisexual) with PCP in NYC. Among these women, three were Hispanic, one was white, and one was Black. Four of the women abused multiple drugs, including cocaine (all four), heroin (three), and mescaline (one). The one woman who did not use illegal drugs was in a stable sexual relationship with a drug-abusing man.[6]

By March 24, 1982, the number of patients with KSOI had risen to 290, with 280 men and 10 women. Among the women, nine were heterosexual and one was bisexual. Approximately 40 percent of the patients had died, with over 60 percent of those with opportunistic infections and 20 percent of those with Kaposi's sarcoma alone succumbing to the disease. Information about intravenous drug use was not consistently collected for all patients, but a question about this was added by the end of 1981. Out of the 157 patients for whom this information was available, 33 reported using intravenous drugs such as heroin, methadone, cocaine, amphetamines, and barbiturates. Heterosexual individuals were more likely to be drug abusers compared to homosexuals ($p < 0.0001$ by chi-square test). The patients' ages ranged from 15 to 58 years with a median of 35. The racial distribution was as follows: 66 percent white, 20 percent Black, and 12 percent Hispanic. Forty percent (115 of 290) of the patients had died. Half of the patients lived in NYC at the time of diagnosis, while one-fourth lived in California. The remaining patients were reported from 17 other states and several countries, including Canada, France, Haiti, Japan, and the United Kingdom.[7]

Key findings from the evaluation of the initial heterosexual patients revealed that about a third of the case-patients had antibodies to cytomegalovirus (CMV), and only two out of ten heterosexual case-patients reported using nitrite inhalants, commonly known as "poppers." These findings effectively ruled out CMV and nitrite inhalants as the primary cause, providing further support for the notion of a new sexually transmitted agent.[8]

The "Tip of the Iceberg"

While logging calls about patients with KS and life-threatening opportunistic infections, I observed that clinicians were spontaneously reporting case-patients of gay men with unusual symptoms. These symptoms included intermittent and prolonged fever of unknown origin, generalized lymphadenopathy, weight loss, and abnormalities in red cells, white cells, and/or platelets, such as aplastic anemia and idiopathic thrombocytopenic purpura. Other forms of cancer, like rare lymphomas, were also reported among gay men. Although these patients did not meet our case definition, their symptoms reminded me of our patient in Pittsburgh, who experienced intermittent fevers, lymphadenopathy, and weight loss for 18 months before being diagnosed with *Pneumocystis carinii* pneumonia (PCP). I documented each patient's case and stored the reports separately.

As time passed, some of these men with non-life-threatening disorders

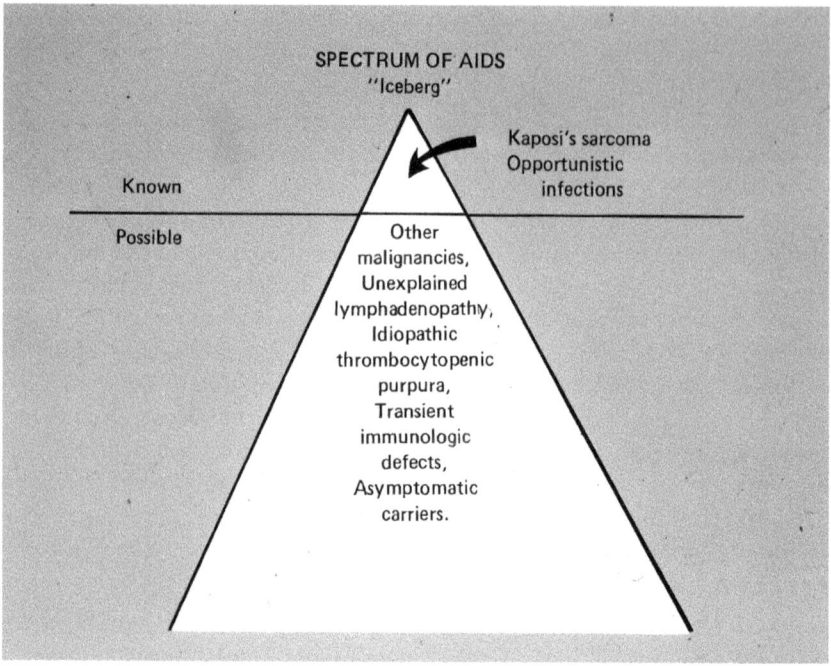

AIDS is the visible "tip of the iceberg." HIV infection manifests across a spectrum from asymptomatic carriers to severe cancers and infections. Numerous individuals with HIV exhibit non-specific signs, remain subclinical, or go unreported (CDC: H. Haverkos, 1982).

were reported again, this time with KS and opportunistic infections. These reports indicated that KS and other opportunistic infections were just the "tip of the iceberg" and represented a broader range of illnesses affecting homosexual men[9] (see figure 1 for visual representation).

Additionally, I received calls from healthcare professionals notifying us about the deaths of previously reported patients. Once a patient was diagnosed with KS and opportunistic infections, their immune suppression persisted, and they generally succumbed to their illness within months or, at most, two to three years after the initial report.

In February 1982, Paul Wiesner, the head of the venereal diseases division at the CDC, appointed five medical officers to serve on the task force for three-month periods. Richard Selik and Peter Drotman were among the recruits who would become long-term contributors to the epidemic response. Richard Selik assumed my role in conducting surveillance, taking over the responsibility. Meanwhile, Peter Drotman and I worked together on several field investigations during the next two years. I welcomed the chance to return to the field, as it provided an

Prisoners in Upstate New York with PCP

In March 1982, Mary Guinan and I went to the Medical College of New York Medical Center to investigate a cluster of case-patients involving male injection drug users who were imprisoned at Sing Sing Correctional Facility in Ossining, New York. These individuals had a history of intravenous heroin and cocaine use prior to their incarceration.

Dr. Gary Wormser, an infectious diseases physician at New York Medical College, diagnosed three white male prisoners with PCP within a month. On review of their prison records, Wormser noticed that the three had been imprisoned concurrently several months earlier at Taconic Correctional Facility in Westchester County, New York. This observation led to the possibility of deciphering the incubation period of PCP by investigating potential linkages between the three men, such as through sexual contact or needle sharing.

However, despite conducting interviews with the three men, as well as the wife of one and the mother of another, no such linkage was evident. It is important to note that the men may have been hesitant to disclose certain information to us due to concerns that it could be recorded in their prison records and potentially used against them in future legal proceedings.[10]

Step 9—As Necessary, Reconsider/Refine Hypotheses and Execute Additional Studies

In early 1982, the CDC organized three studies to further investigate the epidemic. Here are the details of each study:

A. Mary Guinan was assigned to lead the analysis of data collected from heterosexual patients. This study aimed to examine the specific characteristics and risk factors associated with the transmission of the disease in heterosexual populations.[11]

B. Dennis Juranek and I observed that patients with *Pneumocystis carinii* pneumonia (PCP) were dying at a higher rate compared to those diagnosed with Kaposi's sarcoma (KS). Surprisingly, PCP patients reported fewer sexual partners and less use of "street" drugs than KS patients in the case-control study. This led us to question whether there was a single outbreak or two separate epidemics occurring simultaneously. We aimed to determine if the risk factors for PCP and KS were the same. However, due to the limited number of PCP patients available for interview and the higher mortality rate, we recognized the need for a larger sample of PCP patients to conduct a meaningful study.[12]

Peter Drotman (EIS 1979) and I were tasked with evaluating male PCP patients shortly after diagnosis. If a patient reported exclusively heterosexual behavior, the data would be submitted to Dr. Guinan for her study. Conversely, if homosexual or bisexual behavior was reported, the data would be retained for our own study.

C. Jim Curran recruited Bess Miller (EIS 1981), an EIS officer in the chronic diseases division, to conduct a medical chart review of pathology reports from lymph node biopsies performed at seven hospitals in New York City between 1977 and 1981. The object of the study was to investigate whether the syndrome of unexplained generalized lymphadenopathy in gay men was related to KSOI.[13]

These three studies aimed to gather essential data and insights into various aspects of the epidemic, including its transmission patterns, risk factors, and potential connections between different manifestations of the disease.

Field Epidemiology

In Dallas, Texas, I interviewed a 38-year-old white male who had recovered from PCP. He was married, worked in the apparel industry, and had no children. He denied drug abuse and sexual encounters with men. During his annual trade convention meeting in Atlanta, he would visit the hotel bar and engage in consensual vaginal sex with women. He did not engage in paid sexual activities.

In Miami, I interviewed a Hispanic man who had recovered from PCP. He denied engaging in sexual encounters with men and drug abuse. He was married with children but claimed to regularly engage in sexual activities with prostitutes, later referred to as commercial sex workers. The question arose: how could we track these women to determine if they were the source of disease?

How could we ensure the accuracy of reports of individuals who claimed to have exclusively engaged in heterosexual behavior? In the case-control study, I interviewed a 24-year-old man with Kaposi's sarcoma at the apartment he shared with his father. During a subsequent interview conducted by Polly Thomas (EIS 1981), an EIS officer assigned to New York City, the young man admitted to lying during my initial interview. He had been afraid of his father overhearing the conversation in the adjoining room, so he had concealed the truth about his sexual behavior.

Haitian Connection

In March 1982, a cluster of case-patients caught our attention. Seven Haitian-born men were diagnosed with CNS toxoplasmosis, with five residing in Miami, Florida, and one each in New York City and Montreal, Canada. Simultaneously, there were reports of a few men in Port-au-Prince, Haiti, displaying skin lesions resembling Kaposi's sarcoma. To investigate, I traveled to Miami to look into the patients with CNS toxoplasmosis.

In Miami, I reviewed the medical records of eight men and one woman. Among them, six had CNS toxoplasmosis, and one each had PCP, Kaposi's sarcoma, and disseminated cryptococcosis. Unfortunately, seven of them had already died. The sole surviving patient was disoriented and unable to provide an interview due to the condition. Despite attempting to contact the families of the deceased patients, I was unsuccessful. However, I did have a conversation with two Haitian-born physicians who confirmed that their patients were neither homosexual nor injecting drug abusers. These findings convinced me that these patients met our case definition.[14]

Initially, our focus was on identifying a new virus transmitted through sexual behavior and drug use. However, we were puzzled about the cause of the diseases observed among Haitians. Three alternative hypotheses were suggested: malnutrition, mosquitoes, and even voodoo practices.

When attempting to explore these issues with the surviving patient and relatives of the deceased, I faced several obstacles. Firstly, I didn't speak Creole. Secondly, being recognized as a federal agent from the CDC, discussing sensitive topics such as immigration status, homosexual behavior, or voodoo practices was considered taboo. Consequently, I made limited progress in investigating these matters.

Hemophilia A

During our investigation of AIDS among Haitians, we came across an unexpected finding. Three heterosexual men with hemophilia A were reported to have been diagnosed with PCP. Unfortunately, two of them had already died, while the third was in critical condition. Let's look at the details of these case-patients:

1. A 62-year-old resident of upstate New York was diagnosed with PCP in Miami, Florida;
2. a 59-year-old lifelong resident of Denver, Colorado;
3. a 27-year-old lifelong resident of northeastern Ohio.[15]

Hemophilia A is a rare hereditary bleeding disorder characterized by a deficiency of Factor VIII activity. The condition is treated with intravenous administration of exogenous Factor VIII, which is obtained from cryoprecipitate or Factor VIII concentrate. Cryoprecipitate is derived from a single donor's plasma, whereas Factor VIII concentrate is manufactured from plasma pools of numerous donors.

In 1976, there were approximately 20,000 individuals with hemophilia A in the United States.[16] Since it is a recessive, X-linked chromosome defect, the condition is more commonly seen in males than females. Males have one X chromosome, and if it is affected, they develop disease. Females, on the other hand, have two X chromosomes and may be carriers if one of them is affected. Only when both X chromosomes are affected do females display disease, which is rare.

By the end of 1982, we had encountered four additional case-patients with hemophilia A. These included three heterosexual men and a 10-year-old boy, who were diagnosed with an opportunistic infection. The boy lived in Pennsylvania, while the men resided in Alabama, Missouri, and Ohio. It was noteworthy that all of them had received multiple doses of Factor VIII and blood transfusions. The geographic distribution of these hemophilia patients indicated the potential transmission of the virus through commercial blood products rather than sexual contact.[17]

AIDS (Acquired Immune Deficiency Syndrome)

Initially, the new disease was named GRID (gay-related immune deficiency) by Michael Gottlieb. However, as reports of case-patients emerged involving heterosexual men and women, injecting drug users, Haitians, and hemophiliacs, it became clear that the term GRID was not appropriate. At the CDC, we referred to the collection of diseases as KSOI (Kaposi's sarcoma and opportunistic infections). However, this acronym was not particularly catchy or widely recognized.

In September 1982, the CDC introduced the term AIDS (Acquired Immunodeficiency Syndrome) to encompass the range of opportunistic infections and malignancies associated with the condition. This new term was chosen to acknowledge the expanding demographic pattern of affected individuals. The term AIDS sought to capture the attention of both the medical community and the general public, reflecting the urgent need for awareness, research, and public health efforts.[18]

Heterosexual Men and Women

Mary Guinan (EIS 1974) played a key role in organizing interviews and collecting laboratory samples from individuals with AIDS, specifically focusing on "heterosexual" men and women. Guinan's educational background includes a bachelor's degree in chemistry from Hunter's City College in New York and a doctoral degree in physiology/space medicine from the University of Texas, Galveston. While her initial aspiration was to join NASA as an astronaut, she pursued and completed medical school at Johns Hopkins University in Baltimore in 1972. Following an internal medicine residency at Penn State University, Hershey, and an infectious diseases fellowship at the University of Utah, Guinan volunteered to work in the Smallpox Eradication Program in India. She returned to the CDC in 1978, joining the venereal diseases division and becoming a charter member of the KSOI task force in 1981.

By June 1, 1982, a total of 377 patients with Kaposi's sarcoma (KS) or opportunistic infections were reported. Among them, 302 (80 percent) were gay men, 64 (17 percent) were heterosexual men and women, and 11 (3 percent) men with unknown sexual orientation. Out of the 64 heterosexual patients, 31 were interviewed, comprising 24 men and seven women. Among this group, 22 (71 percent) reported using heroin and/or cocaine. Additionally, four patients were Haitian natives, and five had no identified risk factors.[19]

In comparison to gay men, heterosexual men with KS or opportunistic infections were more likely to be Black or Hispanic, married, and reported fewer lifetime sexual partners. In the case-control study, gay men with KSOI reported a median of over one thousand lifetime sexual partners. In contrast, male heterosexual intravenous drug users reported a median of 40 lifetime female partners, Haitian men reported 81 partners, and other men reported 23 partners.[20]

Step 12. Maintain Surveillance to Monitor Trends and Evaluate Control Prevention Measures

By February 1983, the CDC had received reports of 1,000 individuals in the United States who met the case definition for AIDS and were between 10 and 60 years old. Among them, 270 were diagnosed before January 1, 1982 (averaging one case per day), while 730 were diagnosed in the following 13 months (averaging two case-patients per day). Among these patients, 59 were female. PCP was the diagnosed condition in over half of the case-patients, followed by KS in about one-third of the case-patients, and another opportunistic infection in one-sixth of the case-patients. By December 31, 1982, 392 individuals had unfortunately died (39 percent). Case-patients were reported from 32 states and the District of Columbia, with over 80 percent of the case-patients reported from New York, California, New Jersey, or Florida. Among the racial breakdown, 588 patients were white, 271 were Black, 129 were Hispanic, five were classified as other, and six were of unknown race.[21]

Richard Selik (EIS 1978), the head of surveillance activities, developed a hierarchical system of risk classification for the patients. Each patient was assigned to a single category based on their "rank" of risk. The first rank consisted of gay or bisexual men, which also included those who reported injection drug abuse or were of Haitian birth, among other factors. Later, gay men were referred to as men who have sex with men (MSM). The second rank included heterosexual patients who reported injecting drugs not prescribed by a physician. The following table presents the breakdown of the 1,000 patients by sex and risk group.

AIDS Risk Group	Male	Female
Homosexual/Bisexual men	727	0
Injection drug abuser	126	29
Haitian American	45	5
Hemophiliac	7	0
Other	36	25
Total	941	59

Of all the patients, only 61 (6 percent) could not be classified into one of the four major risk groups: homosexual men, heroin users, Haitian Americans, and hemophiliacs. The remaining group, labeled as "other," comprised 36 males and 25 females. Among them, 33 had PCP, 16 had KS, and 12 had other opportunistic infections. Due to inadequate information caused by the patients' death or unavailability for interviews at the time of reporting, some risk factors for these patients were unclear. However, certain emerging risk groups started to surface. For instance, there were five women with PCP who denied injecting drug abuse but were steady sexual partners of male injecting drug abusers. Additionally, two patients with no apparent risk were reported to have received blood transfusions three years prior to the onset of their illness, leading to investigations into the donors of their blood components. This "other" group of patients required increased scrutiny.[22]

The hierarchical system had its strengths in expediting the identification of new groups of patients at risk. Over the following months, we would identify blood transfusion recipients, infants, children, and health care workers with AIDS. By marking these groups and tracking trends over time, we could determine if new risk groups or routes of transmission were emerging.

However, the hierarchical system also presented a challenge: understanding the number of patients in lower-ranked groups. Those listed as injecting drug users included an unknown number of promiscuous heterosexual men and female sex workers. According to this system, all of these patients were classified as intravenous drug users and none due to heterosexual contact. In the summer of 1984, we added heterosexual contact case-patients as rank #5. However, this definition proved to be too restrictive, excluding women reported as prostitutes who couldn't name a specific contact with AIDS or at risk for AIDS, as well as men who had engaged in sexual activity with commercial sex workers but were unaware of their drug use or Haitian origin. For example, the men I interviewed in Dallas and Miami would be placed in the "Other" group, later named persons at no increased risk (NIR).

Although case-patients of heterosexual men and women with AIDS were reported from the early days, their presence was initially overlooked due to various disguises, such as amphetamine and cocaine abusers, partners of non-drug-using commercial sex workers, and Caribbean natives. As we divided them by gender and acknowledged one direction of transmission while denying the other, the use of the hierarchical system contributed to false beliefs that heterosexual transmission of HIV was uncommon and that transmission was significantly higher from male to female than female to male.

Pediatric AIDS

One of the first AIDS case-patients among children was also one of the first attributed to blood transfusion. The patient was a 20-month-old boy from the San Francisco area who developed unexplained immune deficiency and an opportunistic infection after receiving multiple blood transfusions shortly after birth. The boy was delivered by cesarean section at 33 weeks of gestation and remained in the hospital for a month. His medical history was complex, including hepatosplenomegaly at 4 months, hospitalization for severe otitis media at 7 months, and a diagnosis of non-A, non-B hepatitis, now known as hepatitis C, at 9 months. At 14 months, he developed neutropenia, thrombocytopenia, hemolytic anemia, and decreased numbers and function of T cells, which are white cells associated with AIDS. A bone marrow biopsy was sent for culture, and his blood disorders were treated with systemic corticosteroids. Three months later, the bone marrow sample tested positive for *Mycobacterium avium-intracellulare*, an opportunistic infection.[23] Investigation of the blood products received by the infant revealed that one of the donors was a 48-year-old white male resident of San Francisco who was well at the time of donation but was later diagnosed with PCP in December 1981.

When Richard Selik and I reviewed the toddler's medical history, we suggested that his physicians should rule out any possible congenital immunologic defect before considering the child to have AIDS. However, Jim Curran and Harold Jaffe disagreed with our assessment. Around the same time, pediatricians at Albert Einstein College of Medicine in NYC reported four children with opportunistic infections:

Case 1: A 17-month-old Black/Hispanic boy diagnosed with disseminated *M. avium-intracellulare* infection. His mother, an injecting drug user, died of a different opportunistic infection, PCP.
Case 2: A five-month-old Haitian boy with PCP, cryptococcus, and cytomegalovirus infections. The health status of the parents was unknown.
Case 3: A five-month-old Haitian boy with PCP. The health status of the parents was unknown.
Case 4: A five-month-old white girl with PCP. Her mother, a sex worker and injecting drug user, had oral candidiasis and lymphopenia. The mother had two older daughters from different fathers, and both girls were diagnosed with unexplained cellular immunodeficiencies. One of them died of PCP.[24]

In the spring of 1983, Dr. James Oleske and colleagues in Newark, New Jersey, reported eight children with PCP or severe immunodeficiency. The median age of the children was 12 months, and they presented with recurrent fevers, failure to thrive, interstitial pneumonitis, and hepatosplenomegaly. The immune defect observed in these children was similar to that seen in adults with AIDS. Six of the children had parents who reported injecting drugs; one had parents born in Haiti; and another had a mother born in the Dominican Republic, on the other half of Hispaniola, with a shared border with Haiti.[25]

I took the reports as a challenge to my case definition and failed to recognize the emergence of a new risk group—transmission from an

3. Surveillance 45

infected mother to her baby in the womb or during delivery (perinatal transmission). Instead I recommended further tests on the children to rule out congenital or hereditary immunodeficiencies.

Several pediatricians challenged the age restriction on our case definition and expressed their concerns about the delayed recognition of AIDS among infants and toddlers by the CDC. In response, Jim Curran assigned two CDC pediatricians, Martha Rogers (EIS 1981) and Polly Thomas (EIS 1981), to develop a case definition and set up a separate surveillance system for children.[26]

According to the CDC, a case of pediatric AIDS is defined as a child who meets the following criteria:

1. Has a reliably diagnosed disease that strongly indicates an underlying cellular immunodeficiency. The diseases considered indicative of underlying cellular immunodeficiency are the same as those used in defining AIDS in adults, except for congenital infections such as toxoplasmosis or herpes simplex virus infection within the first month after birth, or cytomegalovirus in the first 6 months after birth.
2. Has no known cause of underlying cellular immunodeficiency. Specific conditions that must be ruled out in a child include:
   A. Primary immunodeficiency diseases—severe combined immunodeficiency, DiGeorge syndrome, Wiskott-Aldrich syndrome, ataxia-telangiectasia, graft versus host disease, neutropenia, neutrophil function abnormality, agammaglobulinemia, or hypogammaglobulinemia with raised IgM (immunoglobulin M).
   B. Secondary immunodeficiency associated with immunosuppressive therapy, lymphoreticular malignancy, and starvation.[27]

By December 31, 1984, the CDC reported 7,699 (7,609 + the 90 for pediatric) case-patients of AIDS case among U.S. residents[28] as follows:

Adult/Adolescent

Patient Group*	Males	Females	Total
Homosexual/Bisexual	5,541	—	5,541
IV drug user	1,042	275	1,317
Haitian	221	42	263
Hemophilia	49	0	49
Heterosexual contact†	5	54	59
Blood transfusions	49	41	90

Patient Group*	Males	Females	Total
None of the above	206	84	290
Total	7,113	496	7,609

*Patient groups listed are ordered hierarchically; case-patients with multiple characteristics are tabulated only in the group listed first.
†Heterosexual contact with a person with AIDS or at risk for AIDS.

Pediatric†

Patient Group*	Boys	Girls	Total
Parent with AIDS/or at risk for AIDS	34	30	64
Hemophilia	4	0	4
Blood transfusions	10	2	12
None of the above	5	5	10
Total	53	37	90

*Patient groups listed are ordered hierarchically; case-patients with multiple characteristics are tabulated only in the group listed first.
†Includes patients under 13 years of age at time of diagnosis.

Summary

At first we were aware of a few dozen homosexual men with KS, PCP, and other life-threatening opportunistic infections. As surveillance continued, however, it soon became apparent that AIDS was not confined to homosexual/bisexual men, later designated as men who have sex with men (MSM). Over time, the demographic pattern widened to include injection drug users, prostitutes (commercial sex workers), heterosexual women, Haitian Americans, Caribbean islanders, hemophiliacs, blood transfusion recipients, heterosexual men, infants and children, health care workers, lesbians (women who have sex with women), and transgender people. Patients would be reported from Europe, then Africa, South America, Oceania, and Asia.

The full spectrum of disease would include Kaposi's sarcoma and opportunistic infections but also other malignancies, generalized lymphadenopathy, selected blood dyscrasias, transient immunosuppression, and asymptomatic carriers. AIDS was a progressive disease, death was pervasive, and we were just counting the "tip of the iceberg."

4

National Study of Gay Men

> *March 3, 1983—The Public Health Service pronouncements on AIDS included the first risk-reduction guidelines ever issued by the federal government. The PHS saw fit to offer only two sentences of guidance to gay men eager to avoid the strange new disease despite reams of data collected in the still-unpublished case-control study. "Sexual contact should be avoided with persons known or suspected to have AIDS," the PHS wrote. "Members of high-risk groups should be aware that multiple sex partners increase the probability of developing AIDS."*
>
> *That statement represented the sum total of the U.S. government's attempt to prevent the spread of acquired immune deficiency syndrome among gay men in March 1983, more than twenty months into the epidemic.*
>
> —Randy Shilts, 1987[1]

In December 1981, Harold Jaffe's case-control study yielded preliminary results. We interviewed 60 men to serve as case-patients, but only 50 were eligible for analysis. Unfortunately, seven gay men were interviewed too late in the study, resulting in a lack of controls. Additionally, three case-patients denied engaging in homosexual behavior, leading to their exclusion from the case definition.[2]

The case-patients had an average age of 35 years, ranging from 21 to 53 years. Among the 50 case-patients, 39 had Kaposi's sarcoma (KS), eight had *Pneumocystis* pneumonia (PCP), and three had both conditions. Seventy percent (35 individuals) were residents of New York City, and 76 percent (38 individuals) identified as white. It's worth noting the case-patients were highly educated with a median schooling duration of 16 years.

Obtaining controls for the 50 case-patients presented varying degrees of success. We included 120 gay men who were matched to case-patients based on age, race, and residence. Among those controls, 78 were patients from sexually transmitted diseases clinics, while 42 were participants from private practice. Regrettably, only 23 (46 percent) of the 50 case-patients were able to identify friends who could serve as potential controls, resulting in their exclusion from the analysis. When approaching heterosexual men as potential controls, most declined to participate. Consequently, we only interviewed seven heterosexual men (4 percent), but we ultimately excluded their interviews as well.

Upon first examination of the questionnaire results (see Appendix B), we were immediately struck by the prevalence of sexual behavior, rates of sexually transmitted diseases, and illicit drug use among the participants, as shown in Table 1. Notably, the reported number of lifetime sexual partners among case-patients ranged from under 100 to over 10,000, indicating a wide range of sexual activity.

Both case-patients and controls commonly reported the presence of gonorrhea (86 percent of case-patients), syphilis (68 percent), and non–B hepatitis (48 percent). Furthermore, at the time, certain sexual practices that were considered unconventional, such as "fisting" (inserting one's fist into a partner's rectum) and "rimming" (licking a partner's rectum), were reported in 52 percent and 78 percent of case-patients, respectively.

Some of the data surprised us. For instance, 70 percent of both case-patients and controls report engaging in sexual activity with women, indicating that they were bisexual rather than exclusively homosexual. Additionally, 40 percent of the participants had engaged in sexual intercourse with a female by the age of 18. The age at first homosexual contact was particularly startling, with 20 percent of case-patients and controls reporting engaging in sexual activity with a male or boy by the age of ten; one case even reported his first sexual exposure at the age of two. Moreover, over 50 percent of both case-patients and controls had engaged in sexual activity with a male by the age of 16. These findings suggested that our case definition's lower limit of 15 years was inadequate.[3]

Table 1. Frequency of Selected Variables Among Participants in Case-control Study[4]

Variable	Case-patients (n=50)	Clinic Controls (n=78)	Private Controls (n=42)
Italian, Jewish, or Eastern European ancestry, %	38	22	26
Ever married, %	18	13	7
Gonorrhea, %	86	73	74
Syphilis, %	68	36	36
Hepatitis B, %	14	14	21

4. National Study of Gay Men

Variable	Case-patients (n=50)	Clinic Controls (n=78)	Private Controls (n=42)
Non–B hepatitis, %	48	30	33
Parasitic diarrhea, %	32	15	48
Inhaled nitrites, %	96	96	95
Marijuana, %	88	89	93
Amphetamines, %	70	46	52
Cocaine, %	66	51	60
LSD, %	64	44	45
Heroin, %	10	8	5
Median male sexual partners per year, number	61	27	25
Median proportion of sex partners from bathhouses in past year, %	50	23	4
Median age at initiating regular sex with men, years	19	20	22
Median lifetime sexual partners, number	1,160	370	340
Exposure to feces during sex, %:			
Inserted penis into partner's rectum	98	95	88
Inserted tongue into partner's rectum	78	64	62
Inserted hand into partner's rectum	52	33	38
Exposure to semen or rectal trauma during sex, %:			
Partner's penis in interviewee's mouth	98	99	100
Partner's penis in interviewee's rectum	94	88	95
Partner's hand in interviewee's rectum	18	13	21

Over a hundred discrete variables were more common or prevalent among case-patients than controls, including various sociodemographic measures, previous illnesses, prescription medications taken, illicit drug use, and measures of sexual behaviors. How does one determine which variable or series of variables "cause" the problem?

Keewhan Choi, Ph.D., was the statistician assigned to work with Harold Jaffe. Multivariate analysis is a complex statistical methodology to sort out such a problem. I think of it as a two-step process. Because over a hundred variables were statistically different between case-patients and controls, one first needed to reduce that to a more manageable number for the second step—*logistic* regression. You might remember *linear* regression from high school math: "the sum of least squares." You were given a number of points on a graph and asked to find a line with the "best fit" to describe the data points. Logistic regression determines the "best fit" variable(s) from all the variables entered into the model using a similar summation but a more complex mathematical formula.[5]

National Case-Control Study: Laboratory Results

While we waited for results of the multivariate analysis, the laboratory studies were completed under the supervision of David Morens (EIS 1976) of the viral diseases division. The laboratory component of the case-control study involved the analysis of various sample types.[6]

A total of 167 serum specimens were collected, with 50 from case-patients and 121 from controls. Additionally 170 urine samples were collected, consisting of 49 from case-patients and 121 from controls. Throat swabs were obtained from 160 individuals, with 43 from case-patients and 117 from controls. Rectal swabs were obtained from 136 individuals, including 34 case-patients and 102 controls.

All of these samples were collected at the time of the interviews and were promptly sent to the CDC labs in Atlanta via overnight mail. It's worth noting that heparinized blood samples require timely processing within 24 to 48 hours of collection for immunologic testing. Due to the specific requirements of the procedure and the need for a relatively large amount of blood, only 47 heparinized blood samples, 18 from case-patients and 27 from controls, arrived at the CDC labs within the required time limits and were used for immunologic testing.[7]

Cytomegalovirus was a prime suspect. Antibodies to CMV were found in 100 percent of case-patients and 98 percent of controls. Cytomegalovirus complement fixation titers were significantly higher for case-patients than controls. Cultures of urine and throat swabs yielded CMV in 25 percent of case-patients and 9 percent of controls ($p < 0.05$). DNA restriction endonuclease studies, a way to "fingerprint" each isolate of CMV, were done on 20 samples isolated in cell culture using 10 from patients and 10 from controls. Different restriction endonuclease patterns were found for each of the 20 isolates; there were no matches. There was no evidence to support a unique "new" strain of cytomegalovirus as the cause of AIDS.

The laboratory investigators tested for a variety of viruses, bacteria, fungi, and parasites, and found a few differences between case-patients and controls. Case-patients had a higher prevalence of antibodies to hepatitis A virus; to *Treponema pallidum*, the cause of syphilis; and to Epstein-Barr virus, another herpes virus.[8] They also injected five juvenile chimpanzees with blood and bodily fluids from AIDS patients hoping to induce disease in those animals.[9]

Although the CDC laboratory workers did not find the cause of AIDS, they were able to rule out the prime suspect, CMV, as the primary cause. However, because all samples were collected from case-patients after the onset of illness, one could not decipher if the increases in CMV isolation rates and complement fixation titers were the result of immunosuppression, or acted as a cofactor enhancing immunosuppression induced by the yet-to-be-found causative agent(s).

Immunologic Findings

When compared with controls, patients were found to have significantly lower total lymphocyte and T-lymphocyte counts, specifically lower T-helper cell numbers. Levels of immunoglobulins G and A were significantly higher for patients than controls.[10] These results were expected. Similar data had been reported by Michael Gottlieb and others.

National Case-Control Study: Multivariate Results

One of the reasons the analysis took so long was that Harold Jaffe and Keewhan Choi could not agree on how to group variables for entry into logistic regression. Jaffe argued as a clinician and biologist that specific sex acts do not cause disease, but rather that an infectious agent is spread person to person. Men who do many different acts with multiple partners are at higher risk than men who do only one specific act, e.g., oral sex with fewer partners. Choi, a biostatistician, wanted to use individual variables with the greatest statistical difference from the initial analysis—let the numbers of events "speak" for themselves. As I watched these two scientists wrestle with the data, I tried to imagine the men as artists—Jaffe an "impressionist" and Choi a photographer or one who "paints by numbers."

Many of the individual variables were correlated with each other. For example, the variable "number of male sex partners per year" was highly correlated with 10 of the 31 significant variables of interest, including meeting partners in bathhouses ($p < 0.0001$), history of syphilis ($p < 0.0001$), use of nitrite inhalants ($p < 0.001$), and use of "street" drugs ($p < 0.02$). Jaffe and Choi eventually agreed on 32 different grouped variables to enter into logistic regression. For example, the median number of male sexual partners per year became a single variable that best described a composite of sexual behavior variables. They grouped illicit drug use variables into a single variable, e.g., number of different "street" drugs used. They developed a feces exposure score based on interviewee's putting one's hand (one point), penis (one point) or tongue (one point) into a partner's rectum (maximum 3 points); and a mean sperm exposure and rectal trauma score, inserting one's penis into interviewee's mouth (one point), inserting his penis (one point) or his hand (one point) into interviewee's rectum (maximum 3 points). Lifetime nitrite use was calculated by multiplying total months of use by the average number of days of use per month.[11]

Table 2. Frequency of Selected Grouped Variables Associated with KS and PCP[12]

Variable	Case-patients (n=50)	Clinic Controls (n=78)	Private Practice Controls (n=42)
Number of male sexual partners per year (median)	61	27	25
% of sex partners from bathhouses (median)	50	23	4
Age (years) of regular sex with men (median)	19	20	22
Mean feces exposure score (see text)	2.3	1.9	1.9
Mean sperm exposure and rectal trauma score (see text)	2.1	2.0	2.2
Median number of different "street" drugs used*	6	4	4
% using drugs for enteric parasites†	44	19	50
Lifetime use of nitrite inhalants (median) days	336	168	264

*Includes amphetamines, barbiturates, cocaine, heroin, LSD, marijuana, methaqualone, and phencyclidine.
†Includes use of iodoquinol, metronidazole, paromomycin, and quinacrine (antibiotics for various diarrheal diseases).

As a final compromise, Keewhan Choi and Harold Jaffe calculated linear logistic regression analysis for three data sets: grouped factors, ungrouped factors, and individual variables. They selected only "important" elements, that is, grouped, ungrouped, and individual variables that were highly statistically significant ($p < 0.01$) from a group of related variables.

Table 3. Significant Variables Associated with AIDS in 50 Gay Men as Selected by Linear Logistic Regression Analysis[13]

Variable	Rank* Grouped Factor	Rank* Ungrouped Factor	Rank* Individual Variables
Number of male sexual partners per year	1	1	1
Proportion of sex partners from bathhouses in past year	1	3	—
Syphilis previously	2	—	2
Non–B hepatitis previously	2	—	5
Italian, Jewish, or Eastern European ancestry	3	3	2
Drugs for enteric parasites	3	—	2
Sperm exposure and rectal trauma score	3	3	—
Feces exposure score	3	—	4
Number of different "street" drugs used	4	4	—
Lifetime nitrite use	4	—	—
Age at initiating regular sex with men	—	2	2
Ever married	—	2	5

*Highest-rank variables are most strongly associated with illness. Dash indicates that the variable was not selected.

The final epidemiological results revealed that the variables most strongly associated with AIDS were those related to the number of male sexual partners and meeting those partners in bathhouses, indicating a potential sexually transmitted agent.[14] The utilization of multivariate analysis was particularly impressive as it provided a systematic approach to evaluating a vast number of variables that differentiated case-patients from controls, ultimately identifying the variable(s) that best explained the data.

However, in hindsight, I believe there is an alternative interpretation of these results. The data actually support the idea of a multifactorial cause for AIDS, which suggests that a combination of infectious agents, environmental toxins, and genetic factors collectively overwhelm the immune system or, alternatively, enhance the immunosuppressive effect of a new infectious agent. Subsequently, other infectious agents such as *Pneumocystis carinii*, *Toxoplasma gondii*, and human herpesvirus type 8 (HHV-8) manifest clinically as opportunistic infections and cancers.

This alternate interpretation highlights the complexity of the disease and acknowledges that multiple factors may contribute to the development and progression of AIDS. It emphasizes the importance of considering a comprehensive range of variables and not solely focusing on a single causal factor.

Step 10—Implement Control and Prevention Measures as Early as Possible

During the fall of 1982, while the manuscript was still awaiting clearance by the CDC bureaucracy, Jim Curran was given permission to present preliminary results to the public. The recommendations, based on the available preliminary results, aimed to address the emerging AIDS epidemic and were intended to promote public health and safety.

In his presentation, Curran summarized the findings and put forth two key recommendations:

> To gay men: Curran advised limiting the number of sexual partners. This recommendation aimed to reduce the potential transmission of the suspected sexually transmitted agent and mitigate the risk of acquiring AIDS.
>
> To health departments: Curran recommended the closure of bathhouses. This measure was suggested as a preventive strategy to minimize opportunities for the spread of the disease within a high-risk population.

Jim Curran's presentation sparked an immediate and passionate response from the gay community. The community felt that they were being further stigmatized by the focus on gay men as potential spreaders of a life-threatening sexually transmitted disease. The report's portrayal of gay men as sexually promiscuous, having multiple sexually transmitted infections, and engaging in drug abuse exacerbated the existing stigma. Moreover, recommending the closure of bathhouses generated strong opposition and antipathy toward the CDC.

From our perspective, it was assumed that gay bathhouses facilitated anonymous sexual encounters with multiple partners, thus increasing the risk of transmitting the untreatable and deadly disease. Based on this assumption and supported by the available data, recommending the closure of bathhouses seemed like a reasonable approach. However, many in the gay community viewed bathhouses as symbols of sexual freedom and argued that they provided safe spaces for men to gather and opportunities for AIDS education. The idea of closing the bathhouses was met with resistance and was not open for discussion among several gay leaders.

From an epidemiological standpoint, the presence of bathhouses represented a confounding variable rather than a direct cause of AIDS. Confounding arises when a risk factor for the disease of interest is also associated with the exposure. In this case, shutting down bathhouses would not prevent sexual activity but might instead lead to a shift of such activities to public parks and restrooms. This shift would introduce additional risks, including the potential for physical abuse and legal consequences if reported to the police.

The situation highlights the complex dynamics at play during that time. Our recommendation was based on our understanding of the disease transmission patterns, but failed to consider the broader social and cultural implications of our proposed interventions. The response from the gay community reflected their concerns about stigmatization, infringement on personal freedoms, and the potential unintended consequences of certain interventions.

Nitrite Inhalants and AIDS

For many, the case-control study findings have effectively ruled out nitrite inhalants as a significant contributor to the development of AIDS. Despite case-patients reporting higher exposure to nitrites compared to controls, the study's logistic regression analysis ranked lifetime nitrite inhalant use fourth, indicating it was not a major factor. Moreover, it did not significantly contribute to the ranking of ungrouped factors or individual variables. The CDC considered nitrite inhalant use as a confounding variable rather than a causative factor for AIDS.[15] In fact, in their 1984 budget request to the Department of Health and Human Services, the CDC listed ruling out a role for nitrite inhalants as a cause of AIDS as their primary accomplishment in 1983.

Unsurprisingly, manufacturers of nitrite inhalants responded positively to these results. Joseph F. Miller, representing Great Lakes Products, Inc., expressed relief through a statement in the gay press, acknowledging the government studies had definitively demonstrated the lack of health hazards associated with nitrites. Similarly, W. Jay Freezer, another nitrite manufacturer, along with Dr. Bruce Voeller, a researcher funded by the nitrite industry, urged the CDC to reassure the public about the safety of these products.

First Official CDC Prevention Recommendations

In the March 4, 1983, *MMWR*, the CDC provided an overview of the current trends of AIDS and issued its first official prevention recommendations. By that time, over 1,200 case-patients of AIDS had been reported from 34 states, the District of Columbia, and 15 countries. More than 450 patients had died, and the case-fatality rate for case-patients diagnosed over a year earlier exceeded 60 percent. The affected groups included gay men with multiple sex partners, intravenous drug abusers, Haitians, hemophiliacs, heterosexual women linked to men with AIDS, children, and blood transfusion recipients from donors with AIDS. (Note: Female-to-male transmission was not acknowledged in this list.) The final results from the national case-control study and preliminary findings from the Orange County, California, cluster study indicated that AIDS was caused by a sexually transmitted agent, with the highest rates observed among gay and bisexual men.[16]

Although the exact cause of AIDS was still unknown at that time, the Public Health Service recommended the following prevention measures:

1. Avoid sexual contact with individuals known or suspected to have AIDS. High-risk groups should be aware that having multiple sexual partners increases the likelihood of developing AIDS.
2. As a temporary measure, individuals belonging to groups at increased risk for AIDS should refrain from donating plasma and/or blood. This recommendation applies to all individuals in these groups, regardless of their individual risk levels. Plasma and blood collection centers should inform potential donors about this recommendation. The FDA is in the process of preparing new recommendations for plasma derivative manufacturers and blood collection establishments. This interim measure aims to protect recipients of blood products until specific laboratory tests are available.
3. Studies should be conducted to evaluate the effectiveness of screening procedures in identifying and excluding plasma and blood with a high probability of transmitting AIDS. These procedures should include specific laboratory tests, as well as thorough medical histories, and physical examinations.
4. Physicians should strictly adhere to medical indications for transfusions, and autologous* blood transfusions are encouraged. Autologous blood transfusion involves using an individual's own blood for transfusion.

5. Ongoing efforts should focus on developing safer blood products for use by hemophilia patients.[17]

*Autologous blood transfusion is a process in which a person receives their own blood instead of blood collected and banked from others. For example, patients would donate blood before elective surgery and have that blood provided, if needed, during or after surgery.

Los Angeles Cluster Investigation

David Auerbach (EIS 1981) conducted interviews for the Los Angeles case-patients in the case-control study and discovered that four of the case-patients were sexual partners. Upon learning about this observation, the CDC sent Bill Darrow, a sociologist, to assist Auerbach in gathering the names of sexual partners for all 19 reported case-patients of KS and/or PCP from Los Angeles and Orange counties, California. They conducted interviews with eight surviving patients and close friends of seven out of 11 deceased patients. Sexual partner data was obtained for 13 patients. Within five years of symptom onset, nine out of the 13 patients were found to be sexually connected to each other and/or to a French-Canadian airline steward diagnosed with KS in NYC.[18]

Bill Darrow then traveled to NYC to obtain the names of over 70 sexual partners of the airline steward, eight of whom were reported to the CDC with KS and/or PCP. As the investigation progressed, a total of 40 patients living in ten cities could be linked through sexual contact. It is

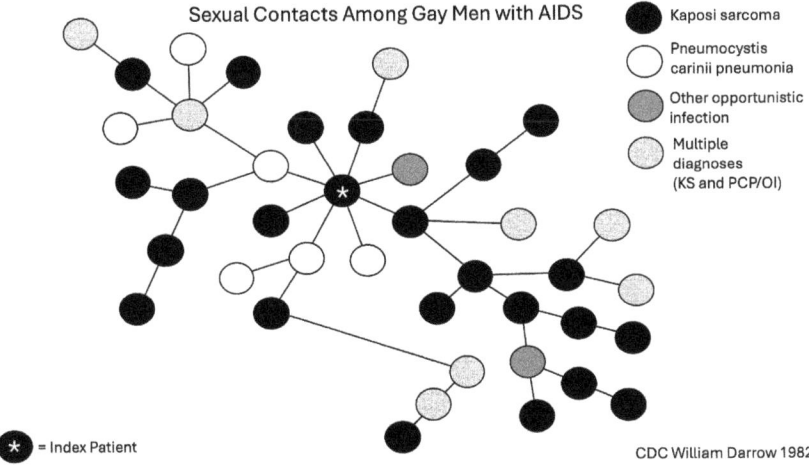

Sexual contacts among homosexual men with AIDS (courtesy David J. Sencer, CDC Museum, William Darrow Collection).

worth noting that three out of the 40 patients were airline stewards. These findings provided further evidence supporting the notion that a sexually transmitted agent was involved, rather than an environmental toxin.[19]

Conclusion

In August 1983, the CDC published the findings of the national case-control study in the *Annals of Internal Medicine*. The study combined epidemiologic data, laboratory results, and analysis of sexual contacts in Los Angeles. Additionally, it considered the development of AIDS among individuals exposed to blood, such as injection drug users and hemophiliacs. Based on these findings, it was concluded that future laboratory studies should focus on identifying an infectious agent that could potentially circulate in the blood or peripheral blood leukocytes, as well as be present in rectal secretions, semen, or other secretions of gay men.[20]

The quest for the AIDS virus was on.

5*

The Search for the AIDS Virus

> *Good afternoon, ladies and gentlemen. The probable cause of AIDS has been found.... Today we add another miracle to the long honor roll of American medicine and science. Today's discovery represents the triumph of science over a dreaded disease. Those who have disparaged this scientific search—those who said we weren't doing enough—have not understood how sound, solid, significant medical research proceeds. From the first day that AIDS was identified in 1981, HHS scientists and their medical allies have never stopped searching for the answers to the AIDS mystery. Without a day of procrastination, the resources of the Public Health Service have been effectively mobilized.... Credit must go to our eminent Dr. Robert Gallo, who directed the research that produced this discovery.*
> —Margaret Heckler, Secretary of Health and Human Services (HHS), April 23, 1984, Washington, D.C.

In October 1981, the CDC conducted a national case-control study that identified the two leading risk factors for AIDS as (1) the lifetime number of sexual partners and (2) meeting partners in bathhouses. Those results suggested that a novel sexually transmitted agent was involved, and retroviruses soon became a target for our search.[1]

Dr. Donald Francis (EIS 1971), CDC Division of Hepatitis and Viral Enteritis, Phoenix, Arizona, was convinced that a retrovirus was the cause of AIDS. He based his assertion on his experiences working on feline leukemia virus, a retrovirus, at Harvard University, under Max Essex, D.V.M., Ph.D.

---

*Chapter 5 adapted from H.W. Haverkos, "Quest for the AIDS virus," *The Pharos* 81 (1) (Winter 2018): 20–27.

Retroviruses

Retroviruses are transmitted as single-stranded enveloped RNA viruses. Upon entry into the target cell (T lymphocytes for HIV), the viral genome is converted into double-stranded DNA by a virally encoded enzyme, reverse transcriptase. The resulting viral DNA is imported into the cell nucleus and integrated into cellular DNA. Once integrated, the virus may become latent, allowing the virus and host cell to avoid detection by the immune system. Alternatively, the integrated viral DNA may be transcribed, producing new single-stranded RNA genomes and viral proteins, which are packaged (enveloped) and released from the cell to infect other cells.

In the 1980s, there were three known subtypes of retroviruses.

1. **Oncoviruses or tumor viruses.** Feline leukemia virus is one such virus that causes leukemia, a cancer of white blood cells, in cats. In the 1960s, several investigators at the National Institutes of Health (NIH) linked an oncovirus, human T-lymphotropic viruses (HTLV-I), to cancers of white cells and bone among humans in Japan and the Caribbean. HTLV-I causes malignant growths of T cells, the same cells depleted in AIDS patients.
2. **Lentiviruses or slow viruses.** No known human diseases had been linked to a lentivirus by 1980, but a few had been identified to affect animals, such as visna virus, which causes encephalitis (inflammation of the brain) and chronic pneumonitis (inflammation of lungs) in sheep. Monocytes and macrophages, types of white blood cells, are the main targets of visna virus.
3. **Spumaviruses or foamy viruses.** These viruses form large vacuoles in infected host cells, but are not associated with disease in humans or animals. Spumaviruses are generally considered laboratory contaminants when found.

At Don Francis's suggestion, Jim Curran invited Dr. Max Essex to come to the CDC in February 1983 to give a lecture on his work on the feline leukemia virus and explain why he and Don Francis thought that a retrovirus was the likely cause of the new syndrome. Francis sent blood samples from our case-control study to Boston to test for antibodies to HTLV-I. Essex found antibodies to HTLV-I in 19 of 75 (25 percent) AIDS patients and two of 336 (0.5 percent) controls, suggesting a possible role for HTLV-I or a related virus.[2]

As the session was winding down, Paul Feorino, a virologist at the CDC attending the session, mentioned that he had isolated a retrovirus in one of the case-control samples, but assumed that it was a lab contaminant, a spumavirus. I nearly jumped out of my seat. Could this be the agent everyone was seeking?

After the meeting, Feorino tried to re-isolate the agent, but without success. Jim Curran asked Don Francis to help the CDC labs develop a comprehensive plan to search for retroviruses. In September 1983, Francis moved from Phoenix to Atlanta to be the CDC's assistant director of viral diseases.

The CDC was also working with Robert "Bob" Gallo at the National Cancer Institute (NCI). He earned a bachelor's degree in biology from Providence College and an M.D. from Jefferson Medical College in Philadelphia. He was among a select group of scientists who first grew T-lymphocytes in 1976, and later identified a new T-cell growth factor, interleukin-2. Those breakthrough discoveries led to his identification of the first retrovirus associated with human cancer, human T-lymphotropic virus (HTLV). In 1982, he received a Lasker Award, considered the highest honor for sciences conferred in the U.S. The award was presented "for his pioneering studies that led to the discovery of the first human RNA tumor virus and its association with certain leukemias and lymphomas."

In September 1981, I met Bob Gallo at a meeting at the NIH. Following a presentation by Jim Curran on the outbreak among gay men, Curran asked Gallo to join our work. Curran suggested that his work on leukemia viruses might be relevant; T cells were affected in KSOI patients. Gallo pointed out that human T-lymphotropic virus type 1 (HTLV-I) caused T cells to proliferate and form a cancer; whatever was causing the new problem was destroying T cells.

Bob Gallo's interest in the epidemic was further stimulated when one of his research fellows identified HTLV-I in two patients with AIDS. One was a 32-year-old African American gay Vietnam veteran living in New York City. He had intermittent fevers, weight loss, lymphadenopathy, and PCP. The second was a 48-year-old African American gay male from Philadelphia with Kaposi's sarcoma and extensive perianal *herpes simplex* virus infection. Could HTLV-I cause AIDS? When Gallo tested the same two patients later in their disease course, he could no longer detect HTLV-I, nor could he find HTLV-I in the next 30 AIDS patients he studied.[3]

A Gathering of Experts in Italy

In the spring of 1983, the CDC received two invitations to attend meetings in Europe. Gaetano Giraldo, an Italian oncologist who associated cytomegalovirus with Kaposi's sarcoma while working in Africa in the 1960s, organized an international conference to discuss AIDS in

Europe and Africa. The second invitation was from the World Health Organization who also wished to hold a meeting on AIDS in Europe. Jim Curran was too busy, so I went to represent the CDC.

Giraldo's meeting was held in Naples, Italy, in June 1983 at the Castel dell'Ovo, a 12th-century concrete fortress overlooking Porto Santa Lucia. The meeting was billed as the first workshop of a European study group on AIDS and Kaposi's sarcoma. Giraldo and his wife, Elke Beth, a scientist with an interest in cancer, hosted the meeting, which was prompted by reports of a new group at risk for AIDS—Europeans returning from Africa.

Giraldo and others speculated that AIDS might be an old illness, endemic in equatorial Africa, and related in some way to cytomegalovirus. The meeting included participants from the U.S. and eight European countries.

I presented the CDC data through April 26, 1983—1,361 case-patients of AIDS reported, of which 40 percent had died. More than 70 percent were gay men, but several other groups of patients had been identified including intravenous drug users, Haitians living in the U.S. and Haiti, hemophiliacs, female and male heterosexual partners of AIDS patients, blood transfusion recipients, and infants and children of high-risk parents.

A New Retrovirus

In the afternoon, Jean-Claude Chermann, a virologist at Institut Pasteur, Paris, reported the isolation of a new retrovirus, lymphadenopathy-associated virus (LAV), from a lymph node biopsy of a gay male with multiple lymphadenopathy. The virus was propagated in cultures of T lymphocytes from a healthy adult blood donor, and umbilical cord blood of newborns. At 15 days in culture, reverse transcriptase activity was detected in the supernatant. A retrovirus was observed on electron microscopy of thin sections of virus-producing lymphocytes; however, its morphology was different from that of HTLV-I and HTLV-II. The core proteins of the new retrovirus were immunologically distinct from the two previously reported human retroviruses.[4]

My wife Lynne and I arrived late for the closing dinner; the French investigators had saved two chairs in the middle of their table. They toasted the CDC for recognizing the new disease and suggesting a viral cause. I toasted them for finding the cause of AIDS.

I asked them to send an LAV sample to the CDC. In turn, we sent blood samples of AIDS patients and controls to France. Unfortunately, the CDC virologists could not identify reverse transcriptase in the sample, and requested a second sample from Paris, which also did not grow.

Blood Recipients and Their Donors

On January 2, 1984, the CDC sent me to Los Angeles to interview blood donors to four pediatric AIDS case-patients attributed to blood transfusions. One of the pediatric case-patients was the son of a prominent Los Angeles lawyer, a major supporter of Ronald Reagan, who demanded an investigation of the blood donors, but the Los Angeles Health Department claimed to not have the manpower to conduct the investigation.

I was given a car, a map of the city, and a list of 42 donors linked to the four children. Over the next two weeks, I interviewed 14 of the donors, and linked each child to at least one gay male blood donor. A few of the donors were already symptomatic with AIDS-related complex.

While in Los Angeles, Michael Gottlieb, the immunologist at UCLA, had identified two unique PCP patients—one was a blood donor linked to a blood transfusion recipient. He wondered if we could grow the virus from them and show that the two viruses were identical, and if that would fulfill part of Koch's postulates. The CDC sent Dr. Paul Feorino to Los Angeles to start viral cultures with fresh blood samples.

In the 19th century, Jacob Henle and Robert Koch formulated the following criteria to establish a causative relationship between a microbe and a disease.

1. The microorganism must be found in abundance in *all* organisms suffering from the disease.
2. The microorganism must be isolated from the diseased host and grown in pure culture.
3. The microorganism should cause disease when introduced into a healthy organism.
4. The microorganism must be re-isolated from the inoculated, diseased host and shown to be the same as the originally inoculated agent.

The blood transfusion recipient was a 38-year-old woman who was diagnosed with PCP a few weeks earlier. When Gottlieb took her history, she told him that she had developed uterine bleeding 12 months earlier and had a hysterectomy. She had received two units of blood from two separate donors at the time of surgery. She was in a monogamous heterosexual relationship, and denied illicit drug abuse. Two weeks after surgery, she developed a transient mononucleosis-like syndrome with fevers and fatigue, consistent with acute HIV infection, but did not seek medical care. In December 1983, she was admitted to a hospital for an acute onset of pneumonia that did not respond to antibiotics, had undergone open lung biopsy, and was found to have PCP.

Gottlieb measured her helper-suppressor ratio and it was low at 0.46 (normal range is 0.9 to 3.7). He contacted the Los Angeles blood bank to see if he could determine the identity of the two blood donors. He found that one of them was a former patient of his, a 24 year-old gay male diagnosed with PCP 10 months earlier. His helper-suppressor ratio was 0.02. The other donor was a healthy male with no apparent risk factors for AIDS.[5]

Identifying the AIDS Virus

On April 23, 1984, Margaret Heckler, President Reagan's secretary of Health and Human Services (HHS), announced that Robert Gallo had found the virus that caused AIDS. She promised Americans that the NIH would have a blood test for the virus in six months [right before the November 1984 elections], and a vaccine in two years.

I was in Atlanta at the time of the announcement and watched it on TV with my colleagues. We were disappointed that Secretary Heckler did not cite the CDC in the announcement. More importantly, there was no mention of the French. It was also unusual for a scientist of Bob Gallo's stature to release a statement to the public prior to publication of results.

The May 4, 1984, issue of *Science* contained four seminal articles from Bob Gallo's group describing their virus, human T-lymphotropic virus type 3 (HTLV-III). The papers documented the two new findings of the NCI. First, they were the first to report the identification of a new retrovirus in AIDS patients, as opposed to a patient with lymphadenopathy, as the French had reported. Second, they identified a cell system for the reproducible detection of the retrovirus from clinical samples. The cells were specific clones of a permissive human neoplastic T-cell line.[6] This cell system provided large amounts of virus for detailed molecular and immunologic analyses and opened the way for the development of a blood test for detection of antibodies to the virus.

In retrospect, the Margaret Heckler proclamation was a political ploy by the Reagan administration in the president's bid for reelection. Promising a blood test in six months meant that a test would be available in October 1984, right before the November elections. The Democratic primaries were ongoing and there was much criticism of Ronald Reagan for apparent lack of progress on AIDS. The primary purpose of the announcement was to shut down the opposition—and it succeeded. However, Bob Gallo's reputation was forever sullied by his silent participation in the event.

Later in the spring of 1984, Paul Feorino and colleagues identified a retrovirus in Michael Gottlieb's blood donor and recipient pair.

The viruses were identical, and the same as LAV reported by the French in 1983. The CDC reported the findings in the July 6, 1984, issue of *Science*.[7] In my opinion, this pair of patients fulfilled Robert Koch's third and fourth postulates of disease causation, specifically demonstrating transmission of an infectious agent to a previously uninfected host with subsequent development of the same disease, then isolating the identical virus.

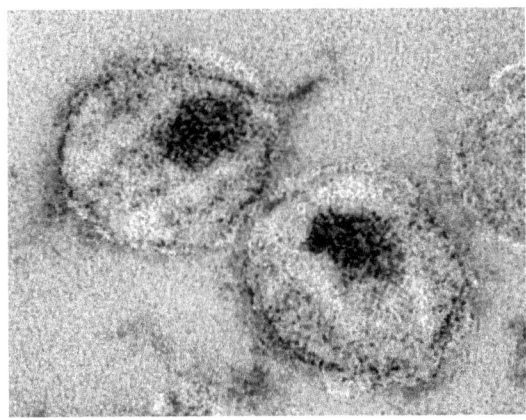

This electron micrograph image depicts the ultrastructural details of a number of HIV particles, or virions (courtesy A. Harrison, P. Feorino, E.L. Palmer, Public Health Image Library).

In the August 24, 1984, issue of *Science*, Dr. Jay Levy, University of California, San Francisco, and colleagues reported isolation of the same retrovirus in 22 AIDS patients and in healthy gay men in San Francisco. The viruses could be propagated in an established adult T-cell line, HUT-78. Levy named the virus AIDS-related virus (ARV).[8]

Strategies to Attack the Virus

We all agreed that a new retrovirus was the cause of AIDS, and strategies to attack the virus were the next steps.

1. Develop a commercially available blood test to screen the blood supply.
2. Develop a vaccine to prevent infection.
3. Develop antiretroviral agents to eradicate the virus.

Shortly after Margaret Heckler's announcement, HHS put out a call for candidate manufacturers to obtain licenses to develop a blood test under the pending patent for Bob Gallo's HTLV-III test. Twenty-five companies applied for licenses, and the HHS awarded non-exclusive, royalty-bearing licenses to seven companies on the basis of experience in working with retroviruses; ability to grow cells in culture for mass production; ability to package, market, and distribute kits in a national system, i.e., millions of assays per year at a reasonable price; and potential for product improvement and refinement.

The FDA worked with the selected companies to facilitate development of candidate donor screening tests. Five companies' tests were licensed by the FDA in 1985:

Abbott Laboratories, Chicago, Illinois
E.I. du Pont de Nemours & Co., Inc., Wilmington, Delaware
Electro-Nucleonics, Inc., Fairfield, New Jersey
Litton Bionetics, Sunnyvale, California
Travenol/Genentech Diagnostics, Cambridge, Massachusetts

Each of the licensed companies pursued a different configuration for an ELISA (enzyme-linked immunosorbent assay) test, but all used a disrupted HTLV-III (virus lysate) as the antigenic substrate—they broke the virus into constituent proteins and tested for antibodies to those inactive pieces of virus.

By late summer of 1984, the manufacturers were ready for clinical trials. The FDA provided a panel of 18 blood samples to evaluate their performance compared to the Bob Gallo prototype test.[9]

Each company was required to demonstrate that their test kits were sensitive enough to detect at least the 1:100 dilutions of sera from patients with AIDS, or in ARC (AIDS-Related Complex), and remain nonreactive in populations presumably unexposed to HTLV-III. To demonstrate performance characteristics, the FDA estimated the sensitivity of each kit by reporting results of studies in which patients with a clinical diagnosis of AIDS were tested, assuming that 100 percent of those patients had antibody to HTLV-III. The specificity of the tests was estimated by testing samples from random blood and plasma donors, assuming a zero prevalence of HTLV-III antibody in those populations.

By December 1984, enough progress was made on the test kits that the Public Health Service developed three provisional recommendations for screening of blood and plasma for HTLV-III antibodies. First, all donated blood and plasma should be tested for HTLV-III antibodies. Second, all positive units must not be transfused or manufactured into other products capable of transmitting agents. Third, the donor should be notified if positive (repeatedly reactive) on the screening ELISA test, or confirmed as positive by another test such as a Western blot.

The ELISA test used antibodies and color change to identify antibodies to HIV. To conduct the test, the sample serum was diluted at least 100-fold and applied to a plate containing HIV antigens. If HIV antibodies were present in the serum, they bound to the HIV antigens. The plate was washed to remove all components not attached to the antigens. A second antibody was then applied to the plate that bound to the person's HIV antibodies, if present; the plate was washed again. The second antibody was chemically linked (conjugated) to an enzyme that converted a substrate to generate a signal that was measured, e.g., color, fluorescence. The plate contained the enzyme in proportion to the amount of second antibody attached to the sample HIV antibodies that bound to the antigens on the plate. The enzyme generated a signal in which its strength was correlated with the amount of HIV-specific antibody that was present in the test sample.

The ELISA test was reported as a number derived as the ratio of the signal strength to a cutoff value representing the upper limit of negative controls.*

On March 1, 1985, the Abbott Laboratories test was licensed by the FDA and immediately used by the American blood banking industry (sensitivity 93.4 percent, specificity 99.8 percent).

On March 7, the Electronucleonics test was licensed (sensitivity 99.6 percent, specificity 99.2 percent).

A third test, developed by Litton Industries, was licensed on April 5 (sensitivity 98.9 percent, specificity 99.6 percent).[10]

Government officials applied to the U.S. Department of Commerce for a patent. On May 28, 1985, HHS was awarded a patent for Bob Gallo's test.

Two additional licenses based on antigens of HTLV-III were awarded in October and November 1985 to du Pont and Travenol, respectively.

A Contentious Situation

In December 1985, the Institut Pasteur filed four lawsuits against the U.S. government. Lawsuits filed with the U.S. Court of Appeals alleged breach of contract, patent interference, damages in the amount of $200 million, and violations of the Freedom of Information Act for review of all NIH laboratory records and memos.[11]

In May 1986, a group of international viral taxonomists declared that all four viruses (Institut Pasteur, NCI, CDC, and San Francisco) reported were identical, and named it human immunodeficiency virus (HIV).[12]

---

*Thanks to Dr. Jay Epstein, a lead scientific reviewer at FDA, for providing his perspective on licensing HIV test kits.

Second Italian Meeting

In June 1986, Gaetano Giraldo held a second European conference on HIV/AIDS, this time in Sorrento, Italy. It would be the first time that Bob Gallo and Dr. Luc Montagnier, French virologist, would appear at a conference together. I was invited to update the epidemiology of AIDS among hemophiliacs and blood transfusion recipients. It was now more than a year since the availability of the Gallo antibody test for screening blood products.

Luc Montagnier named the French virus "Lymphadenopathy-associated virus" in a 1983 report and "Lymphadenopathy AIDS virus" in a 1986 report; both designated as LAV. This may have been to counteract Bob Gallo's claim that he was the first to find the virus in AIDS patients.

Montagnier listed the evidence as to why he considered LAV the cause of AIDS:

> LAV is easily isolated from cultured T lymphocytes of AIDS patients, those with ARC, and asymptomatic carriers from all risk groups.
> LAV replicates exclusively in a subset of T4+ lymphocytes, the same subgroup of cells reduced in AIDS patients.
> The receptor for LAV is associated with the CD4 molecule of T4+ cells.
> LAV can infect non-activated T lymphocytes but only after mitogen stimulation of the cells.
> LAV can also infect and replicate in bone marrow precursor cells.
> Antibodies to LAV were found in some asymptomatic persons in the various high-risk groups indicating infection with the virus.
> LAV is present in blood products, semen, saliva, cervical fluids, as well as in tissue biopsies of spleen, lymph nodes and brain.[13]

Luc Montagnier was allotted 20 minutes for his presentation, but he spoke for almost an hour, leaving no time for questions.

Bob Gallo also gave his 20-minute talk in about an hour. He reviewed his work on AIDS and his virus HTLV-III/LAV (note new dual name of virus). He made four points:

> He and his colleagues had been looking for retroviruses as the cause of AIDS for several years.
> The French found LAV and associated it with a pre–AIDS condition, lymphadenopathy, but Gallo was the first to find HTLV-III/LAV in patients with full-blown AIDS and in various high-risk groups.
> The turning point in AIDS research was accomplished by his laboratory, namely establishing T-cell clones permissive for

5. The Search for the AIDS Virus 69

continuous production of the virus. Large-scale preparation of the virus permitted production of specific reagents and the development of the antibody tests to identify symptomatic and asymptomatic infected persons.

The genome of the virus suggested the relatedness of HTLV-III/LAV to HTLV-I, HTLV-II, and to animal lentiviruses.[14]

I will never forget that evening in Sorrento. On a veranda overlooking the Bay of Naples, dinner tables were set for five. The head table was to include Gaetano Giraldo, his wife Elke Beth, Bob Gallo, Luc Montagnier, and Jean-Claude Chermann. I was seated at a side table with Michael Gottlieb, his wife, and two others. However, when Chermann arrived with a striking red-headed French journalist introduced as his traveling companion, Giraldo was suddenly in a quandary. After whispering at the head table, Giraldo asked if I would take his place. I had met Chermann and other French investigators in 1983 at Giraldo's first meeting and knew Gallo from the NIH. The evening continued pleasantly enough with small talk among the five of us, but escalated into a shouting match between Gallo and Montagnier over various press accounts of comments each had made about the other. All eyes were focused on our table. It was quite tense for several minutes but eventually resolved.

After dinner, Bob Gallo, Jeanne-Claude Chermann, Luc Montagnier, and I met in the hotel bar. Gallo proposed a settlement for the 1985 French lawsuits. First, he and the French scientific team would be declared "co-discoverers" of HIV as the cause of AIDS. Second, the royalties (about $6 million U.S. per year) from the blood tests would be split three ways— one-third to the Institut Pasteur, one-third to the U.S. Department of Health and Human Services (HHS), and one-third put into a trust to support AIDS research in Africa.

On March 31, 1987, U.S. president Ronald Reagan and French prime minister Jacques Chirac agreed that HHS and the Institut Pasteur would share the patent for the HIV blood test, and future royalties would be split in three parts.

However, there were several findings in the NIH laboratory records provided in response to the Freedom of Information Act lawsuit that would disrupt the settlement. On review of electron micrographs of HTLV-III published in May 1984, it was discovered that one of the micrographs was of an LAV sent to the NCI by the French.[15] This "inadvertent" mix-up established that Robert Gallo had used a French virus in his report on AIDS causation.[16] In addition, the Gallo HLTV–III based blood test was based on detecting antibodies against a pool of five viruses, one of which was identified as LAV.[17]

On July 11, 1994, HHS agreed to cede all future patent royalties to the French, and acknowledged that NIH scientists used a virus provided by the Institut Pasteur in developing the AIDS blood test.

In 2008, the Nobel Prize in Physiology or Medicine was divided—one half jointly to Francoise Barre-Sinoussi and Luc Montagnier "for their discovery of HIV," and the other half to Harald zur Hausen, a German scientist, "for his discovery of human papillomavirus causing cervical cancer." Bob Gallo was not mentioned in the announcement.

Acknowledgment: Thanks to Dr. Jay Epstein, a lead scientific reviewer at FDA, for providing his perspective on licensing HIV test kits.

6

HIV Transmission Via Blood

> *July 11, 1982*—An order for pentamidine had come in from Denver. The Pneumocystis victim, the doctors had said, was a hemophiliac.... Because bacteria, protozoa, and one-celled microbes were easily weeded out of the Factor VIII during its preparation process, this meant that GRID was caused by a virus, the only organism small enough to pass through the filters.... Both Lawrence and Evatt [CDC medical officers] knew there would be more GRID case-patients among the hemophiliacs soon and blood transfusion case-patients would follow. Because of their exposure to vast numbers of donors, the hemophiliacs simply had the misfortune to get it first, like the gay men playing on the freeway in the late 1970s.*
> —Randy Shilts, 1987[1]

Dale Lawrence (EIS 1973) was a highly active medical officer at the CDC during the period from the summer of 1982 through the spring of 1983. As a member of the host factors division, he played a pivotal role in evaluating some of the earliest AIDS patients among those with hemophilia and blood transfusion recipients. Additionally, he conducted investigations into the sexual transmission of the virus to spouses. Notably, Lawrence was the first to recognize that the average time interval between HIV infection and the development of AIDS, a critical aspect known as its latency period, was not one to three years, but greater than five years.

AIDS Among Patients with Hemophilia A

In January 1982, a 62-year-old married resident of New York state who had hemophilia A received a diagnosis of *Pneumocystis carinii* pneumonia

---

*Note: This date is wrong and should be sometime in late June 1982 (see text).

(PCP) while in Miami, Florida. This individual regularly used commercial Factor VIII concentrates and had been previously diagnosed with hepatitis B infection. Back in November 1981, he had been admitted for elective knee replacements, but the surgery had to be canceled due to symptoms such as fever, shortness of breath, and increased swelling in his knees. He responded well to antibiotic treatment, prednisone, and an immunosuppressive agent, and was discharged in time for the holidays. Unfortunately, he was readmitted just a week later in severe respiratory distress. An open lung biopsy revealed a large number of *Pneumocystis carinii* organisms. He was promptly treated with intravenous trimethoprim/sulfamethoxazole but passed away two weeks later due to massive gastrointestinal bleeding, shock, and renal failure.[2]

Initially, I did not consider this case as AIDS because of the patient's age (over 60) and recent steroid treatment prior to the PCP diagnosis. However, it was noteworthy as PCP in a hemophiliac had never been reported to the CDC before. In the following weeks, two more men with hemophilia A were reported to have PCP:

- A 59-year-old lifelong resident of Denver, Colorado, with severe hemophilia, experienced gradual weight loss, trouble swallowing, and enlarged lymph nodes starting in October 1980. He received a diagnosis of PCP and CMV pneumonia in May 1982 and passed away on July 5, 1982.
- A 27-year-old resident of northeastern Ohio with severe hemophilia developed symptoms such as fever, fatigue, and a urinary tract infection in July 1981. PCP was diagnosed in October 1981, and he responded well to treatment with trimethoprim/sulfamethoxazole. In February 1982, he was diagnosed with oral candidiasis. He was hospitalized in May 1982 and diagnosed with disseminated *Mycobacterium avium-intracellulare*, another opportunistic infection, and passed away shortly thereafter.[3]

Within a few months, four more case-patients of AIDS were reported among males aged 10 to 55 years with hemophilia A, coming from Alabama, Missouri, Ohio, and Pennsylvania. The geographical distribution of these case-patients among hemophiliacs suggested transmission of a virus through commercial blood products rather than person-to-person contact.[4]

Dale Lawrence and his colleagues in the host factors division at the CDC meticulously reviewed the manufacturer and lot numbers of the clotting factor concentrate used by each patient. Importantly, they found that no patients had received concentrates from the same lot. These findings were compiled into patient reports and shared with both the National

Hemophilia Foundation and the healthcare professionals responsible for the well-being of hemophilia patients.[5]

Hemophilia A, a rare hereditary bleeding disorder, profoundly impairs the blood's ability to clot due to a deficiency in Factor VIII activity. Factor VIII is a crucial protein in the clotting cascade. This condition, which is inherited in a recessive, X-linked chromosomal manner, is considerably more prevalent among men than women. In males, who possess a single X chromosome, the presence of a faulty gene leads to the manifestation of the disease. Females, on the other hand, have two X chromosomes, and they serve as carriers if only one X chromosome carries the defective gene. Full-blown disease symptoms in females occur when both X chromosomes are affected.[6]

Hemophilia A stands as the most common variant of hemophilia, representing approximately 85 percent of the 20,000 individuals affected by hereditary coagulation disorders in the United States during the 1970s. Other forms of hemophilia include hemophilia B (Factor IX deficiency), hemophilia C (Factor XI deficiency), and Von Willebrand disease, characterized by a deficiency in a specific component of Factor VIII.

Before the outbreak of World War II, individuals with hemophilia faced a grim outlook. Most became disabled and unemployable by the age of 20, with an average life expectancy of just 27 years. This disability stemmed from recurrent excessive bleeding into the joints, resulting in mobility challenges and persistent pain. Fatalities were primarily attributed to bleeding episodes within vital organs. However, the 1940s brought significant advancements in transfusion technology, allowing hemophiliacs to receive fresh whole blood or frozen plasma to replace missing clotting factors. By 1960, these breakthroughs had extended their life expectancy to approximately 40 years. Subsequent developments, including the introduction of cryoprecipitate (a substance precipitated from blood at low temperatures) and the availability of self-administered freeze-dried clotting factor concentrates, made of a pooled plasma contributed by hundreds, if not thousands, of donors, had further boosted life expectancy to around 60 years by 1980.[7]

Tragically, the use of pooled plasma concentrates became a conduit for the widespread transmission of HIV to many hemophiliacs in the United States and across the globe. Individuals with all forms of hemophilia and coagulation disorders were treated with the replacement of missing blood factors and, in many instances, blood transfusion. AIDS case-patients were reported among individuals with various congenital bleeding disorders, not only in the United States but also in the Caribbean, Europe, and other nations where factor concentrates were derived from American donors. By 1988, hemophiliacs had the highest prevalence of HIV infection (70 percent) among all known AIDS risk groups, surpassing even that of gay men[8]!

Heterosexual Spread of HIV from Hemophiliacs to Their Wives

Dale Lawrence conducted immunologic studies of hemophiliacs with AIDS to explore the potential for sexual transmission to their wives. Initially, he couldn't find conclusive evidence of transmission from males to females. However, over time, some of the wives developed T-cell dysfunction and later contracted AIDS.[9]

In a 1987 survey of physicians caring for hemophilia patients with AIDS, it was found that 10 percent of the female sexual partners (77 out of 772) were HIV-positive. Among those tested before, during, or after pregnancy, 13 percent (22 out of 167) were found to be HIV-positive. Shockingly, nine out of 13 children born to HIV-positive mothers also became infected.[10]

AIDS Transmission Via Blood Transfusions

Could the as-yet-unidentified AIDS agent be transmitted through blood products from HIV-infected donors? The first documented case of AIDS linked to blood transfusions surfaced in San Francisco in August 1982. It involved a prematurely born Caucasian infant who received multiple blood transfusions during his time in the hospital nursery. At the age of four months, the infant started experiencing fevers and pancytopenia, a condition marked by a drop in all three blood components: red cells, white cells, and platelets. By 20 months of age, the child was diagnosed with *Pneumocystis* pneumonia (PCP).

As I reviewed the child's medical history, I initially suggested that the doctors investigate the possibility of a congenital immunodeficiency. However, my perspective shifted when the Irwin Memorial Blood Bank in San Francisco revealed that one of the donors who contributed blood to the child had recently succumbed to both Kaposi's sarcoma and PCP. This information came from Dr. Arthur J. Ammann (1936–2021), a renowned pediatric immunologist and expert on T-cell dysfunction.[11]

Several other case-patients of blood transfusion recipients contracting PCP emerged from New York City and California. These case-patients could be traced back to high-risk blood donors who subsequently developed AIDS, ARC, or persistent immunosuppression. Here are the details of the first three adult blood transfusion recipients diagnosed with AIDS and linked to a high-risk donor:

- A 64-year-old Hispanic male was diagnosed with PCP in July 1982. He had received 20 units of blood during coronary bypass surgery in January 1981.
- A 56-year-old white female was diagnosed with PCP in August 1982 (Chapter 3). She had received two units of whole blood during a hysterectomy in April 1980.
- A 19-year-old white male was diagnosed with PCP in October 1982. He had received 2 units of packed red cells during surgery following trauma in December 1979.[12]

In November 1982, Jim Curran assigned me the task of visiting the FDA office in Bethesda, Maryland. My mission was to present the three "definite case-patients" of AIDS cited above. During this visit, I had the opportunity to meet with high-ranking officials from the FDA, as well as presidents of prominent organizations such as the American Red Cross and the American Association of Blood Banks, along with other leaders in the field of blood banking.

My primary goal during this meeting was to share detailed patient histories and propose that the blood banking industry seriously consider implementing hepatitis B screening for blood donations. Eighty-eight percent of gay men with AIDS had been found to have antibodies to hepatitis B core antigen. The aim was to identify and exclude hepatitis-infected donors, thus reducing the risk of AIDS transmission to recipients.

However, my proposal was met with a mixture of shock and disagreement from the group. They raised numerous questions and concerns. They wanted to know whether the CDC believed that three case-patients were sufficient to justify such a significant response. They questioned whether other factors might be at play. Some wondered about the health status of the three patients before receiving blood transfusions. There were concerns about the sensitivity and specificity of hepatitis B testing for this unknown agent. Additionally, there were worries about the volume of blood that would be needed to be discarded and the associated costs. The potential impact on the entire blood banking industry was also a source of apprehension.

I found myself questioning why Jim Curran and Bruce Evatt had chosen me to present these findings to the FDA and the blood banking industry. I felt frustrated and uncertain about whether Curran or Evatt might have been better suited for this task.

Following this meeting at the FDA, I returned to Atlanta and reported to my colleagues that our suggestions had not gained much traction.

However, the situation took a turn when Edward N. Brandt, Jr., the assistant secretary of Health and Human Services in Washington, who had oversight over both the CDC and FDA, scheduled a meeting at the CDC in January 1983.

On January 4, the U.S. Public Health Service organized an impromptu advisory meeting at the CDC to address the emerging crisis of AIDS transmission through the blood supply. The primary goal of this meeting was to identify strategies to prevent the spread of AIDS through blood transfusions. Attendees included representatives from various organizations, such as the CDC, the FDA, the NIH, American Association of Blood Banks, American Red Cross, National Hemophilia Foundation, Pharmaceutical Manufacturers Association, and National Gay Task Force. The media was also present, and the meeting was marked by intense discussions and debates.

By this time, Dale Lawrence and Bruce Evatt had collected data on six adult blood transfusion recipients who had developed PCP. They had identified high-risk donors or donors with AIDS or AIDS-related complex in all of these case-patients. These six were clustered in cities with a high incidence of AIDS, such as Chicago, Los Angeles, New York, and San Francisco. It had become evident that a virus similar to hepatitis B was contaminating the blood supply.[13]

During the meeting, I presented the medical histories of these patients, and Jim Curran introduced two possible courses of action for discussion:

1. Implement guidelines to prevent individuals at high risk of AIDS from donating blood.
2. Screen blood donors for hepatitis B virus infection using a test for antibodies to the hepatitis B core antigen, which had shown positive results in 88 percent of gay men with AIDS.

Jim Curran emphasized that AIDS had a latency period of at least one year, and that regardless of any decisions made that day, more case-patients of blood-borne AIDS were likely to emerge over the coming years. Urgent action was needed.

However, instead of focusing on practical solutions, the meeting sparked heated debates among the participants. The FDA and the blood banking industry raised familiar concerns, echoing their objections from our private meeting. The hemophiliac community expressed outrage at the government for failing to warm them about the issue and for the lack of protective measures against the yet-to-be-identified AIDS virus. The gay community felt unfairly targeted and stigmatized as blood donors, questioning why all gay men were being discriminated against when only a select few "fast lane" gays had contracted AIDS.

Unfortunately, by the end of the day, no concrete recommendations were agreed upon, leaving those of us at the CDC deeply frustrated with the lack of progress in addressing the AIDS crisis through blood transfusions.

Don Francis's outrage was palpable, and Matthew Modine, who portrayed him in the movie "And the Band Played On," passionately voiced his frustration, saying:

"How many dead hemophiliacs do you need? How many people have to die to make it cost-efficient to do something about it? A hundred? A thousand? Give us a number so that we won't annoy you again until the amount of money you begin spending on lawsuits makes it more profitable for you to save people than to kill them!"[14]

Simultaneously, the assistant secretary of health expressed disappointment with the outcome of the meeting and applied pressure to high-level officials at the CDC, the NIH, and the FDA to formulate basic recommendations aimed at preventing the sexual and blood-borne transmission of the suspected agent responsible for AIDS. These recommendations were published in the *MMWR* on March 4, 1983.[15]

1. Sexual contact should be avoided with persons known or suspected to have AIDS. Members of high risk groups should be aware that multiple sexual partners increase the probability of developing AIDS.
2. As a temporary measure, members of groups at increased risk for AIDS—gay men, intravenous drug abusers, Haitians, and hemophiliacs—should refrain from donating plasma and/or blood. This recommendation includes all individuals belonging to such groups, even though many individuals are at little risk of AIDS. Centers collecting plasma and/or blood should inform potential donors of this recommendation. The FDA is preparing new recommendations for manufacturers of plasma derivatives and for establishments collecting plasma or blood. This is an interim measure to protect recipients of blood products and blood until specific laboratory tests are available.
3. Studies should be conducted to evaluate screening procedures for their effectiveness in identifying and excluding plasma and blood with a high probability of transmitting AIDS. These procedures should include specific laboratory tests as well as careful histories and physical examinations.
4. Physicians should adhere strictly to medical indications for transfusions, and autologous blood transfusions are encouraged.
5. Work should continue toward development of safer blood products for use by hemophilia patients.[16]

On March 24, 1983, the FDA took further action by notifying all blood collection centers and plasma derivatives manufacturers to quarantine and dispose of any products collected from donors known or suspected of having AIDS. Educational programs were established to inform donors at increased risk for AIDS to stop donating, and donor screening personnel were trained to recognize early signs and symptoms of AIDS. Additionally, the FDA approved a new heat treatment method to inactivate viruses in anti-hemophiliac concentrates. These measures were crucial steps in addressing the AIDS crisis and ensuring the safety of blood and blood products.[17]

As expected, the number of AIDS patients among hemophiliacs in the U.S. increased exponentially, doubling every nine months between 1982 and 1986. AIDS case-patients also surfaced among hemophiliacs in countries that used factor concentrates produced in the United States. Initially, case-patients were reported in the Caribbean and Europe, spreading soon afterwards to hemophiliacs in South America, Africa, Asia, and Australia.[18]

The cumulative count of AIDS patients linked to blood transfusions also surged, doubling every eight months from 1982 to 1986 in the United States. Although the majority of these case-patients reported to the CDC originated in New York and California, by the end of 1986, transfusion-related case-patients tied to high-risk donors were reported from 30 states and several countries across the globe.[19]

Furthermore, HIV transmission occurred between heterosexual partners of blood transfusion recipients with AIDS in both directions, from male to female and from female to male.[20]

Estimating the AIDS Latency Period

Dale Lawrence conducted a unique study focused on blood transfusion case-patients, allowing for a more accurate determination of the AIDS latency period—the time from infection to the diagnosis of AIDS. Assuming that an infectious agent was responsible for the disease, he examined the incubation period (the time from infection to the onset of illness) in the first 11 adult blood transfusion AIDS patients. The results showed a mean incubation period of 18 months, ranging from 4 to 34 months. Additionally, he calculated a mean latency period, which is the time from infection to the diagnosis of *Pneumocystis* pneumonia (PCP), averaging 22 months and ranging from 15 to 34 months.[21]

However, an important epidemiological principle came into play. During an epidemic, it's common to underestimate the true latency period because case-patients with shorter periods between infection and illness are typically reported first. Case-patients with longer incubation periods may not have manifested yet. Dale Lawrence recognized that as the HIV epidemic dramatically expanded from the late 1970s to the early 1980s, the number of recipients of infected blood grew exponentially each year, surpassing the previous year's count. To account for this unequal post-infection observation interval, Dale Lawrence collaborated with Kong-Jung "KJ" Lui, a CDC statistician experienced in hepatitis B virus and blood transfusion issues. They employed a "maximum likelihood probability" approach, and their estimation revealed a "true" latency period of 5.5 years, with a range from 6 months to 11 years.[22]

Subsequently, KJ Lui updated the latency period estimate for adults developing AIDS from blood transfusions to 8.2 years in 1988. He also used data from a cohort of 84 gay men with serological studies documenting the time of HIV seroconversion to calculate an estimate of 7.8 years, with 90 percent confidence intervals ranging from 4.2 years to 15.0 years.[23]

First HIV Antibody Tests Licensed by FDA

In March and April, 1985, the FDA licensed three different HTLV-III ELISA antibody tests with sensitivities ranging from 93.4 percent to 99.6 percent and specificities of 99.2 to 99.8 percent (Chapter 5). These tests marked a crucial step in implementing donor testing within the blood industry, which commenced immediately.[24]

The American Red Cross, a major blood provider in the United States, embarked on extensive testing efforts. They examined over a million units of donated blood within the first four months, discovering that over 10,000 units (1.0 percent) tested positive on the initial test. Of these, 17 percent yielded positive results on repeat testing. Subsequently, all blood donations that tested repeatedly positive were discarded. A specialized experimental test known as Western blot analysis was then employed, resulting in 23 percent of these samples testing positive. These findings led to an estimated prevalence of 38 per 100,000 donors (0.038 percent), meaning that approximately one in 2,500 blood transfusion units were infectious.

Prior to these developments, the Red Cross had already ceased blood collection in San Francisco and New York City several months earlier. The prevalence of donors who tested repeatedly positive on ELISA and Western blot varied by location, with higher rates in Los Angeles and Washington, D.C. (0.11 percent) and lower rates in Boston, Detroit, and Philadelphia (0.03 percent), as well as even lower rates in Portland, Oregon

(0.015 percent), Peoria, Illinois (0.011 percent), and Tulsa, Oklahoma (0.003 percent).[25]

Although it was reported that the Abbott test had a sensitivity of approximately 94 percent, removing less than 0.2 percent of donations resulted in the elimination of about 90 percent of truly infected blood, as per package insert information. Nevertheless, the blood industry recognized the need for further improvement. By the end of 1985, they made the decision to discard all blood that tested positive, even on the first test. Additionally, they actively advocated for the FDA to introduce screening tests with increased sensitivity.

The American Red Cross took proactive measures to contact and evaluate donors who repeatedly tested positive. Notably, 90 percent of those testing positive on the Western Blot were male. In communities where donor notification was initiated, an analysis of the first 41 individuals who repeatedly tested positive on ELISA and Western Blot revealed that 36 of them belonged to high-risk groups. Among these individuals were 30 gay or bisexual men, three recipients of blood transfusions within the past 6 to 30 months, and one each who was a female sex partner of an intravenous drug user, a male with contact with prostitutes in Africa, and someone considered at high risk for non-specified reasons. Surprisingly, most of these 36 individuals were regular blood donors who acknowledged being aware of the definition of high-risk groups but did not perceive themselves as members of such groups. This finding underscored the fact that not only "fast lane" gay men were affected. Any male who had engaged in sex with another male within the last decade was at risk, regardless of their self-identified sexual orientation as "gay," "straight," or "bisexual."[26]

In September 1985, the Public Health Service issued recommendations. They advised that men who had had even a single male sex partner since 1977 should refrain from donating blood. Additionally, they suggested that all commercial sex workers and their customers should wait for at least six months after any commercial encounter before making a blood donation. Some blood banks allowed individuals scheduled for elective surgeries to recruit their own blood donors and even permitted certain patients to donate blood before surgery for their own use.[27]

Legal Response

As the HIV AIDS epidemic unfolded, an increasing number of lawsuits were filed against various entities, including blood suppliers, hospitals, municipalities, and physicians by hemophiliacs and blood transfusion recipients who contracted AIDS. While some of these suits were settled out of court, many went to trial. In these legal battles, a pivotal distinction was whether providing blood or blood components constituted a "service" or a "product." Under traditional product liability laws, products carry an implied warranty, making defendants (such as physicians and the blood industry) liable if the product is deemed faulty. Conversely, if blood provision was considered a service, plaintiffs (the patients) needed to demonstrate negligence on the part of the service provider to establish liability. This was particularly challenging for AIDS patients who received blood before March 1985, as there was no reliable way to test blood for HIV at that time. Nevertheless, lawyers representing patients meticulously examined every step in the blood collection, processing, sale, and transfusion process to determine if providers had been negligent and whether they had taken sufficient measures to minimize risks.[28]

Physicians and the blood industry welcomed the courts' rulings that classified hemophilia concentrates and blood as "services," not "products." However, they recognized the need to improve the education of blood collectors in identifying "high-risk" donors and to closely monitor testing procedures. The blood industry committed to continually reassessing its programs and upgrading its services. Fortunately, over time, more sensitive and specific screening tests for HIV became available.

One lawsuit filed by a hemophiliac patient in France garnered international attention and intensified the ongoing feud between French and American virologists (see Chapter 5). In March 1985, the Gallo HTLV-III based blood became available for use, along with heat treatments for hemophilia factor concentrates. However, Drs. Michel Garetta and Jean-Pierre Allain, directors of the French transfusion centers, initially decided to continue using already collected products and wait for an approved test using the French virus LAV. The FDA licensed such a test on February 18, 1986. In October 1985, the French directors reversed their decision and implemented American recommendations. The number of hemophiliacs in France infected between March and October 1985 remains uncertain, with estimates ranging from five to 50 case-patients. The lawsuit went to trial, and in October 1992, the judges imposed $1.8 million in fines and sentenced Michael Garetta to four years in prison and Jean-Pierre Allain to two years.[29]

Despite the efforts of the blood banking industry, the number of new AIDS case-patients among hemophiliacs and blood transfusion recipients continued to rise over the years (see table). These case-patients persisted well into the 21st century, underscoring the extended latency period of HIV. The average latency period was found to be 8–10 years, contrary to the initial suggestion of 5.5 years by Dale Lawrence and colleagues, with a range spanning from 6 months to 15–20 years.

New AIDS Case-patients Reported Annually Among Hemophiliacs and Blood Transfusion Recipients in the United States (1985–2007)[30]

Year	Hemophiliac	Blood Transfusion Recipient	Total
1985	72	184	256
1986	135	289	424
1987	255	646	901
1988	332	992	1,324
1989	312	829	1,142
1990	357	894	1,251
1991	351	700	1,051
1992	338	650	988
1993*	1,128	1,224	2,352
1994	521	713	1,234
1995	471	576	1,047
1996	340	462	802
1997	248	327	575
1998	223	172	395
1999	165	150	315
2000	117	249	366
2001	106	220	326
2002	90	267	357
2003	85	222	307
2004	92	196	288
2005	79	160	239
2006	54	132	186
2007†	46	110	156
Total, 1982–2007	5,979	10,466	16,445

*From 1993 onward, it is challenging to interpret data because of changes in the AIDS case definition.

†Starting in 2008, CDC grouped risk groups, including hemophiliac, blood transfusion, and perinatal transmission AIDS case-patients, under "Other."

A Positive Note

While the initial response from the blood industry was hesitant, once the HIV blood test became available, they promptly adopted its use and

6. HIV Transmission Via Blood 83

actively advocated for the approval of more sensitive and specific tests by the FDA. The federal response to HIV infections transmitted through blood transfusions and hemophilia factor concentrates has had a profound impact.[31]

This response included several key measures:

1. Donor education materials: The blood industry introduced donor education materials to inform potential donors about the importance of safe blood donation practices.
2. Specific deferral questions: Specific questions were incorporated into the donor screening process to identify high-risk donors effectively.
3. Advancements in HIV donor testing: Continuous advancements in HIV donor testing technology significantly improved the safety of the blood supply.

As a result of these efforts, the risk of HIV infection from one in 2,500 transfusion units before HIV testing was introduced in 1985 has been substantially reduced. Current estimates suggest a remarkably low risk of one transmission in 1.5 million units transfused.[32]

Furthermore, the development of viral inactivation procedures for hemophiliac factor concentrates derived from pooled plasma has further enhanced the safety of these products. A solvent/detergent treatment method has effectively eliminated lipid membrane enveloped viruses from pooled plasma products.[33]

Importantly, over the past two decades, there have been no documented transmissions of HIV, HBV (hepatitis B virus), or HCV (hepatitis C virus) through U.S. licensed blood products. In addition to HIV, donated blood is now screened for a range of infectious diseases, including Chagas disease, hepatitis B virus, hepatitis C virus, human T-cell leukemia virus types 1 and 2, West Nile virus, and syphilis. With these safety measures in place, we now have significantly safer blood products available, and the blood service industry has successfully adapted and thrived.[34]

7

Workplace Transmission Concerns

> *Meanwhile, the doctors [in NYC] fell into little groups, seizing on the implications of GRID in hemophiliacs. First gays, then intravenous drug users, and now hemophiliacs. Those are the major risk groups for hepatitis B. They also knew that there was another risk group for hepatitis B: doctors, nurses, and health care workers. Hospitals were now vaccinating their entire staff with the new hepatitis B vaccine in the first move toward eliminating that dreaded disease from the profession. Would GRID be the encore? Many doctors wondered aloud that afternoon whether the next risk group to be described in the MMWR would include themselves.*
> —Randy Shilts, 1987[1]

In the fall of 1982, there was no evidence yet of AIDS transmission to hospital workers from patient contact or clinical specimens. However, AIDS spread among groups like gay men, drug users, and hemophiliacs similar to hepatitis B virus (HBV). HBV causes hepatitis, cirrhosis, and liver cancer worldwide through mucosal surface contact (like sex) or parenteral exposure (like drug injection).

Healthcare workers (HCWs) contracted HBV through blood and fluid exposure. We recommended "blood and bodily fluid" precautions for HCWs when identifying hemophiliacs as an AIDS risk group, like those in place for hepatitis patients.[2]

I was impressed with the CDC's proactive approach, mirroring HBV precautions, even before any AIDS case-patients attributed to healthcare contact. Back then, we didn't routinely wear gloves for blood work or fluid handling during research. Luckily, I had no needlestick incidents while working with participants. Once, a control subject fainted while I drew blood, but no accidents or fluid contact occurred.

In November 1982, we issued initial recommendations to prevent the transmission of a suspected virus to healthcare workers, even though the specific virus was not yet identified. Over the next five years, we gradually refined and updated these precautions.[3] It wasn't until August 1987 that we recommended "universal precautions," urging all healthcare workers to apply preventive measures for all patients, irrespective of perceived risk, particularly in settings where there was potential exposure to blood and bodily fluids.[4]

Step 10—Implement Control and Prevention Measures as Soon as Possible

In the November 5, 1982, *MMWR*, the CDC addressed the potential transmission risk of an unidentified agent, possibly AIDS, among healthcare workers. It was suggested that this agent could spread similarly to HBV, particularly through contact with blood and bodily fluids from hospitalized AIDS patients or individuals in high-risk groups exhibiting symptoms like chronic generalized lymphadenopathy, unexplained weight loss, and prolonged fever, later designated as AIDS-related complex (ARC).[5]

The CDC recommended several precautions when caring for AIDS patients:

1. Avoid injuries from contaminated sharp instruments and refrain from contact with open skin lesions.
2. Wear gloves when handling blood specimens, blood-soiled items, bodily fluids, excretions, and contaminated surfaces.
3. Use gowns when clothing may be soiled with bodily fluids, blood, secretions, or excretions.
4. Wash hands after removing gowns and gloves and before leaving AIDS patient rooms. Immediate handwashing is essential if they come into contact with blood.
5. Label blood and other specimens prominently with warnings like "Blood Precautions" or "AIDS Precautions." Contaminated specimen containers should be cleaned, and all blood specimens should be double-bagged for transport.
6. Promptly clean up blood spills with disinfectant solutions, such as sodium hypochlorite.
7. Items soiled with blood should be placed in labeled impervious bags for disposal or designated infectious waste bags. Disposable items should be incinerated, and reusable items reprocessed as per hospital policies.

8. Needles should not be bent after use and should be disposed of in puncture-resistant containers. Recapping needles should be avoided to prevent injuries.
9. Prefer disposable syringes and needles. If reusable syringes are used, they should be decontaminated before reuse.
10. Isolate severely ill patients in private rooms, especially those with poor hygiene due to conditions like profuse diarrhea or altered behavior.

These precautions aimed to reduce the risk of potential transmission. Similar recommendations were made for laboratory workers handling clinical specimens and individuals involved in studies with experimental animals inoculated with materials from known or suspected AIDS case-patients. Overall, these guidelines represented early efforts to protect healthcare workers and researchers during the early stages of the AIDS epidemic.[6]

The initial recommendations for AIDS precautions faced several challenges. Firstly, identifying patients with AIDS or at risk in the emergency room or hospital was difficult. Secondly, the guidelines overlooked crucial areas like dental care, hemodialysis, necropsy, outpatient care, and surgery, where hepatitis B transmission had occurred. Thirdly, these precautions unintentionally reinforced the AIDS stigma. Some healthcare workers refused to treat AIDS patients or high-risk individuals, contributing to discrimination against these groups. This fear among healthcare workers led to increased discrimination against gays, drug users, and immigrants, highlighting broader societal issues.

Healthcare Workers with AIDS

By the end of 1982, AIDS case-patients were reported among gay healthcare workers, but no case-patients were reported without any risk factors. However, in May 1983, a 32-year-old Black male hospital housekeeper in Baltimore, with no apparent AIDS risk factors, was diagnosed with *Pneumocystis* pneumonia (PCP) and sadly passed away a week later. In February 1982 he had experienced a needle-stick injury while disposing of a used needle. Although there were no known AIDS patients in the hospital in February, it was known that a homosexual male had undergone a lymph node biopsy in that same clinic in June 1982.

The housekeeper had been working in the ambulatory surgery area since August 1981, handling surgical equipment often contaminated with blood and rarely wearing gloves. While it couldn't be definitively proven that he contracted AIDS through occupational exposure, it couldn't be ruled out either.

In the July 15, 1983, *MMWR*, the CDC documented similar case-patients. One involved a male nurse's aide in New York City with a history of needlestick injury but no known AIDS patient care. The other case-patients included a female hospital laundry worker in New Jersey and a male private-duty nurse in Miami, both with PCP and no documented needlestick injuries. These case-patients raised concerns about the transmission of AIDS to healthcare workers outside known risk groups, emphasizing the need for better understanding and precautions in healthcare settings.[7]

The source of AIDS in these four healthcare workers was never definitively determined, but their PCP diagnoses in AIDS-prevalent urban areas raised concerns. By then, AIDS was believed to result from a virus transmitted through sexual contact, exposure to contaminated blood and bodily fluids, and transfusions months before symptoms appeared. The healthcare workers weren't directly linked to AIDS patients but might have been exposed to asymptomatic carriers or early-stage AIDS case-patients.

These case-patients prompted various reactions within the healthcare community. Some adopted safer practices, like wearing gloves not only with AIDS patients but also for all procedures in hospitals. Janitors and laundry workers were advised to wear gloves when handling potentially contaminated materials.

However, not all responses were positive. Some healthcare workers questioned the risks versus benefits of invasive procedures on seemingly terminally ill AIDS patients. Sadly, a few refused care to gay individuals or those of Haitian descent, displaying discrimination.

Phlebotomists faced difficulties drawing blood while wearing gloves, raising safety concerns. Rising needlestick injuries fueled fear and anxiety among healthcare circles.

These reactions illustrate the multifaceted response of healthcare workers to the emerging AIDS crisis. While some adopted safer practices, others displayed discrimination and fear.

CDC's Hospital Infections Branch

Jim Curran assigned two crucial tasks to the CDC's Hospital Infections Branch:

1. The first task involved updating the August 1982 occupational risk guidelines and including healthcare outside the hospital

setting. These guidelines were originally designed to offer recommendations and precautions for healthcare workers (HCWs) amid the emerging AIDS crisis. Revisions became necessary due to evolving information, increasing case-patients, and a better understanding of the disease's dynamics.[8]

2. The second task was to establish a surveillance system to monitor and record occupational exposures among healthcare workers who interacted with AIDS patients. This surveillance was essential for collecting data on potential risks and incidents related to HCWs' interactions with AIDS patients.[9]

To achieve these objectives, the Hospital Infections Branch reconvened the group that had originally developed the recommendations for healthcare workers in August 1982. This group worked on updating and expanding precautions for a broader range of healthcare professionals, including those in dental care, autopsy, and mortician services. These precautions were extended to three specific patient groups: AIDS patients; individuals with chronic lymphadenopathy, unexplained weight loss, or unexplained fever; and all hospitalized patients with "possible" AIDS. This comprehensive approach aimed to protect healthcare workers and the public from potential AIDS transmission in diverse healthcare settings.[10]

For Dental Care Personnel:

1. Personnel should wear gloves, masks, and protective eyewear during dental or surgical procedures.
2. Instruments used in patients' mouths should be sterilized.[11]

For Persons Performing Necropsies or Providing Morticians' Services:

1. Deceased persons should be identified as belonging to one of the specified patient groups, with this information staying with the body.
2. During postmortem examinations, personnel should wear double gloves, masks, protective eyewear, gowns, waterproof aprons, and waterproof shoe coverings. Contaminated instruments and surfaces should be treated as potentially infective.
3. Morticians should evaluate their procedures to prevent exposure of personnel to body fluids, following infection control measures.[12]

The impact of these recommendations varied among healthcare professionals. Dentists, for example, were not accustomed to wearing gloves during procedures before the AIDS crisis. However, after the guidelines expanded to include dental care precautions, many dentists adopted glove usage consistently to enhance safety for themselves and their patients.

In contrast, implementing recommendations for morticians presented unique challenges. Communication gaps made it difficult to inform morticians when a patient had an AIDS diagnosis, leading to various issues. Some morticians refused to serve AIDS patients due to fears of exposure, and in other case-patients, family members learned about the diagnosis from the mortician rather than from healthcare workers. This highlighted the need for improved communication protocols and sensitivity in handling AIDS case-patients, even after a patient's passing.

For Optometrists, Ophthalmologists, and Eye Care Professionals:

The CDC issued recommendations in the August 30, 1985, *Morbidity and Mortality Weekly Report*. These measures were prompted by the isolation of HIV in the tears of an AIDS patient without eye abnormalities. To enhance infection control and prevent potential HIV transmission in eye care settings, the following precautions were advised:

1. Professionals were encouraged to wear disposable gloves during eye exams.
2. Thorough hand washing between patient examinations was emphasized to reduce cross-contamination risk.
3. Rigorous disinfection after each patient encounter of all instruments and equipment in contact with the eye, including contact lenses used for fittings, was recommended. These measures aimed to ensure no HIV transmission risk through contaminated instruments.[13]

The National Cooperative Needlestick Study

In August 1983, the CDC launched the National Cooperative Needlestick Study, a prospective cohort study to enroll HCWs who had needlestick injuries or mucous membrane exposures to AIDS or related illnesses. The study aimed to monitor these HCWs' health for three years, checking for potential AIDS-related symptoms every six months.

By December 31, 1983, 51 HCWs were enrolled, including 24 nurses (47 percent), 9 physicians (18 percent), and others with varying patient contact. Most were from New York, Texas, Pennsylvania, or New Jersey. Needlestick injuries and cuts with sharp instruments comprised 81 percent of exposures, and none of the participants exhibited AIDS symptoms at that time.[14]

In 1983, French researchers discovered a new retrovirus, later confirmed as the cause of AIDS by American virologists in 1984. In 1985, the FDA approved a commercial HIV blood assay. HIV was found in various bodily fluids, and antibodies to HIV were detected in asymptomatic individuals from high-risk groups and those with AIDS or ARC. This indicated an infectious carrier state where individuals could harbor the virus without symptoms, complicating HIV/AIDS transmission and control efforts.

With HIV antibody tests available, investigators could detect HIV antibodies without waiting for AIDS symptoms. A study involving 1,758 HCWs found 26 (1.5 percent) testing positive for HIV antibodies. Among these, 23 (88 percent) were high-risk group members. Of the three HCWs without high-risk factors, one was tested anonymously, while the other two case-patients were reported in the September 27, 1985, *MMWR*.[15]

Patient 1: A female healthcare worker had needlestick injuries in November 1983 and March 1984 while drawing blood from AIDS patients. In November 1984, she tested positive for HIV antibodies, but no earlier sample existed for comparison. By June 1984, she had developed persistent lymphadenopathy, followed by intermittent diarrhea in August 1984. She denied high-risk factors for AIDS. Her longtime partner initially tested HIV-negative but had the virus detected in his lymphocytes in April 1985, though subsequent tests were negative.[16]

Patient 2: A male lab worker sustained a hand cut processing leukemia patient blood in December 1983 and had a needlestick injury processing platelets in August 1984. By early 1985, he had cervical lymphadenopathy and tested HIV-positive in April 1985. HIV was isolated from his blood lymphocytes in September 1985. He reported 12 lifetime female partners, none believed to have AIDS or be at increased risk.[17]

These case-patients stressed the need for HIV testing and surveillance among healthcare workers, including those not traditionally seen as high risk. They also highlight the challenges of understanding HIV transmission and the virus's asymptomatic carrier state.

Recommendations for Child Care

The case of Ryan White, one of the first school children diagnosed with AIDS in 1984, brought significant national attention to HIV transmission and discrimination in educational settings. In response, the CDC issued recommendations in the August 30, 1985, *MMWR* to address HIV transmission risks while ensuring access to education and childcare for HIV-infected children.[18] Key recommendations included:

1. Decisions about the appropriate setting for HIV-infected children should be based on comprehensive evaluations of their behavior,

neurologic development, physical condition, and expected interactions in that setting.
2. Most school-aged HIV-infected children should attend school and participate in activities without restrictions to normalize their lives and provide equal access to education.
3. Some preschool-aged or neurologically handicapped children with HIV, who lack control over secretions, display problematic behavior, or have uncovered, oozing lesions, may require more restricted environments tailored to their needs.
4. Care involving exposure to an infected child's body fluids and excrement, such as feeding and diaper changing, should be performed by individuals aware of the child's HIV status and the potential transmission modes.
5. Schools and day-care facilities, regardless of HIV-infected children, should adopt routine procedures for handling blood or body fluids. This includes prompt surface cleaning with disinfectants and the use of disposable towels or tissues. Cleaning personnel should avoid exposing open skin lesions or mucous membranes to blood or bodily fluids.

These recommendations aimed to balance public health protection with access to educational and childcare services for HIV-infected children, reducing unnecessary restrictions and combating HIV/AIDS stigma. Ryan White's case and the CDC's guidance played a vital role in raising awareness about HIV/AIDS and fighting associated discrimination.[19]

Updated Recommendations for Preventing HIV Transmission in the Workplace

In a November 1985 report, the CDC issued recommendations to prevent HIV transmission in different settings[20]:

1. Healthcare workers (HCWs), including students and hospital personnel, were urged to receive education on HIV epidemiology, transmission modes, and prevention at work. Adherence to prevention recommendations, especially after needlestick or scalpel injuries during procedures, was crucial to minimize transmission risk.
2. Personal service workers (PSWs) like barbers, hairdressers, and tattoo artists, with close client contact and skin-penetrating instruments, were advised to learn about HIV transmission,

emphasizing hygiene and disinfection. They were encouraged to use disposable or thoroughly cleaned instruments to prevent potential HIV transmission.
3. Food service workers (FSWs), such as cooks and waitstaff, were advised to prevent hand injuries while preparing food and to discard potentially blood-contaminated food to avoid HIV transmission through contaminated food.

These recommendations aimed to protect individuals across various work settings by promoting awareness, hygiene, and safety to minimize the risk of HIV transmission. The CDC also addressed the possibility of HCWs transmitting HIV to patients and planned to provide recommendations on HIV testing for HCWs performing invasive procedures. These guidelines reflected the evolving understanding of HIV/AIDS and the importance of prevention across different job contexts.[21]

Update: Child Care

In February 1986, the CDC reported a case involving a mother who seemingly contracted an infection while caring for her son. Her son, born in February 1984, had a congenital intestinal abnormality diagnosed at four days old. He underwent numerous surgeries, spent 17 months in the hospital, and received blood from 26 different donors. One of these donors, in May 1984 (prior to HIV testing of donors), was a 34-year-old woman who tested HIV-positive in January 1986.[22]

The mother was intimately involved in her son's care, extensively handling his blood, feces, saliva, and nasal secretions. Her caregiving tasks included drawing blood, removing IV lines, emptying and changing ostomy bags, and more, often without consistent glove use or immediate handwashing. She did not report any needlestick injuries or skin lesions on her hands.

In March, June, and October 1985, she donated blood (not given to her child), testing negative in March and June but positive for HIV in October 1985. Subsequent tests in December 1985 confirmed her HIV-positive status, although she remained asymptomatic. Her T-cell function showed a marginal decrease in December 1985.

In response, the CDC stressed the importance of healthcare workers wearing gloves and gowns when exposed to children's blood and bodily fluids, underscoring the need for infection control measures in such settings. This case highlighted the potential for HIV transmission in healthcare settings, even without reported needlestick injuries or symptoms in the infected individual.[23]

The National Cooperative Needlestick Study: Results

As of December 31, 1985, a project enrolled 966 healthcare workers with the following breakdown:

- Nurses: 572 (60 percent)
- Physicians and medical students: 155 (16 percent)
- Laboratory workers: 97 (10 percent)
- Phlebotomists: 52 (5 percent)
- Respiratory therapists: 41 (4 percent)
- Other healthcare workers: 21 (2 percent)
- Loss to follow-up: 28 (3 percent)

About 78 percent were female, averaging 40 years in age, from various states, with New York, New Jersey, California, and Pennsylvania being common origins.[24]

Information on source patients was available for 597 exposures, with 88 percent having the CDC-defined AIDS and 12 percent having AIDS-related complex. Among AIDS case-patients, 68 percent were homosexual/bisexual men, 13 percent were injecting drug users, and others had lower percentages.

Notably, a commercial HIV blood assay became available in March 1985, testing 48 percent of participants. Two individuals (1.65 percent) tested positive, both exposed through needlestick injuries from AIDS patients.[25]

1. A female nurse tested HIV-positive nine months after a needlestick injury contaminated with blood and feces from an AIDS patient. Her male partner, also HIV-positive, declined interviews, raising potential heterosexual transmission.
2. Another female healthcare worker experienced a deep needlestick injury with visibly contaminated equipment. She developed symptoms consistent with primary retroviral syndrome, subsequent illnesses, and tested HIV-negative nine days post-injury but positive on days 184 and 239. Her husband remained HIV-negative.[26]

By 1987, the CDC had documented four HIV infections among 1,215 healthcare workers following needlestick or mucous membrane exposures. Ten more case-patients were reported, with six in the U.S. and four internationally. Additionally, the CDC identified six more HIV infections linked to blood or bodily fluids exposure through a literature review.[27] These findings highlighted ongoing HIV transmission concerns in healthcare settings, especially through occupational exposures.

HIV Transmission from a Dentist to Six Patients

In December 1989, the first known cluster of HIV/AIDS infections resulting from exposure to an infected dentist was reported in Florida. The case involved a 21-year-old woman diagnosed with PCP, despite having no known risk factors for HIV/AIDS. She had mentioned having two teeth extracted by a dentist, later discovered to be a bisexual male with AIDS, about two years prior.

Approximately four weeks after the dental procedure, she sought medical care for a sore throat, consistent with primary retroviral infection symptoms. In June 1989, she developed oral candidiasis and sadly passed away in September 1990.

The dentist had been diagnosed with Kaposi's sarcoma in September 1987 and also passed away in September 1990. Genetic sequence analysis of both their viruses showed a striking similarity.[28]

The State Health Department's investigation identified five more HIV-infected patients who had received dental care from the same dentist, and their viral sequences were genetically related.[29] This case highlighted the potential for HIV transmission in healthcare settings, even through dental procedures.

In August 1987, a critical shift occurred in AIDS prevention recommendations for healthcare workers, personal service workers, and food service workers. "Universal" precautions were introduced, advising all workers to apply preventive measures with every patient, regardless of perceived risk, in settings involving potential blood or bodily fluid exposure.[30] This marked a transformative step toward comprehensive infection control. The timeline below summarizes the evolution of these recommendations.

MMWR Date	Target Groups	Source Patients	Inciting Event
11/5/1982	Clinical/laboratory hospital staff	AIDS/ARC	Resemblance to HBV transmission
7/15/1983	Alert: Initial reports of HCWs infected	AIDS/ARC	AIDS among HCWs
9/2/1983	Dental care personnel, morticians, dieners	AIDS/ARC	Recommendations for allied HCWs
8/30/1985	HCW performing eye exams (optometrists, opticians)	HIV-infected patients	HIV grown from tears
8/30/1985	Schools and foster care of children	HIV-infected children	Ryan White
11/15/1985	HCW, PSW, and FSW	All patients/clients (routine use)	HIV transmission reported

MMWR Date	Target Groups	Source Patients	Inciting Event
11/15/1985	Patients treated by HIV-infected HCW	HIV-infected HCW performing invasive procedures	HIV transmitted from surgeon/dentists to patients
2/7/1986	Childcare providers	HIV-infected children	Child-to-mother HIV transmission reported
4/11/1986	HCW performing invasive procedures	HIV-infected HCWs	Question raised about HIV testing of HCW
4/18/1986	Update for dental care personnel	All patients (routine use)	Recognition that dentists exposed to additional pathogens
6/13/1986	Dialysis unit workers	HIV-infected patients	Special concerns of dialysis units
8/21/1987	All HCW, PSW, and FSW	All persons (universal precautions)	Compilation of CDC recommendations
7/27/1990	Alert: Initial report of a patient infected by HCW	HIV-infected dentist	HIV transmission from HCW to patient

A Case Report

After finishing my morning clinic and en route to my job at the National Institute on Drug Abuse (NIDA), the head nurse approached me with a request to see a patient transferred from the ER. The patient, a 22-year-old nurse, had experienced a needlestick injury while drawing blood from an AIDS patient; she was just starting her job at Walter Reed Army Medical Center. Overwhelmed and fearful, she had received prompt care in the ER, including wound cleaning, HIV testing, and a prophylactic two-drug regimen within an hour of the incident.

I provided reassurance, explaining that while the risk of HIV transmission in such case-patients was low, it wasn't nonexistent. We decided to monitor her health over six months, discussing potential medication side effects. To safeguard her boyfriend's well-being, I advised her to inform him and recommended seeking emotional support from a family member or trusted friend.

She returned to the clinic a week later, thankfully tolerating the medications well, with her hand wound healing. She had also shared her experience with her supportive father and informed her boyfriend, though they would separate during this challenging period.

I am pleased to report that at the critical six-month mark, she remained HIV-negative, despite the emotional toll on her personal life.

Conclusion

Developing recommendations to prevent HIV transmission among diverse groups, including healthcare employees, personal service providers, food service workers, and family members, was a lengthy and challenging process. Even before identifying the cause of AIDS, efforts were underway to anticipate HIV transmission in the workplace and offer initial guidance.

It took nearly five years to establish "universal precautions" for HIV prevention. Unfortunately, during this period, fear among healthcare workers and the public increased, leading to heightened stigma and discrimination against those affected by HIV/AIDS.

It's crucial to note that the mechanisms for hepatitis B virus (HBV) infection in healthcare workers are similar to HIV transmission. Both viruses can be transmitted from infected healthcare workers to patients, albeit rarely. However, HBV transmission rates in the workplace are higher than HIV. For instance, the risk of HIV transmission through a single needlestick exposure is about 0.3 percent, whereas HBV's risk ranges from 6–30 percent, significantly greater. Fortunately, there's an effective HBV vaccine for healthcare workers, unlike HIV.[31]

Continuously improving preventive measures and education in healthcare settings on HIV and HBV transmission are essential to protect both patients and workers. This effort can reduce fear, stigma, and discrimination while promoting a safe, supportive environment for all involved.

8

Haitian Connections*

> *During the final weeks of March 1982, the pace quickened in the labyrinthine corridors of the red brick Building 6 of the CDC in Atlanta.... The latest crisis had started with sporadic reports to the CDC's parasitic disease division of toxoplasmosis in Haitians, first in Miami and then in New York City. At first parasitologists thought this was some problem unique to the malnourished refugees who had come from the most impoverished nation in the Western Hemisphere. Others remembered reports of strange case-patients of toxoplasmosis among gay men in the early case-patients.*
> —Randy Shilts, 1987[1]

In March 1982, I conducted evaluations on several patients with opportunistic infections across multiple locations—Florida, Texas, and upstate New York. I then returned to Atlanta to present a paper at the annual Epidemic Intelligence Service (EIS) conference. This paper described our case definition and the active surveillance system we had in place.

During this time, Jim Curran approached me and requested that I withdraw my paper. He asked me to go to Miami, Florida, where a pathologist had reported two male Haitian immigrants with central nervous system toxoplasmosis. There were also other patients with CNS lesions of undetermined diagnoses in Miami. The Miami pathologist sent samples to experts across the country, including pathologists at Stanford University. These experts confirmed the diagnosis of CNS toxoplasmosis in five of the Miami patients. Furthermore, they reported two additional case-patients of Haitian refugees with toxoplasmosis, one from Montreal and another from New York City, to the CDC parasitology division.

---

*Chapter 8 adapted from H.W. Haverkos, "Caribbean Connections." The Pharos 82 (1) (Winter 2019): 36-43.

In Miami, I conducted a thorough review of the medical records of nine patients. Among them, six had CNS toxoplasmosis, one had *Pneumocystis carinii* pneumonia (PCP), one had Kaposi's sarcoma (KS), and one had disseminated cryptococcosis. My assessment led me to believe that these patients met the criteria outlined in our case definition.[2]

Additionally, I had conversations with two Haitian-born physicians who confirmed that their patients did not fit the profile of being either gay or injecting drug users.

Following Jim Curran's request, I joined a team of scientists from the National Institutes of Health (NIH) on a trip to Haiti. The team was led by Dr. Richard Krause, who served as the director of the National Institute of Allergy and Infectious Diseases (NIAID). It also included three other physician-scientists: Cliff Lane, Tom Quinn, and Al Saah (who had previously been part of the Epidemic Intelligence Service in 1976).

Upon our arrival in Haiti, we were greeted by an American-born diplomat and offered coffee while our luggage cleared customs. We were then transported to our hotel, where we were informed that we could request anything we desired, including female companionship.

During our time in Haiti, we made several presentations to groups of doctors at the university hospital and were granted permission to examine patients. One significant encounter occurred in an open ward located in a poorly lit section of the hospital. Among the seven patients presented to us, one was a 50-year-old white male government employee who exhibited symptoms of esophageal candidiasis and oral thrush. He was married with five children and initially denied engaging in homosexual behavior. However, a medical resident was able to elicit a history of homosexual activity from the patient on the night before our visit. The resident explained that the patient would not be seen by the visiting American doctors if he denied his homosexual history. Sadly, when we arrived at his bedside, the patient was unresponsive and unable to communicate. We were unable to confirm his sexual history. On physical examination, we observed that his skin and mucous membranes were dry, and when we attempted to pinch his skin, it tented—a clear indication of severe dehydration. When we questioned the resident about the lack of intravenous fluids, he informed us that IV fluids were not part of routine care at the hospital. It was the responsibility of the patient's family to obtain the necessary materials from a local pharmacy. Tragically, the patient passed away the following day.

Another patient we encountered was a Black woman in her twenties, reportedly a sex worker, who had a severe genital infection caused by herpes simplex virus (HSV). Upon uncovering her at the bedside, we observed vesicles and pustules affecting her genital area. It was surprising to see her in an open ward, as standard protocol in the United States would have

8. Haitian Connections

mandated placing her in a private room with wound and skin precautions in effect. These precautions include measures to protect the wound from contamination by healthcare workers, as well as to safeguard healthcare workers from exposure to HSV and other infectious agents. This typically involves handwashing; wearing masks, gowns, and gloves before entering the patient's room; and the careful removal and disposal of these items in a closed container, followed by handwashing before moving on to the next patient.

With the assistance of the Haitian medical residents, we discussed antiviral treatments for HSV infection. I shared information about my work with interferon but did not recommend it for this patient, as I believed that a virostatic agent would have limited impact on such an extensive HSV infection.

The last patient we encountered was a gay male with multiple infections, including pulmonary tuberculosis (TB). He had only been started on anti–TB medications three days prior to our visit. In the United States, he would have been placed in a private pressurized room, where air pressure could be adjusted to protect staff from TB exposure. Unfortunately, such facilities were not available in Haiti.

During our trip, we had the opportunity to meet Dr. Jean Pape*, an infectious diseases clinical researcher who had a remarkable background. Dr. Pape was born in Haiti and graduated with a degree in biology from Columbia University in 1971. He went on to earn a medical degree from Cornell University Medical College in 1975. Dr. Pape's work was supported by the Rockefeller Foundation, and he was conducting research on infants with diarrheal disease, a significant cause of mortality in Haiti and other developing regions. He shared with us the impressive outcomes achieved through the implementation of oral rehydration therapy and careful patient monitoring.

Dr. Pape guided us through a large room with 24 beds under a cement roof, and we continued to an open-air patio where additional infants were lying on individual cots.

While we were engaged in patient care, Dr. Richard Krause held discussions with hospital administrators. The Haitian doctors sought financial support to study the increasing number of patients with AIDS. They also requested expensive laboratory equipment, such as lymphocyte cell sorters for measuring T-cell functions and medications for the treatment of viral infections. Most notably, the Haitian physicians urged Krause to

---

*Thanks to Jean William "Bill" Pape, M.D., for providing his perspective on AIDS among Haitians, and for his lifelong compassionate service to the Haitian people.

remove Haitians from the CDC's list of AIDS risk groups. They questioned why the entire nation of Haiti should be labeled as a risk group. However, Krause conveyed that he couldn't modify this designation and deferred to me as the CDC representative, leaving me in a somewhat challenging position.

When queried about the CDC's classification, I clarified that there might be something unique or different among Haitians that could help in identifying the cause of the new disease and devising strategies to prevent it within all three affected groups: gay men, injecting drug users, and Haitians. I encouraged them to explore potential risk factors among their patients. They repeatedly emphasized the hardships they faced due to this designation. I assured them that I would communicate their concerns to my superiors.

Upon our departure from the hospital, the clinical staff, for a few days, refused to provide care to patients without utilizing the protective measures I had recommended. After spending ten days in Haiti, we were driven to the airport, where our bags were unceremoniously thrown out of the taxi, and we were left to fend for ourselves. It was apparent that our visit had not met their expectations, and tensions persisted.

Upon my return to Atlanta, I conducted a thorough review of case report forms from national surveillance and the travel histories of gay men participating in our national case-control study. In this analysis, I discovered a small number of gay men with AIDS who had reported vacationing in Haiti. Some of these individuals had also reported engaging in sexual activities with men and/or boys during their trips.[3]

In the October 20, 1983, issue of the *New England Journal of Medicine* (*NEJM*), Dr. Jean Pape and his colleagues provided a summary of clinical findings from 61 previously healthy Haitians who had been diagnosed with either Kaposi's sarcoma (15 case-patients), opportunistic infections (45 case-patients), or a combination of both (1 case) in Haiti between June 1979 and October 1982. Of these case-patients, 52 (85 percent) were men, and tragically, 54 of them (89 percent) had passed away. Notably, nine of the male patients (17 percent) reported engaging in bisexual behavior, with a few reporting sexual encounters with American men in Miami and New York City. While three men and two women reported prior blood transfusions, none reported illegal drug use. One-third of the male patients were from Carrefour, a popular vacation destination known for commercial sex work, and 71 percent of the patients reported a previous sexually transmitted infection. Dr. Pape suggested that there might be a strong bias against homosexuality in Haiti and that the connections between American gay men and Haitian bisexual men might have been underestimated.[4]

Meanwhile, clinicians had reported ten Haitian American heterosexual men residing in Brooklyn, New York, who presented with opportunistic infections and immunologic defects similar to those seen in gay men with AIDS. These men ranged in age from 24 to 39 years old, and sadly, six of them had already passed away by the time of publication in *NEMJ*. All of them denied engaging in gay sexual behavior or injection drug use.[5]

At the request of Jim Curran, I conducted an investigation into a Haitian American individual who had been diagnosed with PCP as far back as 1959. I visited Kings County Hospital in Brooklyn and met with one of the coauthors of the case history reported in 1961. This raised the intriguing question of whether AIDS might have been occurring unnoticed for more than 20 years.

The patient in question was a 49-year-old black man admitted on June 8, 1959, with complaints of a persistent three-month cough. His chest X-ray revealed diffuse haziness, which was consistent with PCP but not unique to it. His white blood cell counts ranged from 10,800 to 62,000 cells per cubic millimeter, an unusual finding for an AIDS patient. Tests for common bacteria, tuberculosis, and common fungi all returned negative results. He was treated with isoniazid, streptomycin, tetracycline, and corticosteroids but sadly passed away on the 20th day of his hospitalization. Subsequent autopsy confirmed the presence of PCP. The patient had been born in Haiti and had immigrated to New York City as a teenager in 1927, where he worked as a shipping clerk in an apparel factory.[6]

Despite these intriguing historical findings, I was unable to conclusively confirm a diagnosis of AIDS. The use of steroids before the diagnosis of PCP was a disqualifying factor, and the elevated white blood cell counts were atypical for an AIDS patient. The mystery surrounding the emergence of AIDS continued to deepen.

Missed Clues

I shifted my focus to evaluate hemophiliacs and blood transfusion recipients. In doing so, I overlooked important clues regarding Haitians and heterosexual transmission. In late 1982, researchers at Albert Einstein College of Medicine in the Bronx, along with their colleagues, reported four noteworthy case-patients:

- A 17-month-old Black/Hispanic male with a disseminated *M. avium-intracellulare* infection. His mother, an injecting drug user, had succumbed to PCP.
- A five-month-old Caucasian female with PCP, whose mother

was both a commercial sex worker and an injecting drug user. The mother exhibited oral candidiasis and lymphopenia and had another daughter who had previously died from PCP.
- Another five-month-old, this time a Haitian male, presented with PCP, cryptococcus, and cytomegalovirus (CMV) infections. Unfortunately, we lacked information about the health status of the parents.
- A second five-month-old Haitian male also had PCP, with no information available about the parents' health.[7]

I initially failed to recognize the Haitian connection in these reports and considered them as a challenge to my existing case definition. I questioned whether it was possible to rule out congenital or hereditary immunodeficiencies.

Clinicians in Newark, New Jersey, later reported eight children, with a median age of 12 months, who suffered from PCP or severe immunodeficiency. One of these children had parents born in Haiti, and another had a mother born in the Dominican Republic, a nation which shares the island of Hispaniola with Haiti. Six of the children's parents admitted to injecting drugs. The children displayed recurring fevers, failure to thrive, interstitial pneumonitis, and hepatosplenomegaly. Their immune defect closely resembled that seen in adults with AIDS.[8]

In July 1981, I had established the original CDC definition of AIDS, which included the following criteria:

1. Biopsy-proven KS and/or culture or biopsy-confirmed life-threatening opportunistic infections that were at least moderately predictive of immunosuppression.
2. The affected person was between the ages of 15 and 60 years.
3. There was no prior evidence of underlying immunosuppression, such as a cancer diagnosis, organ transplant, or the use of steroids or other immunosuppressants.

Some pediatricians questioned the age restrictions in our case definition and wondered why the CDC was slow in recognizing AIDS among infants and children. As a response, Curran assigned two CDC pediatricians to develop a case definition specifically for pediatric patients and set up a separate surveillance system.[9]

In the January 4, 1984, issue of *NEJM*, pediatricians in Miami reported 14 infants with AIDS, with 12 having Haitian-born parents and two having non–Haitian parents who were injecting drug users.[10] The undeniable Haitian connection became apparent.

Case-Control Studies

The CDC initiated a case-control study within the Haitian American community residing in Miami and New York City. The study defined a "case" as a patient diagnosed with AIDS who was born in Haiti and had previously been hospitalized at either Jackson Memorial Hospital in Miami or Downstate Medical Center in NYC. "Controls" were individuals of Haitian origin, both men and women, selected from hospital wards, outpatient clinics, and private physician offices associated with the two hospitals. Controls were matched to case-patients based on sex, age, and city of residence, and those with underlying cancers, immune suppression, chronic medical conditions, or HIV-positive status were excluded from the study.[11]

The interviews were conducted confidentially by five trained interviewers proficient in both Creole and English. These interviews covered the individuals' time spent in the U.S. and the last five years of their life in Haiti. Laboratory tests were carried out to assess immune function and detect sexually transmitted and mosquito-borne infections. A standardized questionnaire was developed and translated into Creole. This questionnaire explored various aspects related to the transmission of infectious agents, including living conditions, occupation, medical history, sexual history, use of folk healers, history of tattoos, involvement in voodoo practices, and the date of arrival in the U.S. The questionnaire was designed to obtain detailed information on topics such as homosexuality and blood transfusions through specific questions about sexual activities, including commercial sex work with tourists.

Between March and December 1984, a total of 45 men and 10 women with AIDS, along with 242 controls, were interviewed. Of these, 37 patients and 164 controls were in Miami, while 18 patients and 78 controls were in NYC. Of the 51 case-patients in whom blood was drawn, 49 (96 percent) were found to be HIV-positive, whereas 10 out of 218 (5 percent) controls tested positive for HIV when blood was drawn and were subsequently excluded from further analysis.

The analysis of data was performed separately for men and women. Among the male patients, one was identified as gay, and one female patient had received a blood transfusion. None of the patients admitted to injecting drugs, having hemophilia, or engaging in sexual contact with AIDS patients. However, male patients were more likely to report sexual contact with commercial sex workers and a history of gonorrhea and/or syphilis. Female patients were more likely to have received offers of money for sex and to have friends who were voodoo priests. Based on these findings, the CDC concluded that the case-patients resulted from heterosexual transmission.[12]

Additionally, Dr. Pape and colleagues conducted a case-control study in Haiti, interviewing 93 men and 35 women with AIDS, along with 112 age- and sex-matched controls who were either siblings or friends of patients. They identified known risk factors for 43 percent of patients, including 33 bisexual men, one intravenous drug abuser, and five men who had received blood transfusions. Among female patients, 14 reported previous blood transfusions, and two were spouses of men with AIDS. Two variables, the number of heterosexual contacts and the receipt of intramuscular injections, showed significant differences. Dr. Pape concluded that the earliest case-patients were likely bisexual men who had connections to American gay men vacationing in Haiti, followed by transmission to others in Haiti through heterosexual contact.[13]

A New Risk Factor

The Haitian study not only confirmed the CDC's initial link to heterosexual transmission but also identified a new risk factor, which was the receipt of intramuscular injections with reusable needles. Over the five-year period before the onset of symptoms, a striking 89 percent of patients had received intramuscular injections, compared to 66 percent of controls. Patients received a higher number of injections per year and were more likely to get these injections from non-medical sources. It was common practice in Haiti for individuals to receive intramuscular injections of antibiotics or vitamins when they felt unwell.[14]

By May 1985, the CDC removed Haitians as a major risk group. Subsequently, the CDC's surveillance team identified five men with AIDS born in Barbados, Jamaica, St. Vincent, and Trinidad with no known risk factors, along with case reports of AIDS from other Caribbean Islands. As a result, the term "Haitian" was removed from the CDC reports and replaced with "born in the Caribbean."[15]

In 1985, Jim Curran assigned Ken Castro (EIS 1983) to investigate an agricultural community, Belle Glade, located on Lake Okeechobee, 45 miles west of West Palm Beach, Florida. This was prompted by an unusually high rate of reported AIDS case-patients in the area with no identified risk factors. The community saw an influx of thousands of migrant farm workers, including American Blacks, British West Indians, Haitians, and Hispanics during sugarcane and vegetable harvesting seasons.

The investigation began by interviewing surviving AIDS patients, inquiring about known risk factors for HIV transmission, including contact with other AIDS patients or individuals at risk for HIV infection. If patients were deceased, family members or known sexual contacts were interviewed. They identified risk factors for 66 of 73 male patients and 19 of 20 female patients. Notably, nine of the patients were born in Haiti. Of the patients, 35 men and 7 women, were linked through heterosexual contact with a person with AIDS or someone at an increased risk for AIDS. Additionally, 21 patients were injecting drug users, and 17 men identified as homosexual or bisexual.[16]

Subsequently, three seroepidemiologic studies were conducted between February and October 1986. A standardized questionnaire, available in English, Spanish, and Haitian Creole, explored various topics, including living conditions likely to result in increased exposure to insects. Three populations were recruited: a randomly selected group of 877 participants approached door-to-door, 115 participants who requested HIV testing (non-randomly selected), and 28 clinic attendees being evaluated for potential HIV infection. Participants were also asked to volunteer for various tests, including HIV infection, sexually transmitted diseases, and insect-borne infections.[17]

HIV-seropositive individuals were found to be more likely to originate from Haiti and/or have lower incomes, more sexual partners, and more syphilis and hepatitis B infections. Seropositive men were more likely to report sex with men, sex with commercial sex workers, injection drug use, and gonorrhea. Seropositive women were more likely to have given birth to children with different fathers, have been paid for sex, have engaged in sex with injection drug users, have gonorrhea, have received blood transfusions, and have tattoos. Importantly, there was no evidence to suggest transmission by insects.

The CDC's conclusion that the high cumulative rate of AIDS in Belle Glade was primarily due to heterosexual contact and intravenous drug use marked a significant development. In August 1986, the CDC transferred patients born in the Caribbean with no known risk factors from the undetermined category to heterosexual contact case-patients. The CDC and the World Health Organization (WHO) subsequently issued reports designating three categories of AIDS transmission worldwide[18]:

1. Pattern I countries, such as those in North America and Europe, where male homosexuality and injecting drug use were predominant risk factors.
2. Pattern II countries, such as those in the Caribbean and sub-Saharan Africa, where heterosexual transmission was believed to play a major role, and transmission from mother to child was common.
3. Pattern III countries, such as Eastern Europe, the Middle East, Asia, and most of the Pacific, where case-patients occurred

primarily among individuals who had traveled to endemic areas and had sexual contact with commercial sex workers or gay men.

By March 1988, 136 countries had reported a total of 84,526 AIDS case-patients. Haiti, in particular, reported 912 case-patients, ranking first among Caribbean nations and one of the top 15 countries worldwide for AIDS case-patients.[19]

Haitian Americans played a crucial role in shedding light on the early clusters of AIDS patients linked to heterosexual transmission. This phenomenon was fueled by three key risk factors: social discord, commercial sex work, and drug abuse. Social discord often occurred when men and women were separated from each other due to various social conditions, including immigration, seasonal farm or mine work, cross-country trucking, and military deployment.

Haiti, as a mountainous country in the West Indies, occupies the western third of the island of Hispaniola, located between Cuba and Puerto Rico in the Caribbean Sea. It is recognized as the world's oldest Black republic and is also one of the poorest countries in the Western Hemisphere.

The Duvalier family's rule played a significant role in shaping Haiti's history. Francois Duvalier, known as Papa Doc, was elected president of Haiti in 1957. He declared himself president for life and governed the country as a dictator. Upon Papa Doc's death in 1971, his son, Jean-Claude Duvalier (Baby Doc), who was just 19, succeeded him and continued to rule as a dictator. The regime controlled the armed forces and operated a secret police force known as the Tonton Macoute, named after a bogeyman figure from folklore who abducted children in the night.

In the early 1970s, many Haitians left their homeland due to poor economic conditions and harsh treatment by the secret police. Economic and political conditions worsened over the following decade, leading to a massive migration of Haitians to New York City and South Florida at the same time that HIV was introduced into North America.

The Haitian HIV connection highlighted the immigration pattern in which men would often establish themselves in a new land before returning to retrieve their spouses. This migration pattern brought heterosexual transmission of HIV infection into sharp focus.[20]

AIDS Worldwide

The impact of HIV/AIDS on a global scale has been devastating. According to WHO, more than 35 million lives were lost to HIV/AIDS worldwide between 1981 and 2013, and as of the end of 2013, 36.7 million people were living with HIV infection. Certain key populations, including men who have sex with men, female sex workers, users of injection drugs, truck drivers, fishermen, and military personnel, have been disproportionately affected by the disease around the world.[21] The sentinel patients among Haitians living in Haiti and the United States played a crucial role in recognizing international HIV transmissions, particularly through heterosexual behaviors.

To summarize, the first case-patients of AIDS in Haiti were identified in 1978–1979, which coincided with the recognition of AIDS among gay men in New York and California. Jean Pape suggested that HIV was introduced into Haiti either by gay tourists or by bisexual Haitians returning from the United States and then spread to heterosexual individuals in Haiti. It's worth noting that we can also connect heterosexual Haitian Americans in Miami to white, Black, and Hispanic heterosexual drug users in Belle Glade, Florida. From there, HIV likely spread through South Florida and continued to spread throughout the U.S.[22] The Haitian connections, while significant, are likely not unique, as similar HIV networks exist worldwide.

While many historians favor the hypothesis that AIDS originated in Africa, Jean Pape's research did not establish a direct link between the earliest AIDS case-patients in Haiti and Africa.[23] He noted that around a hundred Haitian professionals, primarily teachers, had gone to Africa, particularly Zaire (now the Democratic Republic of Congo), in the late 1960s to escape the dictatorship of Francois Duvalier. However, very few of them returned to Haiti, and none were among the earliest case-patients of AIDS.

In essence, the HIV/AIDS pandemic has a complex and multifaceted origin, and the contribution of various populations and factors, including those observed in Haiti and the Haitian American community, has played a significant role in our understanding of the disease's transmission dynamics.

9

Out of Africa?

> *Recent reports have also identified another group at risk of developing AIDS and opportunistic infections, namely equatorial Africans living in France, Belgium, or in their native country. This important observation leads [one] to consider that this syndrome is an old illness, endemic in equatorial African regions, with a recent epidemic expression in the western civilization due to pertinent cultural changes in a selected population of our society.*
> —Gaetano Giraldo, 1984[1]

In 1983, the CDC received two European invitations. Dr. Gaetano Giraldo invited Jim Curran to speak at an AIDS conference in Italy. Simultaneously, the World Health Organization in Geneva, Switzerland, requested Curran's assistance in preparing for their first AIDS meeting. Due to Curran's busy schedule, I represented the CDC.

In June 1983, I attended the First Workshop of the European Study Group on AIDS in Naples, Italy. Organized by Gaetano Giraldo, the meeting emphasized Giraldo's research linking cytomegalovirus to Kaposi's sarcoma in Uganda in the 1970s. It also suggested AIDS was an ancient disease endemic in Africa. At this meeting, I first learned about the French retrovirus, lymphadenopathy-associated virus (LAV), and the existence of another at-risk group for AIDS: heterosexual Africans living in Belgium, France, or their home countries.

Between May 1979 and April 1983, 16 previously healthy Black Africans and one Caucasian Greek native, who had lived in Zaire for two decades, were admitted to hospitals in Brussels, Belgium. They displayed signs of multiple opportunistic infections and/or Kaposi's sarcoma. Most were Zairian tradesmen, students, or diplomats living in Belgium with their families. All identified as heterosexual and denied engaging in homosexual behaviors or injection drug abuse. Tragically, ten of them had already succumbed to their illnesses. Among the survivors, three had Kaposi's sarcoma, four had *Pneumocystis* pneumonia (PCP), six had cryptococcosis, three had central nervous system toxoplasmosis, and five had herpes simplex virus (HSV) infections. Many faced simultaneous or sequential life-threatening infections, including disseminated CMV infection, candidiasis, and tuberculosis. Eleven also had rare parasitic infections, uncommon in the United States, such as schistosomiasis, amebiasis, ascaridiasis, and filariasis.[2]

In early 1983, Joe McCormick (EIS 1973) learned about these Belgian AIDS case-patients at a viral hemorrhagic fever conference in Virginia. McCormick was well-acquainted with Zaire, having served in the Peace Corps there in 1965–1966, when Zaire was known as the Congo, and participated in the CDC's investigation of the 1976 Ebola outbreak in Zaire and southern Sudan. He contacted a colleague from the Ebola outbreak who now worked at the Zaire Ministry of Health, seeking permission to visit Kinshasa.[3]

In September 1983, Belgian physician Peter Piot approached Richard Krause, director of the National Institute of Allergy and Infectious Diseases (NIAID), during an infectious diseases meeting in Vienna, Austria. Piot sought funding to visit Kinshasa, and Krause immediately agreed, enlisting Tom Quinn, a top NIAID infectious diseases physician-scientist. Upon sharing his plans with the U.S. Public Health Service leadership, Krause was encouraged to collaborate with Joe McCormick of the CDC, who had already established contacts with the Zaire Ministry of Health. The team convened in Antwerp, Belgium, before embarking on their journey to Kinshasa in October 1983.[4]

A History of the Belgian Congo

In 1885, King Leopold II of Belgium assumed control over what is now known as the Democratic Republic of the Congo, or Congo (Kinshasa). During his rule, he governed with an iron grip, resorting to brutal tactics like amputating hands, fingers, and feet or holding families hostage if villagers failed to meet the rubber tax demands. These atrocities prompted global outrage, eventually leading to the Belgian government taking over administration of the region in 1908.

By 1959, discontent with Belgian rule had grown, resulting in riots. On June 30, 1960, Belgium granted the colony its independence. However, the process was marred by ongoing unrest, forcing many Belgian officials to leave the country. Meanwhile, educated individuals from the villages relocated to the capital, which was initially named Leopoldville but later renamed Kinshasa in 1971.

This mass migration of educated villagers to the capital created a

An Expedition to Kinshasa, Zaire

During a three-week visit by Joe McCormick, Peter Piot, and Tom Quinn, the multinational team visited hospitals in Kinshasa and identified 38 newly admitted patients with the CDC-defined AIDS. Among them, 32 had opportunistic infections but not Kaposi's sarcoma (KS), five had KS along with other opportunistic infections, and one had KS alone. Profound weight loss and severe chronic diarrhea were prominent clinical features. Thirty-one patients had oral and/or esophageal candidiasis, ten had chronic mucocutaneous HSV infections, and five had cryptococcal meningitis. Pulmonary tuberculosis was suspected in four patients, resembling the pattern of diseases we had observed in Haiti.

These case-patients were found at Mama Yemo University Hospitals in Kinshasa and two smaller hospitals in the area. Immunologic measures were consistent with AIDS patients elsewhere. Surprisingly, none of the patients reported homosexual behavior or intravenous drug abuse. Male patients (median age 41.4 years) were older than females (median age 28.4 years), with 18 of 20 men married compared to four of 18 women. Among male patients, 13 out of 15 reported more than one female sex partner before illness onset, with a median of seven female sex partners (range 1–100). Eight of 16 men reported a history of sexually transmitted diseases. Six of eight female patients reported more than one sexual partner, with a median of three male sexual partners (range 1–5).

The team identified two AIDS clusters among heterosexual partners in Kinshasa. One cluster included a married male and four of his sexual partners, with the index case being a woman who died of cryptococcal meningitis in 1980. Another cluster involved three men and two women, with the index case being a 30-year-old married woman who died in 1981. Her husband died in 1982, and two other male partners died in 1983. The wife of one male lover also died in 1983, suggesting heterosexual transmission.[5]

Piot, Quinn, and McCormick reported these findings and argued for further investigation. This led to the establishment of Projet SIDA, a collaborative effort between American, Belgian, and Zairian clinicians and researchers to study the emerging pandemic in central Africa.[6]

In November 1983, Jim Curran offered me the lead position in Zaire for a three-year term. However, I had to decline the opportunity. The thought of relocating my family to Africa was daunting, especially considering the risk of malaria, with no effective treatments available for young children at that time. Our son Daniel was four and daughter Katie was two. Colleen was born two years later. Convincing my wife, Lynne, to embrace the idea was a considerable challenge, considering she had never experienced a third-world country and was deeply committed to her private practice in Atlanta.

Projet SIDA (French for AIDS Project)

Projet SIDA began officially in June 1984 at Mama Yemo Hospital in Kinshasa, Zaire, with the collaboration of clinical researchers from the United States, Belgium, and Zaire. Their mission was to investigate HIV infection/AIDS, with the CDC as the major funder, contributing about $2.5 million to the final $4 million annual budget. Additional funding came from NIAID ($1 million) and the Institute of Tropical Medicine, Belgium (about half a million dollars equivalent). Jonathan Mann, a CDC alumnus (EIS 1975), led the project, with Henry "Skip" Francis from NIAID and Robert Colebunders from Belgium joining Zairian physicians Bosenga Ngali and Eugene Nzilambi.

Between July 1984 and March 1985, Jonathan Mann's team conducted city-wide, hospital-based active AIDS surveillance in Kinshasa. They identified 190 patients (102 men and 88 women) aged 11–54, with 89 percent between 20 and 49 years old. Notably, none reported homosexual activity. Among the 97 married individuals, one-third had previous marriages. Patients came from diverse backgrounds. Clinically, case-patients were marked by severe weight loss (98 percent with a median loss of 33 percent body weight) and chronic diarrhea (71 percent). About 41 percent had recognizable opportunistic infections, including candida esophagitis (57 case-patients), cryptococcal meningitis (nine), disseminated KS (four), and chronic HSV infection (two). Unfortunately, death rates were not reported. An additional hundred or so HIV-infected patients had "slims" disease—significant weight loss, chronic diarrhea, and unexplained fevers lasting over a month.[7]

Projet SIDA faced several challenges. First, inadequate health infrastructure and resources meant that infectious disease surveillance was virtually nonexistent. Second, the CDC's widely used AIDS definition, requiring advanced laboratory support, was impractical in these settings. For example, while 63 percent of AIDS patients in America and Europe developed PCP, only 14 percent of African patients diagnosed in Europe had it. In Africa, where diagnostic capabilities were limited, PCP didn't even rank among the most common opportunistic infections. Instead, these included oral candidiasis, cryptococcal meningitis, probable cytomegalovirus chorioretinitis, cryptosporidiosis, and mucocutaneous HSV infection.[8]

Projet SIDA's initial findings suggested that Zaire, Central Africa, and, to a lesser extent, neighboring East and Southern African countries were the hardest-hit by HIV infection. HIV was detected in areas previously considered free of the virus. Other researchers across sub-Saharan Africa also found HIV infection among hospitalized patients, hinting at heterosexual transmission. However, distinguishing between recent virus introductions and awareness of a persistent endemic disease remained challenging due to limited data.[9]

1991: Collapse of Projet SIDA

Despite their accomplishments, conflicts plagued the Projet SIDA investigators in Zaire. The Ministry of Health demanded that Jonathan Mann inform patients that their blood was tested for malaria, not AIDS. This compelled the team to abandon the principle of "informed consent" for research participation. Additionally, the Zairian government reprimanded Dr. Kapita Bila, a Zairian researcher, for discussing AIDS case numbers from Zaire at the First International AIDS meeting in Atlanta in April 1985. The Health Minister in Zaire was adamant about keeping AIDS data collected in the country confidential.

Internally, the international team faced disagreements about their mission's focus. The Zairian government sought help with HIV infection prevention and research training for their healthcare professionals. Conversely, the CDC aimed to conduct extensive surveillance and determine the prevalence of HIV infection in Kinshasa and the surrounding region. The NIH brought costly laboratory equipment to study virology and immunology. When the CDC identified HIV among local blood donors, Zaire advocated universal testing, akin to practices in the United States and Europe. However, the CDC claimed insufficient funds for this. Eventually, Germany stepped in to finance universal testing of all blood donors in Kinshasa.

In 1991, civil unrest erupted in the Zairian capital, marked by gunfire near the team's compound. American and Belgian researchers evacuated the country, and funding ceased. Two years later, Henry "Skip" Francis, a leader of the Projet SIDA team, was sent by the NIH to retrieve some laboratory equipment, but most medical records and stored blood and tissue samples were lost.[10]

9. Out of Africa?

World Health Organization (WHO) Meetings on AIDS

In July 1983, the second part of my European trip involved assisting the WHO in planning their inaugural meeting on AIDS in Europe. My journey took me from Naples, Italy, to Geneva, Switzerland. I expected to deliver a lecture to WHO staff detailing how we set up surveillance and conducted our investigation (see Chapter 2 for the 12 steps). However, my time was unexpectedly consumed when I was given the curriculum vitae of European investigators funded by the WHO and asked for recommendations on who should be invited to the meeting, which I found rather unproductive.

The WHO's meeting on AIDS convened in Aarhus, Denmark, on October 19–20, 1983. European investigators from 15 countries reported a total of 267 AIDS case-patients as defined by the CDC. Seven countries reported 10 or more case-patients, with France (94 case-patients), Germany (42), Belgium (38), the United Kingdom (24), Switzerland (17), Denmark (13), and the Netherlands (12) being the most affected. While most European patients were identified as homosexual men, France and Belgium reported case-patients among African natives or former residents of sub-Saharan Africa, including women. Tom Quinn, who attended the meeting, reported on his recent expeditions to Haiti and Zaire. It was recognized that the transmission patterns in Western Europe resembled those in the United States, with high-risk groups including homosexual men with multiple partners and intravenous drug users. However, in the Caribbean and Equatorial Africa, the ratio of female to male patients was much higher, suggesting different modes of transmission.[11]

Subsequently, the WHO held a follow-up meeting in Geneva on November 22–25, 1983. During this meeting, 38 European participants requested WHO support and coordination for research in various epidemiological settings.[12] Over the next two years, WHO organized several meetings and decided to launch global AIDS surveillance. To accomplish this, they needed to develop a case definition, a standardized data collection process, and a patient report form to organize data by time, place, and person (see Chapter 2).

For global AIDS surveillance, the WHO established not one but two case definitions:

1. The first, the WHO/CDC AIDS definition, aligned with the CDC's definition of AIDS in adults and children, requiring the exclusion of all known causes of cellular immunodeficiency. HIV testing could confirm an AIDS diagnosis, intended for use in countries

with appropriate diagnostic resources, including access to HIV testing.[13]

2. In October 1985, Joe McCormick of the CDC organized a meeting in Bangui, Central African Republic, to develop a "provisional" AIDS case definition suited for resource-limited developing countries. This "Bangui" definition focused on clinical criteria in the absence of advanced diagnostic resources. It required at least two major signs and one minor sign, with major signs including significant weight loss, chronic diarrhea, or prolonged fever, while minor signs encompassed symptoms like persistent cough or herpes zoster. Kaposi's sarcoma or cryptococcal meningitis were also sufficient for an AIDS diagnosis.[14]

The Bangui definition aimed to capture more AIDS case-patients in Africa but faced limitations due to the lack of background data on "slim" disease and opportunistic infections.[15]

In August 1985, the WHO initiated global AIDS surveillance, requesting countries to report the number of patients meeting their AIDS case definition(s). This system relied on passive, voluntary reporting, lacking individual case report forms, which hindered verification, differentiation of definitions used, identification of duplicate reports, creation of data summaries, development of epidemic trends, or measurement of mortality rates. In my view, the system had inherent flaws from the outset.

Worldwide AIDS Surveillance Results

By November 14, 1986, 77 countries had reported a total of 34,448 AIDS case-patients to the WHO Global Control Programme on AIDS (CPA). Reporting was voluntary, with data collected through various channels, including regional surveillance systems, national committees, epidemiologic newsletters, and official sources.[16]

Table 1. AIDS Case-patients Reported to WHO by Continent as of November 14, 1986[17]

Continent	Total AIDS Case-patients Reported	Year of First Report/ Diagnosis	Countries Reporting Case-patients	Countries Reporting Zero Case-patients
Africa	1,069	1982	10	5
Americas	29,273	1979	33	11
Asia	68	1980	9	4
Europe	3,694	1980	23	4

Continent	Total AIDS Case-patients Reported	Year of First Report/ Diagnosis	Countries Reporting Case-patients	Countries Reporting Zero Case-patients
Oceania	344	1982	2	0
Total	34,448	1979	77	24

In Africa, 10 countries reported AIDS case-patients, with Tanzania (462), Zambia (217), and the Central African Republic (202) having the highest numbers. Five African countries reported zero case-patients: Comoros, Ethiopia, Gambia, Mauritius, and Nigeria (Table 2).

Table 2. AIDS Case-patients Reported to WHO as of November 14, 1986, Top Ten Countries[18]

Country	Number of AIDS Case-patients	Population—1985 (in millions)	Rate Per 100,000
USA	26,566	240.7	11.0
France	997	55.4	1.8
Canada	755	25.9	2.9
Brazil	754	136.8	0.6
Germany	715	77.6	0.9
United Kingdom	512	56.4	0.9
Haiti	501	6.4	7.8
Tanzania	462	21.8	2.1
Italy	367	56.9	0.6
Australia	322	15.8	2.0
Total	34,448	4,831.0	0.7

However, despite known AIDS case-patients in Zaire and other African nations, identified through published reports, the governments of Zaire and 38 other African nations had not reported anything at all to WHO, highlighting significant gaps in reporting.

Dr. Jonathan Mann Leaves Projet SIDA to Lead WHO AIDS Program

In June 1986, Jonathan Mann, the lead investigator of Projet SIDA, was recruited by WHO to establish the Global Programme on AIDS in Geneva, Switzerland. In 1987, Dr. James Chin, chief of the infectious diseases section at the California State Department of Health Services in Berkeley, was enlisted by Mann to oversee global surveillance. By 1988,

Chin and Mann would provide updates on AIDS case-patients reported worldwide and describe global disease patterns.[18]

Table 3. AIDS Case-patients Reported to WHO as of October 31, 1988[19]

Continent	Number of Case-patients	Countries Reporting One or More Case-patients	Countries Reporting Zero Case-patients
Africa	19,141	45	6
Americas	88,233	42	2
Asia	281	22	16
Europe	15,340	28	2
Oceania	1,119	5	9
Total	124,114	142	35

Jim Chin and Jonathan Mann acknowledged the challenge of determining when and where HIV infection originated but identified three global transmission patterns:

> Pattern 1: Notable in the United States, Western Europe, Australia, New Zealand, and parts of Latin America. HIV spread rapidly from the late 1970s among individuals engaging in high-risk behaviors, such as men with multiple male partners and injecting drug users. The male-to-female ratio ranged from 10 to 15 to one.
>
> Pattern 2: Prevalent in sub–Saharan Africa and Latin America, particularly in the Caribbean. Most case-patients involved heterosexual transmission with a roughly equal male-to-female ratio. HIV transmission began in the 1970s and occurred through sexual contact and needle reuse in healthcare settings.
>
> Pattern 3: Observed in Eastern Europe, northern Africa, and all of Asia. HIV likely arrived in the 1980s through interactions with infected residents or travelers from Pattern 1 or Pattern 2 countries.[20]

Although these patterns generally aligned with the data, they perpetuated the impression that heterosexual transmission in Africa and the Caribbean was somehow different. WHO suggested that HIV infections were primarily transmitted male to male, male to female, or through needle sharing for drug injection, with female-to-male transmission considered rare.[21]

1991: World Health Organization Discontinues AIDS Surveillance

In 1991, WHO discontinued its AIDS surveillance program. Jim Chin recognized the limitations of this passive surveillance system, which had a distorted timeline. Instead, he provided estimates and short-term projections of AIDS case-patients using a model developed by WHO. Additionally, he estimated HIV prevalence by continent, relying on numerous surveys for Africa, Asia, and the Pacific, as well as estimates from national and regional experts for North America, Europe, and Latin America (including the Caribbean). Notably, no estimates were available for Oceania.[22]

Table 4. Reported and Estimated Cumulative AIDS Case-patients and Estimated HIV Prevalence Worldwide by December 31, 1991[23]

Region	Cumulative AIDS Case-patients Reported	Cumulative AIDS Case-patients Estimated	Estimated HIV Prevalence
Africa	129,060	970,000	6,000,000
North America	208,089	260,000	1,000,000
Latin America	44,888	145,000	1,000,000
Asia	1,254	10,000	More than 1,000,000
Europe	60,195	85,000	500,000
Oceania	3,189	5,000	Not reported
Total	446,681	1,475,000	About 10,000,000

The significant difference between WHO's estimates of HIV infection in Africa and North America, with Africa's numbers exceeding North America's by over sixfold, raised questions. People wondered why this didn't lead to a proportional increase in death rates across Africa. Were these estimates accurate, or did they imply a bias suggesting that AIDS originated in Africa, thus inflating the numbers there?

Jim Chin left WHO in 1992 amid disputes over travel restrictions. In his memoirs, he criticized his own HIV prevalence estimates for Africa, Latin America, and Asia as grossly exaggerated. He pointed out that HIV serological surveys mainly focused on urban areas, including hospitalized patients with fevers and commercial sex workers, rather than random samples of the population. Chin then applied the percentages from these biased surveys to entire African and Latin American populations.[24]

Questions also arose about the accuracy of HIV testing in Africa, primarily relying on a single assay with limited confirmatory testing, such as the Western blot. The sensitivity and specificity of HIV antibody tests were initially determined using blood from subjects in the United States. However, uncertainties remain regarding the test characteristics in Africa. What was the false-positive rate when using a single ELISA assay among Africans?[25]

First Documented AIDS Patient

The recognition of AIDS in Africa aligns temporally with its occurrence in North America, but a few case reports suggest earlier African infections. The earliest known African AIDS case involved a Danish female physician who died in Denmark in December 1977. She had worked in northern Zaire from 1972 to 1975 and later in Kinshasa from 1975 to 1977. Experiencing recurrent diarrhea, fatigue, and lymphadenopathy, she was hospitalized in 1976 in Africa and later in Denmark with severe dyspnea, lung issues, and oral candidiasis. Autopsy revealed *Pneumocystis* pneumonia (PCP), but her sexual history was omitted from the report.[26]

Determining the precise onset and location of the first AIDS or HIV case-patients in Africa is challenging. Notably, chronic, life-threatening diarrheal diseases known as "slim disease" surged in Kinshasa in the late 1970s and in Uganda and Tanzania in the early 1980s. A significant rise in esophageal candidiasis was observed in Rwanda in 1983. Cryptococcal meningitis case-patients in Kinshasa increased sevenfold during 1978–1984 compared to 1953–1977. While AIDS might have occurred earlier in Africa, it likely remained rare until the late 1970s and early 1980s, mirroring the pattern in the United States and Haiti.[27]

The Earliest HIV Infections Documented in Africa

The earliest evidence of HIV infection in Africa comes from retrospective serologic surveys. Samples from Burkina Faso in 1963 and Uganda in 1972–1973 showed weakly HIV-positive results in children. However, the reliability of these findings has been questioned due to assay interpretation challenges, freeze/thaw effects on samples, and unknown test sensitivity/specificity in malaria-endemic areas.[28]

More compelling evidence comes from blood samples collected during Joe McCormick's investigation of an Ebola outbreak in northwestern Zaire in 1976. In 1985, he tested 659 stored serum samples and found 0.8 percent positive for HIV antibodies; HIV was isolated from one.

9. Out of Africa?

Follow-up showed three individuals had died with AIDS-like illnesses, and two remained seropositive and healthy. The positive viral culture was from a woman who died in 1977.[29]

In 1986, the CDC conducted a serosurvey in the same Zaire and south Sudan region, using cluster sampling.[30]

Table 5. Prevalence of HIV Antibody in Selected Groups in Zaire and South Sudan[31]

Group	Prevalence Number Positive/ Total (%)	95% Confidence Interval
Healthy persons (1976)	5/659 (0.8)	0.1–1.4
Healthy persons (1986)	3/389 (0.8)	0–1.6
Pregnant women (1986)	3/136 (2.2)	0–4.7
Female prostitutes (1986)	32/283 (11.3)	7.6–15
Hospitalized patients with one or more clinical criteria of AIDS (1986)	6/31 (19.4)	5.5–33.3

Joe McCormick's research indicates that HIV infection remained stable in rural Zaire for an extended period, with traditional village life posing a low risk of transmission. However, the onset of independence in central Africa in the 1960s triggered urbanization, bringing about social and behavioral changes that may have facilitated HIV transmission.[32]

A Second HIV Type in West Africa Linked to Old World Monkeys

Two types of Human Immunodeficiency Virus (HIV) cause AIDS in humans: HIV-1 and HIV-2. HIV-2 was identified in West Africa and discovered simultaneously by Max Essex's Harvard team and Luc Montagnier's French group.[33] Compared to HIV-1, HIV-2 typically has a longer latency period, lower viral loads, and lower mortality rates. Genetically, HIV-2 is 50 percent different from HIV-1 and more closely related to a virus in African green monkeys called simian immunodeficiency virus (SIVagm).[34]

HIV-1 has several groups: M (main), N, O, and P, which further divide into subtypes or clades. These subtypes can combine to form circulating recombinant forms (CRFs).[35] HIV-1 Group M is the most widespread variant, subdivided into nine distinct subtypes: A, B, C, D, F, G, H, J, and K. In North America and Europe, subtype C (HIV-1-M type C) is most prevalent, accounting for 47 percent of global infections. Subtype B (HIV-1-M type B) represents 12 percent, and subtype A (HIV-1-M type A) comprises 10 percent of infections.[36]

Origins of HIV

AIDS is widely considered a zoonosis, a disease transmitted to humans from animals, with HIV-1 having a close relationship to the retrovirus simian immunodeficiency virus (SIVcpz), primarily found in chimpanzees in central and southern Africa. SIVcpz is believed to be the precursor of HIV.[37]

The transmission of SIVcpz from apes to humans is associated with two main hypotheses. The "cut hunter" hypothesis suggests that the hunting, handling, and keeping of non-human primates for research or pets have led to frequent human exposure to infected bodily fluids of chimpanzees and other primates, resulting in cross-species transmission of retroviruses, which has been documented in captivity.[38]

Another theory, proposed by British journalist Edward Hooper, suggests that SIVcpz entered humans inadvertently through an oral live polio vaccine produced at the Wistar Institute in Philadelphia. According to Hooper, this experimental vaccine was created using chimpanzee kidney cells and was administered orally to children in central Africa and other regions from 1957 to 1960.[39] Hooper pointed out that another monkey virus, simian virus 40 (SV40), was discovered contaminating experimental polio vaccines given between 1955 and 1963. However, SV40, a small DNA virus, has not been conclusively linked to cancer in humans.[40] The Hooper hypothesis faced strong opposition from the research community at the Wistar Institute, who argued that experimental oral polio vaccines worldwide were primarily developed in kidney cells from rhesus monkeys rather than chimpanzees.[41]

The earliest HIV-1 genome, belonging to Group M subtype C, was found in formalin-fixed paraffin-embedded tissues collected in Kinshasa, Zaire, in 1966, suggesting that HIV-1 likely had existed among humans in sub–Saharan Africa for decades.[42]

It's plausible that SIV crossed into humans multiple times in the last century, with some strains persisting in rural sub–Saharan communities. As European colonists left central Africa, urbanization caused social disruption, driving men to cities for work while leaving women behind. This led to a surge in prostitution, facilitating HIV spread in African cities and subsequently reaching Europe. In New York City, following the Stonewall riots of 1969 and the emergence of the gay liberation movement, HIV-1 found a conducive environment to spread rapidly.

9. Out of Africa?

Although Edward Hooper may not have pinpointed the initial introduction of SIV into humans, he raised valid concerns. The U.S. alone houses over 30,000 non-human primates for research purposes, with primate tissues often used for vaccine and medication development and testing. Recognizing the potential hazards of invasive animal research is essential.[43]

10

Nitrite Inhalants and Kaposi's Sarcoma

> *Man's mind cannot grasp the causes of events in their completeness, but the desire to find those causes is implanted in man's soul. And without considering the multiplicity and complexity of the conditions any one of which taken separately may seem to be the cause, he snatches at the first approximation to a cause that seems to him intelligible and says: "This is the cause!"*
>
> —Leo Tolstoy, 1869[1]

Step 9—As Necessary, Reconsider/Refine Hypotheses and Execute Additional Studies

In December 1981, Dennis Juranek and I conducted a review of the initial data printouts from the national case-control study (Chapter 4). We observed that patients with Kaposi's sarcoma (KS) demonstrated higher levels of sexual activity compared to those with *Pneumocystis carinii* pneumonia (PCP). The study included 50 case-patients, out of which 39 patients had KS, three had both KS and PCP, and only eight had PCP alone.[2] However, interviewing the PCP patients proved challenging as many were hospitalized and seriously ill, with some even succumbing to the disease before we could reach them. In contrast, individuals with Kaposi's sarcoma typically presented with skin lesions, received outpatient diagnoses, and had lower mortality rates following diagnosis.

To determine if the risk factors for PCP were similar to those for KS, we realized the need to evaluate more gay men with PCP. Dennis Juranek and I developed an addendum protocol, employing the same questionnaire as Harold Jaffe's study. Peter Drotman and I took on the task of identifying clusters of PCP patients and promptly conducting interviews after their diagnosis. If the patients identified themselves as heterosexual, we forwarded the data to Mary Guinan for her study (Chapter 3). Conversely, if the patients identified as gay, we retained the data for our KS versus PCP study.

Several intriguing observations from national surveillance prompted further investigation. Notably, over 90 percent of KS diagnoses occurred in gay men, making them 23 times more likely to develop KS compared to injecting drug users, Haitians, and hemophiliacs. Haitians, on the other hand, were 12 times more likely to experience opportunistic infections other than PCP, primarily CNS toxoplasmosis, in comparison to the other three patient groups. We hoped that our KS versus PCP study could shed light on these puzzling observations and provide valuable insights into the differences between the two conditions.

Results: KS Versus PCP Study

Enrollment in our study was concluded in October 1982, at which point we had a total of 87 patients available for analysis. Among them, 47 had KS, 20 had PCP, and 20 had both KS and PCP. The patient distribution was as follows: 55 from the Jaffe case-control study, 13 from the Auerbach Los Angeles cluster investigation, and 19 interviewed by Peter Drotman or myself outside New York and California (Table 1). The median age of participants was 35 years, ranging from 21 to 53 years. Among the participants, 69 (79 percent) were white. Forty-three patients (49 percent) resided in New York, 17 (20 percent) in California, and 27 (31 percent) in other states. Notably, no significant differences in age and race were found among the different diagnostic categories. However, patients with PCP were more likely to live outside New York and California ($p < 0.01$).[3]

Dennis Bregman, a senior statistician at the CDC, and Paul Pinsky joined our project. In the initial analysis, we looked at different factors one by one to see how they related to the patients. We found that patients with KS alone or both diseases were more likely to use various "street" drugs like amphetamines, barbiturates, cocaine, ethyl chloride, LSD, methaqualone, and nitrite inhalants compared to patients with PCP alone. Patients with KS alone or both diseases also had higher incomes, engaged in more receptive anal sex, and met sexual partners in bathhouses. Patients with KS alone had more sexual partners in the last year, a higher prevalence of non–B hepatitis (later identified as hepatitis C virus), and were more likely to use marijuana. Notably, there were no significant differences between patients with KS alone and those with both diseases (Table 1).[4]

We then conducted a multivariate analysis to identify which variables (factors) could effectively distinguish between the three groups of patients.

We used a stricter criterion ($p < 0.01$) instead of the usual $p < 0.05$ to select these variables for further analysis. The variable that stood out as the most significant in differentiating the disease groups was the total number of days of nitrite use. This variable was more powerful in distinguishing the groups than any other factors we examined (Table 2).[5]

We also noted that higher incomes were associated with KS alone and both diseases. This might suggest that these patients had the means to travel, meet distant sexual partners, afford more "street" drugs, and/or possibly participate in exclusive bathhouse clubs.

Table 1. Frequency of Selected Variables Among 87 Gay Men with KS, PCP, or Both[6]

Variable (percent)	KS (n=47)	PCP (n=20)	Both (n=20)	P < 0.05
Income > $20,000 in past year	48	11	47	†‡
Use of illicit substances				
Marijuana (ever)	98	80	95	†
(> 720 days*)	53	35	45	NS
Nitrite inhalants (ever)	98	95	95	NS
(> 384 days*)	57	10	68	†‡
Ampules (ever)	75	70	60	NS
(> 57.6 days*)	38	16	45	NS
Labeled bottles (ever)	87	65	80	NS
(> 121.2 days*)	38	37	53	NS
Unlabeled bottles (ever)	77	35	75	†‡
(> 182.4 days*)	36	5	58	†‡
Any drug intravenously (ever)	19	10	20	NS
Used five or more different "street" drugs	62	30	75	†‡
Previous illnesses				
Gonorrhea	89	80	85	NS
Syphilis	74	55	60	NS
Hepatitis B	13	20	15	NS
Non-B hepatitis	46	15	30	†
Sexual activity				
> 100 male sex partners in year before illness	61	30	55	†
Any sex partners from bathhouses in year before illness	85	60	90	†‡
Any receptive anogenital intercourse in year before illness	98	80	95	†
(> 26.2 episodes*)	57	20	53	†‡

*Median number of days or episodes reported by those patients who reported drug use or sexual activity.
†Comparison of KS vs. PCP.
‡Comparison of both KS and PCP vs. PCP alone.

Table 2. Significant Variables Associated with KS Versus PCP Among 87 Gay Men as Selected by Linear Logistic Regression Analysis and Ranked by Level of Statistical Significance[7]

KS vs. PCP	Both vs. PCP	Both vs. KS
Nitrite inhalant use	Nitrite inhalant use	No variables selected
Receptive anal intercourse	Income	
Income		
Bathhouse partners		
Marijuana use		
Unlabeled nitrite use		

Laboratory Results

The methods employed for sample collection and laboratory analysis in our study were consistent with those used in Jaffe's study. We conducted various analyses, including tests of immunologic parameters such as T-helper cell counts, T-helper/ T-suppressor cell ratio, and serologic tests for cytomegalovirus (CMV), Epstein-Barr virus, hepatitis A virus, and syphilis. However, no significant differences were observed in any of these analyses.[8]

Our particular focus on cytomegalovirus arose from its potential association with KS, as initially noted by Gaetano Giraldo. Giraldo had observed herpes-type viral particles on electron microscopy in KS tissues among African patients in the 1970s. Among the five known herpes viruses at that time, Giraldo suggested that the nucleic acid segments were most consistent with CMV. The results of our cytomegalovirus studies, categorized by disease manifestation, are presented in Table 3.

Table 3. Results of Laboratory Tests for Cytomegalovirus (CMV) Among Gay Men with KS, PCP, or Both Diseases[9]
[Number positive/number tested (%)]

Test for CMV	KS	PCP	Both
Serology			
IHA* titer > 1:8	39/39 (100)	14/14 (100)	13/13 (100)
IHA titer > 1:2048	22/39 (56)	9/14 (64)	6/13 (46)
CF† titer > 1:8	21/39 (54)	14/14 (100)	13/13 (100)
CF titer > 1:64	30/38 (79)	8/14 (57)	8/13 (62)
Viral isolation	8/38 (21)	6/12 (50)	2/10 (20)

*IHA = Indirect hemagglutination—a test for both IgM and IgG antibodies to CMV
†CF—Complement fixation—a test for IgG antibodies to CMV

In my opinion, this study shed light on the fact that the risk factors for KS and PCP were not identical, which raised several intriguing questions. Were there two simultaneous epidemics occurring? Or was there a single epidemic of immune deficiency with additional factors accounting for the diverse manifestations of AIDS? Were nitrites a direct cause of KS, or were they merely a confounding variable for another virus or toxin that triggered KS? Moreover, CMV was linked not only to KS but also to PCP. Did CMV play a contributory role in inducing the immunosuppression characteristic of AIDS? Or did it simply reactivate as an opportunistic infection following immunosuppression? These findings startled me, as until then, the focus had been on searching for a new virus to explain the epidemic. It prompted me to reconsider my initial assumptions.

The notion of nitrites serving as a potential cause of KS appeared plausible. Nitrite use was more prevalent among gay men compared to heterosexual individuals, and KS was significantly more common in gay men with AIDS than in injection drug users, hemophiliacs, or Haitians. Nitrites are typically inhaled, and KS lesions primarily appeared on the nose, face, and upper extremities. Laboratory testing had already established that nitrites were carcinogenic and could affect blood vessels, which aligned with the fact that KS is a cancer of the blood vessels. This biological plausibility reinforced the association between nitrite use and KS.

These observations and considerations expanded my perspective and prompted me to reevaluate the role of the new virus, HIV, in explaining the epidemic. My focus shifted toward exploring additional factors, including nitrites and cytomegalovirus, as potential contributors or cofactors in the development of Kaposi's sarcoma (KS) and AIDS.

A Hypothesis for the Cause(s) of AIDS

Based on our findings, we proposed a multifactorial model to explain the diverse manifestations of AIDS. According to this model, the natural progression of the syndrome began with immune dysfunction, likely resulting from the infection of T-helper cells by a novel human retrovirus, acting as an initiator. Subsequently, one or several cofactors would determine which opportunistic infections or cancers each patient would develop. Based on our KS versus PCP data, we suggested that nitrite inhalants played a "promoting" role in the development of KS. New or reactivated infections with PCP, tuberculosis, or toxoplasmosis served as promoters for those specific conditions.[10]

In July 1983, I prepared the results of our study to present at the upcoming AIDS Activity meeting. The group had grown exponentially over the past two years, much like the epidemic itself. Initially, our weekly meetings consisted of just a few individuals gathering in Jim Curran's office, with data written on the blackboard. However, the meetings had now transitioned to a large classroom, attended in person by approximately 50 individuals, with an additional dozen or so participating via telephone from locations like New York City and Phoenix. The expansion of the group reflected the increasing urgency and importance of addressing the AIDS pandemic.

The association between nitrite inhalants and KS faced skepticism, particularly from Jim Curran, who raised several valid concerns. One concern was the potential biases introduced by studying patients from different cities at different times. It was important to ensure that any observed associations were not influenced by these factors. Curran also questioned the possibility of interviewer or recall bias, as well as the potential differences in interviews with PCP patients due to fatigue. Additionally, he questioned whether a case-comparison study was the optimal approach to test the hypothesis. On the other hand, Harold Jaffe invoked "Occam's razor," which emphasizes the importance of simplicity in explanations, suggesting that we should focus on finding the virus rather than getting distracted by side hypotheses.

After the presentation, I received unfortunate news. The timing of our findings couldn't have been worse. The CDC hierarchy had just submitted their 1984 budget request to the Reagan administration, listing the ruling out of nitrites as the cause of AIDS as their top accomplishment.

To address Curran's concerns, we conducted further analyses. We stratified the amount of nitrite use for each patient based on various variables, including the number of different male sex partners, state of residence, onset of illness, length of patient survival, initial study, sex of interviewer, and location and duration of the interview. Astonishingly, in every analysis performed, the amount of nitrite use was consistently higher among patients with KS or both diseases compared to those with PCP alone.[11] These robust results provided strong evidence for the association between nitrite use and KS.

I was disappointed when both Jim Curran and Harold Jaffe declined to be coauthors on the report despite their involvement in the study. Additionally, I was informed by Curran that the paper had to undergo CDC-wide clearance before it could be submitted for publication, and that I was not allowed to present the findings outside the CDC until it was cleared. Following these instructions, I submitted the paper for review and awaited a response.

In June 1984, I transferred to the National Institutes of Health (NIH) and assumed the role of a health science administrator in the National

Institute of Allergy and Infectious Diseases (NIAID). In December 1984, the CDC issued a call for abstracts for the first International Conference on Acquired Immunodeficiency Syndrome (AIDS), scheduled to take place in Atlanta in April 1985. Encouraged by the acceptance of the abstract for an oral presentation at the conference, I assumed it constituted approval, and submitted the manuscript to the *Annals of Internal Medicine*. However, it was promptly rejected. Subsequently, I submitted the paper to the *American Journal of Medicine*, but it was also rejected. Finally, on February 19, 1985, I submitted the paper to the quarterly journal *Sexually Transmitted Diseases*.

The process of trying different journals and facing rejections was disheartening, but I persisted in seeking publication and disseminating what I thought were important findings.

In April 1985, I attended the Atlanta AIDS conference, where over 2,000 scientists from around the world gathered. The conference had multiple presentations happening simultaneously, and I had the opportunity to deliver a 10-minute presentation in an epidemiology section. Approximately 60 scientists were in attendance, and I felt that my presentation went well.[12]

In the same session, Dr. Andrew Moss, an epidemiologist from California, shared the results of his ongoing case-control study on risk factors for AIDS in San Francisco. Moss's findings were significant. He discovered that patients with KS, when compared to those with opportunistic infections, were more likely to report a high number of sexual partners, engage in analingus, use large quantities of nitrite inhalants, consume recreational drugs via non-intravenous routes, and receive metronidazole therapy for intestinal parasites. The multivariate analysis of his study revealed that the variable most strongly associated with KS was the use of more than four "hits" of nitrite inhalants per night of use.[13] Dr. Moss confirmed our results!

In October 1985, our paper titled "Disease Manifestation Among Homosexual Men with Acquired Immunodeficiency Syndrome: A Possible Role for Nitrites in Kaposi's Sarcoma" was published.[14] Unfortunately, the paper generated little scientific interest.

Andrew Moss faced similar challenges in publishing his results. His paper was rejected by multiple journals and eventually published in the *American Journal of Epidemiology*, but not until June 1987.[15]

Nitrite Inhalants (see Chapter 2)

Nitrite inhalants, including alkyl nitrites such as amyl, butyl, and isopropyl nitrites, are colorless or yellow liquids with high volatility. They are esters of nitrous oxide and are known for their fruity odor, often described as unpleasant. These substances have earned the nickname "poppers" due to the sound produced when glass capsules containing amyl nitrite are crushed. The vasodilatory effect resulting from the inhalation of amyl nitrite vapors was first described in 1859 and subsequently reported by T. Lauder Brunton, a Scottish medical student, in 1867. Brunton's report highlighted the clinical application of amyl nitrite in providing relief for angina pectoris.

Following his graduation from Edinburgh University, Brunton promoted the use of amyl nitrite during his postgraduate training across Europe, including a period spent in Vienna, coinciding with Moritz Kaposi's care for his first case-patients of hemangiosarcoma. By the 1890s, amyl nitrite had become the preferred treatment for heart-related chest pain worldwide. Later, physicians used amyl nitrite as a diagnostic test for heart murmurs. In the United States, amyl nitrite was initially marketed by prescription in 1937. Its use became so widespread that the FDA allowed over-the-counter purchases starting in 1960. Around the same time, it was discovered that gay men, adolescents, and young adults in the United States and Europe were using amyl nitrite as an aphrodisiac to prolong penile erection and facilitate anal intercourse.

In 1968, the FDA reinstated amyl nitrite as a prescription-only medication. Subsequently, an underground market for illicit amyl nitrite and other nitrite derivatives, primarily butyl nitrites, emerged. These products were often sold as "room odorizers" under various brand names, such as Rush and Hardware.[16]

My Scientific Reputation Plummets

I vividly remember the incident that greatly impacted my scientific reputation. In November 1984, Dr. Anthony Fauci was appointed as the director of NIAID. During the NIAID holiday party that same year, I mustered the courage to approach Dr. Fauci while we were in the line at the buffet. I asked if I could have a meeting with him to discuss my hypothesis regarding the role of nitrites in KS. To my surprise and dismay, he turned to face me and said in a volume that everyone in the room could hear, "Harry, I know your hypothesis, and you're wrong!" His words stung deeply, and unfortunately, we never had the opportunity to meet and discuss our paper.

On the other hand, Dr. Robert Gallo played a different role in this journey. Despite not agreeing with my hypothesis, he invited me to speak at his annual NCI Division meetings. He demonstrated an open-mindedness that allowed for dialogue and sharing of differing views with the numerous scientists attending his meetings. Furthermore, Dr. Luc Montagnier supported the notion of a multifactorial cause of AIDS and proposed mycoplasma infections as potential cofactors.[17]

Regrettably, the person who had the most damaging effect on my reputation was Peter Duesberg, a biochemist at the University of California at Berkeley. He claimed that my research "proved" the causative role of nitrite inhalants in Kaposi's sarcoma and that HIV was merely an "innocent" bystander in AIDS pathogenesis. Duesberg attributed AIDS to drug abuse in the Americas and Europe, as well as poverty in Africa and the Caribbean region.[18] Consequently, I found myself unfairly grouped with Duesberg as an "HIV denialist," which had a detrimental impact on my standing within the scientific community.

In reflecting on the general reaction to our hypothesis, Jon Cohen, an editor at *Science*, summarized it as "It's the virus, stupid!"[19] This sentiment captured the prevailing belief that HIV was the primary cause of AIDS, overshadowing alternative hypotheses and making it challenging for my work to gain recognition.

I, however, remain determined to pursue this lead. In Chapters 16 and 17, you will find further information on cofactors in AIDS. Similarly, the causes of various chronic diseases, as well as conditions like health disparities and the opioid crisis, may be complex and multifactorial, much like the intricate etiology of Tolstoy's European War of 1812. As the late H.L. Mencken astutely remarked, "For every complex problem, there is an answer that is clear, simple, and wrong." HIV is necessary, but not sufficient to cause AIDS.

11

Early Attempts at Treatment

> *In Larry Kramer's play* The Normal Heart, *the character Felix asks, "Do you think they'll find a cure before I ... How strange that sounds when you say it out loud for the first time!" The play debuted in 1985 when no effective therapy of any sort had been discovered to address the underlying immune deficiency caused by HIV. Physicians made heroic efforts to treat symptoms and prolong the lives of AIDS patients, but the eventual outcome was uniformly bleak, the more so because for the first few years of the epidemic, people hoped that a sizable proportion of those with AIDS would recover, as had always been the case in earlier epidemics. But no one with full-blown AIDS survived.*
> —Victoria A. Harden, 2012[1]

In July 1981, Jim Curran enlisted me to establish a surveillance system targeting Kaposi's sarcoma and opportunistic infections. As part of this role, I was responsible for reviewing the CDC records specifically related to the drug pentamidine isethionate. The objective was to identify case-patients of *Pneumocystis carinii* pneumonia (PCP) in individuals without any known underlying immunosuppressive conditions.

As a public health service, the CDC maintained stocks of various drugs used for treating life-threatening infections, even if their usage was infrequent. In November 1967, the Parasitic Diseases Drug Service submitted a Notice of Claimed Investigational Exemption for pentamidine isethionate to the FDA. This meant that certain drugs, like pentamidine, had not yet fulfilled all the requirements for FDA approval but were sought after by clinicians when approved drugs for life-threatening diseases proved ineffective. Our patient E.M. in Pittsburgh with PCP serves as a reminder of this need (Chapter 1). Consequently, any inquiries regarding pentamidine directed to the manufacturer or the FDA were redirected to the CDC, effectively making the CDC the exclusive access point for pentamidine in the United States.

To ensure prompt delivery of pentamidine to physicians, the CDC strategically stockpiled the drug at multiple airports across the country. Additionally, a member of the Parasitic Diseases team, which I was part of at that time, was available 24/7 to handle requests from clinicians seeking the drug.

During my review of the case reports, I noticed a lack of comprehensive clinical data regarding the effectiveness of pentamidine. This discovery led Dennis Juranek and me to decide on conducting a study to determine the response rates of PCP among AIDS patients, and to compare it with individuals who developed PCP but had preexisting immunosuppressive conditions. We enlisted the assistance of Dr. Walter Hughes, an international expert on PCP from St. Jude Children's Research Hospital in Tennessee, to contribute to the study's design. To initiate this study, we developed a protocol and concise one-page report form. We then distributed these materials to physicians at 28 medical centers who had previously requested pentamidine for PCP case-patients occurring after January 1, 1979.[2]

Overall, our goal was to fill the gap in knowledge regarding the effectiveness of pentamidine as a treatment for PCP. By gathering comprehensive data from diverse sources and collaborating with experts in the field, we aimed to enhance our understanding of the response rates to this life-threatening condition in different patient populations.

Ultimately, the study involved physicians from 19 medical centers who reported a total of 328 biopsy-confirmed case-patients of PCP. Out of these case-patients, 282 patients who received a minimum of four days of therapy with either intravenous pentamidine or trimethoprim/sulfamethoxazole, which are the first-line treatments for PCP, were included in the analysis.[3]

The patients were divided into three distinct groups for further examination:

A. Group A consisted of 101 patients with AIDS.
B. Group B comprised 31 immunosuppressed adult patients, including organ transplant recipients and cancer patients.
C. Group C included 150 pediatric cancer patients, predominantly children with acute lymphocytic leukemia.

Table 1. Demographic Characteristics and Outcome Measures by Group, and Survival Rates by Therapy and Group[4]

	Group A (n=101)	Group B (n=31)	Group C (n=150)
Age (years)			
Mean	38.4	43.9	7.0
Range	20–56	16–70	0–21

	Group A (n=101)	Group B (n=31)	Group C (n=150)	
Sex (percent)				
Male	97.0	67.7	63.1	
Female	3.0	32.3	36.9	p<0.01
Race (percent)				
White	59.4	74.2	94.0	
Black	21.5	12.9	5.3	
Other	18.8	12.9	0.7	p=NS
Residence				
New York	69.3	32.3	0.0	
California	22.8	22.6	0.7	
Other	7.9	45.1	99.3	p<0.01
Outcome				
Discharged Alive/Discharged*	60/99 (62%)	15/31 (52%)	125/150 (83%)	p=NS
Alive > 30 days/followed 30 days	76/99 (77%)	20/31 (65%)	120/150 (80%)	p=NS
Alive > 90 days/followed 90 days	59/93 (63%)	18/31 (59%)	112/150 (75%)	p=NS
Relapse/Alive > 30 days	17/76 (20%)	0/18 (0%)	13/120 (11%)	p=0.06
Therapy				
TMP/SMZ alone	40/44 (91%)	17/26 (68%)	31/33 (94%)	
Pentamidine alone	2/2 (100%)	---	76/87 (87%)	
Both, sequentially	22/30 (73%)	2/4 (50%)	9/19 (47%)	
Both, simultaneously	12/23 (77%)	1/2 (50%)	4/11 (36%)	p<0.05

*Patient excluded if alive but still hospitalized at time of report. Chi-square testing probability (p) value.

Remarkably, our study revealed no significant differences in survival rates over a 90-day follow-up period between AIDS patients and adults with known causes of immune deficiency. However, we observed some notable distinctions among the groups. AIDS patients experienced a delay in diagnosis, with a median of 25 days for Group A, compared to 5 days for Group B and 6 days for Group C. Furthermore, AIDS patients required a longer duration of therapy, with a median of 18 days for Group A, compared to 14 days for Group B and 19 days for Group C. Additionally, AIDS patients exhibited a higher rate of relapse, suggesting a more insidious disease onset and persistent immune deficiency.[5]

The study found that treatment failure with trimethoprim/sulfamethoxazole was an unfavorable prognostic indicator. Survival outcomes were similarly affected when pentamidine was added or substituted after trimethoprim/sulfamethoxazole failure. Follow-up of AIDS patients treated with trimethoprim/sulfamethoxazole and/or pentamidine through national surveillance indicated that 75 percent would succumb within one year of initial PCP diagnosis, and 90 percent within two years.

These findings led us to conclude that improvements in outcomes would necessitate the development of new anti–*Pneumocystis* drugs or the ability to reverse or prevent immunosuppression.

It is important to acknowledge certain limitations of this study. Despite reporting a substantial number of PCP case-patients, the sample size remained relatively small, precluding meaningful statistical analyses for several crucial variables, such as dosage and duration of therapy. Additionally, retrospective studies inherently carry biases. Therefore, we recommended the need for randomized prospective studies to determine the optimal treatment approach for PCP.[6] Notably, this study provided me with an entrée for a job at the National Institutes of Health.

During the PCP study, I had the privilege of collaborating with Henry Masur, a renowned advocate for treatments targeting opportunistic infections. Masur's academic journey began with an undergraduate degree from Dartmouth College in 1968, followed by an M.D. from Weill Cornell Medical College in 1972. After completing a medical residency at Cornell, he embarked on an infectious diseases fellowship in 1975, where he focused his research on *Pneumocystis carinii* and other protozoal diseases. In 1979, he encountered his first AIDS patient and published a report on this patient and ten others in the *New England Journal of Medicine* (*NEJM*) in December 1981. In 1982, he was recruited to the critical care medicine unit at the NIH.

On June 23, 1983, the NIH held a conference to discuss their work on AIDS. During this conference, Henry Masur presented the case-patients of 53 AIDS patients with opportunistic infections, including cytomegalovirus (31 patients), candidiasis (29), PCP (26), *Mycobacterium avium-intracellulare* (15), cryptococcosis (8), herpes simplex (7), cryptosporidiosis (5), *Toxoplasma* encephalitis (5), and herpes zoster (4). The researchers explored both standard chemotherapy for these infections and methods to restore the compromised immune system.[7]

The findings indicated that antimicrobial treatments were generally effective for life-threatening conditions such as candida esophagitis, cryptococcal meningitis, PCP, and mucocutaneous herpes simplex disease. However, these infections often recurred despite treatment. On the other hand, serious infections like disseminated cytomegalovirus, cryptosporidiosis, and disseminated *Mycobacterium avium-intracellulare* remained untreatable with the available regimens.

For instance, the study revealed that approximately 70 percent of PCP patients survived the initial infection, but the organism persisted in their lungs even after 14 to 28 days of treatment with pentamidine or trimethoprim-sulfamethoxazole. The researchers also observed an unusually high incidence of adverse events with trimethoprim-sulfamethoxazole, with 30 percent of patients experiencing hypersensitivity rashes and another 30 percent developing severe leukopenia (low white blood cell count). This raised questions regarding the potential effectiveness of a longer course of therapy or the combination of pentamidine and trimethoprim-sulfamethoxazole.

In treating AIDS-related disseminated cytomegalovirus disease, intravenous acyclovir or vidarabine yielded disappointing results. The quantity of circulating cytomegalovirus was not diminished, and organ dysfunction, such as chorioretinitis (inflammation of posterior layers in the eye), showed no improvement.

Masur concluded that progress in treating AIDS-related infections would necessitate the development of new antimicrobial agents or interventions capable of reversing the immune suppression characteristic of AIDS. This conclusion echoed with our PCP therapy study.[8]

Rebuilding the Immune System

Anthony Fauci and his associate, Cliff Lane, collaborated at the NIH to address the failing immune system in AIDS patients. They conducted experiments with various agents, including interferons, which are natural proteins produced by host cells in response to viral infection and other pathogens (Chapter 1). Interferons have antiviral, anticancer, and immunomodulating effects by impeding viral replication and preventing the spread of infectious agents to surrounding cells. Initial tests on AIDS patients showed mixed results, with some experiencing improved immune systems while others saw declines.

One of their most notable experiments involved bone marrow transplantation between identical twins, where one twin was infected with HIV and the other was not. Fauci hypothesized that because their genetics were identical, a bone marrow transplant would not be rejected and could potentially "cure" the patient. Initially, the transplanted cells led to an improvement in immune function, but the effects were temporary. Eventually, the implanted T cells became infected, leading to the development of Kaposi's sarcoma, progressive cytomegalovirus infection, recurrent bouts of PCP, and eventual death.[9]

Tony Fauci and Cliff Lane also explored the use of interleukin-2, a natural protein previously isolated by Bob Gallo. They treated 12 AIDS patients with a highly purified form of human interleukin-2. Although no clinical responses were observed, several measures of immune function improved, including increased reactivity in skin tests and more normalized numbers of circulating T-suppressor cells and serum immunoglobulins. The NIAID continued studying interleukin-2 for the next two decades before discontinuing its use.[10]

Interferon and Chemotherapy for Kaposi's Sarcoma

Researchers at the intramural National Cancer Institute (NCI) focused on exploring different treatments for Kaposi's sarcoma and lymphomas at the Clinical Center. Interferon showed promise in treating KS in AIDS patients. Investigators at Memorial Sloan Kettering in NYC and the University of California, San Francisco, reported a 49 percent response rate for KS lesions with interferon therapy. However, the response rates with interferon at the NIH were approximately 25 percent. The NCI investigators attributed the lower response rate to the fact that they were dealing with later-stage KS patients who had lower T-helper cell counts at the start of therapy.

All three groups, including oncologists in Bethesda, New York, and San Francisco, had previously attempted using "standard" anticancer chemotherapies like adriamycin, bleomycin, and vinblastine. Unfortunately, these treatments yielded disastrous results. Although some skin lesions regressed with chemotherapy, the resulting immunosuppression, compounded by HIV, led to numerous severe opportunistic infections and deaths.[11]

From Atlanta to Bethesda, Maryland

My contract as an epidemic intelligence officer was to end on June 30, 1984. In order to explore job opportunities, I started making some calls in January. One was to Henry Masur at the NIH in hopes of finding a clinical job. Masur informed me that he didn't have any positions available, but he mentioned that Robert Edelman was looking for someone to work in the extramural program at NIAID. The focus of the work was on treatments for opportunistic infections and the development of animal models of disease. Intrigued by the opportunity, I reached out to Dr. Edelman, and he kindly invited me for an interview.

Robert Edelman was the chief of the Clinical and Epidemiologic Studies Branch at NIAID, which is part of the NIH. His role involved collaborating with clinical researchers at various medical schools and universities around the world to study the epidemiology of infectious diseases and develop new treatments and vaccines. He had a special interest in AIDS research and was responsible for developing research programs to

11. Early Attempts at Treatment

study this emerging disease. One of his notable initiatives was the Multicenter AIDS Cohort Study (MACS), which involved recruiting and following a cohort of 5,000 gay men across five sites. Edelman was currently looking for someone to organize and coordinate clinical trials for the development of new AIDS treatments.

During my conversation with Dr. Edelman, I had the opportunity to share details about my previous activities at the CDC, with a particular emphasis on my involvement in the PCP therapy project and my plans to conduct a similar study on treatments for *Toxoplasma* encephalitis. I also mentioned my experiences at the University of Pittsburgh, where I conducted studies on interferons for herpes simplex virus and papillomavirus infections, as well as my work on pneumonias among organ transplant recipients and cancer patients.

Robert Edelman told me that two former EIS officers, Dick Kaslow (EIS 1971) and Al Saah (EIS 1976), were working with him coordinating the MACS. He also introduced me to another former EIS officer, Karl Western (EIS 1967), who had previously worked in parasitology at the CDC and was now heading NIAID's international program. His expertise and contributions were highly valued at NIH.

My final interview of the day was with Dr. Richard Krause, the NIAID director and a senior member of our group visiting Haiti in May 1982 (Chapter 8). Dr. Krause offered me a position on the spot, and I gratefully accepted.

Now, the challenge was to convince my wife Lynne, a pediatrician, that we should move to Maryland. She had established herself and was content with her role in a four-doctor pediatric practice in Atlanta. Lynne had even been considering a larger home in a more affluent part of Atlanta closer to her practice. Nevertheless, despite the whirlwind of events, she ultimately agreed to the move, showing her unwavering support for my career.

NIH Meeting of Extramural Scientists

In April 1984, Robert Edelman organized a meeting in Bethesda, bringing together extramural scientists funded by NIAID who were working on treating opportunistic infections. During the meeting, Edelman introduced me as an incoming medical officer and administrator who would be working with them. The grantees, esteemed figures in academia, presented their latest research findings. Among them were notable individuals such as Don Armstrong from Memorial Sloan Kettering Cancer Center, focusing on pentamidine therapy for PCP; John Bartlett from the

Johns Hopkins University School of Medicine, researching cytomegalovirus in AIDS; Alice Clark from the University of Mississippi Medical Center, investigating candidiasis; Walter Hughes from St. Jude Children's Research Hospital, studying PCP; Pearl Ma from St. Vincent Catholic Medical Centers of New York, exploring cryptosporidiosis; Henry Murray from Weill Cornell Medicine College, investigating interferon for *Mycobacterium avium-intracellulare* (MAI); and Charles Rinaldo from the University of Pittsburgh School of Medicine, studying cytomegalovirus.

On April 23, 1984, Margaret Heckler, President Ronald Reagan's secretary of Health and Human Services, made a significant announcement (Chapter 5). She revealed that Robert Gallo had discovered the virus that causes AIDS. Heckler promised that within six months, American medicine would have a blood test for the virus, and within two years, a vaccine. This discovery opened new possibilities for developing antiviral treatments to combat the opportunistic infections and cancers associated with AIDS.

Soon after Heckler's announcement, Richard Krause, the head of NIAID, resigned from his position to become the dean of the Emory University School of Medicine in Atlanta. This was the first indication I had that there was tension between NIAID and NCI. Bernie Talbot, M.D., was appointed as the acting director in Krause's absence.

In June, my family relocated to Rockville, Maryland. My role at the NIH was to find treatments that would help AIDS patients, including playwright Larry Kramer's tragic fictional character, Felix, to stay alive. This move marked a significant step in my mission to contribute to the fight against AIDS.

12

A Health Science Administrator at the National Institutes of Health (NIH)

> *The stone baronial mansions for the NIH director and the directors of the most eminent of the institutes stand on grassy knolls, like the stately campus homes of college presidents. That's what they like to call the NIH grounds, a campus. Here, removed from the demands of commerce, scientists are given the freedom to undertake undirected research. Pure science. That means nobody can tell them what to do. The scientists follow their own interests, and, it is hoped, they will stumble across discoveries that will benefit humankind.*
>
> —Randy Shilts, 1987[1]

On Monday, June 4, 1984, I began my role as a health science administrator at the NIH, specifically within the Clinical and Epidemiologic Studies Branch of the Microbiology and Infectious Diseases Program (MIDP) at the National Institute of Allergy and Infectious Diseases (NIAID). My supervisor, Dr. Robert Edelman, graduated from Washington University Medical School in St. Louis. He furthered his training with an internship in pathology and internal medicine at Johns Hopkins Hospital in Baltimore, followed by a fellowship in preventive medicine at Case Western Reserve University in Cleveland.

In 1968, during the Vietnam War, he joined the United States Army and served at the Medical Research and Development Command in Washington, D.C. By 1976, he had achieved the rank of lieutenant colonel and transferred his commission to the U.S. Public Health Service. His assignment within NIAID was to focus on the development of vaccines for malaria, pertussis, viral hepatitis, and the search for treatments for diarrheal diseases. In 1981, he was appointed as the chief of the Clinical and

Epidemiological Studies Branch. A year later, he was handpicked by Richard Krause to oversee extramural research concerning infectious disease aspects of AIDS.

Dr. Edelman entrusted me with three key areas of AIDS research:

1. Enhancing treatments for the opportunistic infections associated with AIDS.
2. Defining the comprehensive spectrum or natural history of HIV infection, which would be used in clinical trials.
3. Developing animal models of infection for testing treatments and vaccines.

Dr. Edelman informed me that attendance at a "program officers" orientation in September was mandatory. This orientation was designed to provide insight into the ethical and legal responsibilities associated with being a health science administrator, as well as an understanding of how NIH prioritizes, coordinates, and funds research.

As a health science administrator, my role involved:

- Identifying research areas deserving increased funding emphasis and crafting statements to solicit grant or contract applications in those areas.
- Offering technical support to applicants throughout the application process and their research activities.
- Conducting site visits to evaluate the adequacy of research and training facilities.
- Serving as a representative for agency programs when interacting with the scientific community, other federal agencies, and Congress.

During our conversation, I shared my interests and goals with Bob Edelman. Specifically, I expressed my desire to attain clinical and research privileges at the clinical center. Additionally, I outlined my plans to undertake a national retrospective review of treatments for toxoplasmic encephalitis, contribute to the MACS, investigate heterosexual transmission of HIV, and explore the potential role of nitrite inhalants in the development of Kaposi's sarcoma.

Bob Edelman acknowledged that it was unusual, though not unheard of, for an "extramural" scientist like myself to work at the Clinical Center. I informed him that Richard Krause had assured me a clinical appointment if I were to transfer from the CDC. To pursue this appointment at NIH, he advised me to get in touch with Henry Masur. In relation to my review of therapy for *Toxoplasma* encephalitis, Edelman supported my intentions but pointed out that I would need to develop a protocol and submit it to the NIH Institutional Review Board for approval.[2]

12. A Health Science Administrator at the NIH   141

Regarding the MACS, Edelman informed me that he had hired two former CDC EIS officers, Richard Kaslow and Al Saah, to work on epidemiologic studies of AIDS. He assured me that they would welcome my input into the project. I had met Dr. Saah in Haiti in June 1982 (see Chapter 8).

When we discussed the topic of heterosexual transmission of HIV and the undercounting of case-patients in the CDC surveillance, Edelman displayed interest. We both questioned why a sexually transmitted virus was not spreading significantly among the heterosexual population. However, he appeared less enthusiastic about my idea concerning nitrite inhalants and Kaposi's sarcoma. He reminded me that infectious diseases fell under the jurisdiction of NIAID, while drug abuse and cancer were the responsibilities of the National Institute on Drug Abuse (NIDA) and the National Cancer Institute (NCI), respectively.

Before concluding our conversation and heading to his next meeting, Edelman advised me to review the NIAID AIDS research grants portfolio, introduce myself to others in our division, and explore the abundant opportunities available at the NIH.

During that first day at NIH, I had a brief encounter with Dr. Bernie Talbott, who was serving as the acting director of NIAID. Talbot expressed concerns about NIAID facing criticism from both the gay community and the Reagan administration due to perceived slow progress on AIDS. He emphasized his support for any initiatives, including attending relevant meetings that could help improve NIAID's reputation. While I didn't inquire further about the reasons behind Richard Krause's resignation, I had heard rumors during my time at the CDC and expected to gather more information in the coming weeks.

It was widely known within the infectious diseases community that Richard Krause was a closeted homosexual man, and the gay community had high expectations of him. However, Krause often cited NIH's slow pace of operation and the federally mandated grant review process as reasons for the delay in progress. He explained that it typically took a minimum of 14 months from the conception of a grant application to its approval and funding, assuming the application was exceptional. More commonly, applications required revisions and amendments before being accepted and funded. Krause's remarks also implied that many clinicians caring for gay men and individuals with AIDS, who were overwhelmed by the dire situation, lacked sufficient research experience to compete effectively for NIH funding. Naturally, these comments stirred controversy, especially among physicians in New York and California who were dealing with a high volume of AIDS patients and needed support.

Later that day, I had a meeting with William "Bill" Jordan, the director of the Microbiology and Infectious Diseases Program (MIDP) and Bob Edelman's superior. Dr. Jordan was well-known for his annual report on vaccine development, known as "The Jordan Report." He expressed dissatisfaction with Margaret Heckler's statement that the Public Health Service would have a blood test in six months and a vaccine in two years. While he believed that Bob Gallo would develop a functional blood test quickly, he considered creating a vaccine within two years a challenging task. The National Institute of Allergy and Infectious Diseases, particularly MIDP, had the primary responsibility for developing an AIDS vaccine. Jordan questioned whether Secretary Heckler truly understood the complexities involved in discovering and testing such a vaccine.

During our conversation, Jordan mentioned reported case-patients of AIDS among army servicemen at Walter Reed Army Medical Center in Washington, D.C. As an advisor to the Department of Defense on infectious diseases, he requested my assistance in reviewing patient reports and attending meetings with him. I enthusiastically accepted his request, and we will delve further into this topic in Chapter 14.

The NIAID AIDS Research Portfolio

My initial task involved reviewing the portfolio of grants and contracts related to AIDS that were funded by the Institute, as well as those expected to receive funding by September 30, 1984. At that time, there were already 74 activated grants totaling $17 million, with an additional 28 grants worth $4 million projected to be funded by the end of the fiscal year. These awards were distributed among 58 different principal investigators in 21 states and the District of Columbia.

Approximately half of the grants were focused on immunology and were managed by project officers in the Allergy, Immunology, and Transplantation Program. The other half concentrated on infectious agents and were overseen by the MIDP. However, I had heard that NIAID's AIDS portfolio faced criticism from the gay community due to what was seen as creative accounting of grants. For example, the institute counted general immunology research studies as AIDS-related, even when there was no direct link to AIDS patients. Additionally, some clinical research trials for treating opportunistic infections only included organ transplant recipients and cancer patients, excluding AIDS patients from participation. Grants aimed at investigating various infectious agents as potential causes of AIDS, such as adenovirus, candidiasis, cytomegalovirus, and parvoviruses, were reclassified as research on treatments for opportunistic infections.

Overall, I was impressed by the number of grants and the quality of the scientific work. However, I identified several significant issues. First, we lacked awards specifically for studying HIV itself, and later I discovered that our intramural scientists did not have access to Bob Gallo's virus. Second, the majority of national experts and NIAID-funded researchers studying opportunistic infections like PCP, candidiasis, and cytomegalovirus were not based in New York or California but in Alabama, Mississippi, Pennsylvania, Tennessee, and Texas. Physicians in New York City and San Francisco were in dire need of assistance in caring for their terminally ill patients. I questioned how we could bring these different groups together, a topic we will explore further in Chapter 15.

Thirdly, there was an imbalance in the number of grants focusing on various fungi as potential causes of AIDS. I learned that Kenneth Sell, the director of NIAID's intramural science program, strongly believed that a toxin released by a fungus was responsible for the immunosuppression characteristic of AIDS. Since the clinical use of cyclosporine, a fungal derivative, to clinically suppress transplanted organ rejections, such a conjecture has some rationale.[3] Consequently, he recommended several studies on fungi for funding. When the NCI internally proposed HTLV-III as the cause of AIDS to the Reagan administration, Ken Sell and Richard Krause opposed it, favoring their fungal hypothesis. This situation highlighted the ongoing tension between NCI and NIAID, and this confrontation may have been the final catalyst for Krause's "resignation."

Anthony Fauci and the "Intramural" Program at NIAID

After submitting my medical school transcripts, clinical credentials, publication list, and letters of recommendation, I successfully obtained clinical and research privileges at the Clinical Center. One of the most remarkable experiences during my time at NIH was the opportunity to participate in rounds with Anthony Fauci, a Cornell Medical School graduate from 1966. Fauci had joined NIH in 1968 as a clinical associate at NIAID and, in 1980, became the chief of the Laboratory of Immunoregulation.

Tony Fauci conducted daily rounds, checking on his patients, and generously invited students, residents, and staff to join him once a week for "teaching rounds." His presence was truly inspiring, known for his brisk pace, rapid speech, and quick thinking. He displayed exceptional clinical expertise and mastery during rounds.

On one memorable occasion, Fauci explained the intricate interactions of HIV with various components of the immune system, such as T cells, B cells, and macrophages, using a vivid analogy. He likened the immune system to an orchestra with its diverse instruments, with the T-lymphocyte acting as the conductor. He then illustrated how, in the case of HIV, the conductor (T-helper lymphocyte) is "kidnapped right before the performance." Consequently, the sounds produced by the orchestra (the various immune system components) became discombobulated. While each instrument may function properly on its own, the lack of coordination leads to a disrupted harmony within the immune system.

Tony Fauci's ability to simplify complex concepts with such analogies left a lasting impression. His teaching style deepened our understanding of the intricate workings of the immune system and the impact of HIV infection.

During one of my sessions at the Clinical Center, I had the opportunity to attend a meeting of the NIAID intramural laboratory scientists, led by Kenneth Sell. Dr. Sell had requested HTLV-III from Bob Gallo. However, Gallo asked for an agreement that would grant him authorship on resulting manuscripts and the right to review the paper before submission in exchange for sharing the virus with NIAID. Sell found this request outrageous and refused to sign the contract. Consequently, Gallo declined to provide the virus to NIAID. Additionally, I learned that the French had sent samples of LAV to NIAID, but, like the samples sent to the CDC, it did not grow in the NIAID lab.

In November 1984, Anthony Fauci assumed the position of director of NIAID, a role he would hold for nearly 40 years, marking a significant milestone in the institute's history.

History of the National Institutes of Health (NIH)

During my initial weeks at NIH, I became acquainted with its illustrious history, dating back to the era of Joseph Kinyoun. Dr. Kinyoun, a physician in the Marine Hospital Service, founded the Hygienic Laboratory in Staten Island, New York, in 1887. Trained in Germany under Dr. Robert Koch, Kinyoun made significant contributions to microbiology. He achieved the distinction of being the first American to successfully culture *Vibrio cholera* in a laboratory setting and played a pivotal role in establishing a microbiology training program in the United States.[4]

In 1930, the laboratory was renamed the National Institute of Health (singular), and Congress authorized fellowships to support research in basic sciences and medicine. In 1937, NIH relocated to Bethesda, Maryland, thanks to a generous land donation from Luke and Helen Wilson.

During this period, NIH expanded its influence by initiating an extramural program that offered grants to non-federal scientists at various institutions to conduct cancer research.

The backdrop of World War II revealed some fascinating historical details. The Selective Service found that a staggering 43 percent of potential draftees were unfit for general military service, with common causes of rejection including defective teeth, rheumatic heart disease, and syphilis.[5]

In 1948, Congress established several institutes, including the NIAID, within the National Institutes of Health (now plural). In 1953, the NIH opened a clinical center on the Bethesda campus, making it the largest clinical research center globally by the time of my arrival.[6] The NIH's mission is to conduct and support cutting-edge research and research training in the field of biomedical research. Approximately 10–15 percent of the NIH research budget is allocated to intramural research, while the remainder is distributed to universities, medical schools, and research organizations across the United States, and sometimes internationally. These extramural grants and contracts are only awarded after competitive peer review.

For instance, my research fellowship at the University of Pittsburgh from 1979 to 1981 was funded by the NIH. As a health science administrator at this prestigious institution, I found myself in a unique position to contribute to significant discoveries that could benefit AIDS patients. The abundant resources, talented researchers, and state-of-the-art facilities at the NIH offered immense potential for groundbreaking advancements in AIDS research and patient care.

13

The Multicenter AIDS Cohort Study (MACS)

The natural history of a disease is concerned with all aspects of its manifestations, from beginning to end, and the circumstances surrounding its occurrence. Natural history requires the skills of the clinician, the scientist, the epidemiologist. I recognized that we would need to study many patients for a long time, from beginning to end, if we were to learn about the full complexity of AIDS, the variation in the course of the disease from one patient to the next.
—Richard Krause, 1988[1]

Working at NIAID was a significant improvement in terms of working conditions compared to my experience at the CDC. At NIAID, I had the privilege of being assigned an office with a window. In contrast, during my time at the CDC, I occupied six offices—two were shared with other officers, and two others were originally designed as animal facilities, complete with sliding "slats" on the doors for researchers to observe rodent activities.

The dress code at NIH was notably more formal, requiring a suit and tie, as opposed to the more relaxed attire of slacks and a collared shirt, with or without a tie, at the CDC.

NIH proved to be a scientific wonderland, hosting numerous conferences and daily institute grand rounds, often presented by Nobel laureates. The environment also provided ample time for staying updated with the latest medical journals and classic articles. It was during my time at NIH in the summer of 1984 that I finally had the opportunity to delve into topics such as the legal status of gay men in America, the Alfred Kinsey report, and the Stonewall Inn riots through extensive reading.

Homosexuality and the Law

Once our legal system was established following the American Revolution, "sodomy" became illegal in all 13 former colonies. The specific acts classified as "sodomy" were rarely explicitly defined in the law, but generally included any sexual acts considered immoral or unnatural, such as oral sex, anal sex, and bestiality. While these laws applied to heterosexuals and homosexuals, the majority of convictions were against homosexual men.

By 1960, homosexual behavior was a felony in all 50 states, the District of Columbia, U.S. territories, and most countries worldwide. It was punishable by imprisonment and/or hard labor, and castration was occasionally imposed. The harshest penalties in the U.S. were in Idaho, where a conviction for homosexuality could result in a life sentence, and in Michigan, where the first offense carried a maximum of 15 years in prison and a life sentence for a subsequent conviction. In certain African and Asian countries, the death penalty for homosexuality was still in effect.

In 1962, Illinois became the first state to decriminalize consensual homosexual sex, although solicitation for sex remained illegal. From 1971 to 1983, a total of 26 states repealed their laws, including California in 1976 and New York in 1980.[2]

Alfred Kinsey and Sexual Behavior

Alfred Kinsey, a professor at Indiana University, Bloomington, conducted a survey in the 1940s with 6,300 volunteers, including 5,300 white men (84 percent of the sample), about their sexual histories.[3] The survey classified sexual behavior as heterosexual or homosexual based on the type of physical or "psychic" stimulation that led to orgasm. According to Kinsey's findings, 69.4 percent of sexual experiences were attributed to heterosexual sources (such as coitus and petting), 24 percent to solitary sources (masturbation and nocturnal emissions), 6.3 percent to homosexual contact (such as mutual masturbation, manual contact, oral sex, and anal sex), and 0.3 percent to relations with animals.

Kinsey reported that 37 percent of interviewees had some gay experience between adolescence and old age. However, he acknowledged that his sample was biased because it included inmates of prisons and reform schools, which may have had higher rates of homosexual behavior due to isolation from the opposite sex. Kinsey also encouraged men who reported exclusively homosexual behavior to recruit their contacts for the study, which may have skewed the results.

Kinsey found a wide range of estimates on the incidence of homosexual behavior in the literature, ranging from 1 percent to 100 percent. The estimates varied depending on the definition of gay behavior and the source of the estimates. For example, the U.S. military reported that about

1 percent of males were rejected by draft boards or identified and discharged during active service due to homosexuality. On the other hand, some psychoanalysts and promiscuous homosexual males estimated that 100 percent of the male population were homosexual or bisexual.

After reviewing all the data, Kinsey concluded that 8 percent of adult males were exclusively homosexual and that 18 percent of men had some homosexual experience between the ages of 16 and 55 years.[4]

Gay Rights Movement

The 1960s witnessed various social revolutions in America, including the civil rights movement, feminism, opposition to the Vietnam War, and the gay rights movement. Many credit the start of the gay revolution to the Stonewall Inn riots, which lasted five days following a police raid in New York City.[5]

On June 28, 1969, police officers raided the Stonewall Inn, arresting both employees (for operating without a liquor license) and drag queens (cross-dressing was illegal in New York at that time). Instead of dispersing, as was typical during police raids, gay men and women fought back. They gathered in Christopher Park, blocked traffic, and prevented paddy wagons from leaving while barricading police cars from entering. The situation escalated when a police officer assaulted a drag queen, leading to the crowd throwing coins at the police and using a broken parking meter to barricade them inside. The riots continued for the following four nights.

In the aftermath of the riots, several gay rights groups emerged, including the Gay Liberation Front and the Gay Activists Alliance. One of the initial targets of the movement was the American Psychiatric Association (APA).[6]

In the first edition of the APA's *Diagnostic and Statistical Manual of Mental Disorders* (*DSM-1*, 1952), homosexuality was classified as a mental illness, and doctors considered all homosexuals incapable of leading happy and productive lives. Shockingly, treatments such as castration, electric shock therapy, hysterectomy, and lobotomy were used in attempts to "cure" homosexuality. However, following the Stonewall riots, gay activists engaged with mental health therapists and initiated a dialogue. This marked the first time that many psychiatrists had conversations with successful homosexual men and lesbians. In the *DSM-3*, published in 1980, homosexuality was declassified as a mental disorder, with the recognition that there was no credible evidence that could change sexual orientation and that it did not need to be changed from a mental health perspective.[7]

By 1981, the gay rights movement had made progress on various fronts, but sodomy laws were still in effect in over half the states, and some foreign countries imposed the death penalty for homosexuality. The emergence of GRID (gay-related immunodeficiency), later known as AIDS, further highlighted the legal and social issues faced by the gay community, leading many closeted gay men to come out to their families, friends, and foes. Conducting research in this population would prove to be challenging.

Dr. Richard Krause

Dr. Richard Krause (1925–2015) served as the director of the National Institute of Allergy and Infectious Diseases (NIAID) from 1975 to 1984. During his tenure, he played a pivotal role in investigating the origins of the AIDS virus through field studies in Haiti (Chapter 8) and Projet SIDA in Zaire (Chapter 9). However, his most significant contribution to the fight against AIDS was the establishment of the Multicenter AIDS Cohort Study (MACS).

Richard Krause graduated from Marietta (Ohio) College in 1947 and later earned his medical degree from Case Western Reserve University School of Medicine in 1952. While in medical school, Krause took an 18-month leave to contribute to the prevention of rheumatic fever. Following medical school, he pursued further training in internal medicine at Barnes Hospital in St. Louis and completed a research fellowship at Rockefeller University. During his time at Rockefeller, he continued his groundbreaking research on streptococcal pharyngitis and rheumatic fever. Notably, he successfully immunized rabbits with streptococcal polysaccharides. In recognition of his remarkable achievements, Krause was elected to the U.S. National Academy of Sciences in 1977.

During our work in Haiti in 1982, Dr. Krause engaged in extensive discussions regarding the findings of Harold Jaffe's case-control study.[8] Both Krause and I acknowledged the likelihood of a sexually transmitted infectious agent as the cause of AIDS. Krause believed that the next logical step was to conduct a cohort study involving asymptomatic gay men to define the incubation period and natural progression of the disease.

Krause shared fascinating insights into his medical school days, when he participated in a team of researchers who followed a cohort of 1,000 children hospitalized with acute rheumatic fever, chorea (a brain disorder characterized by muscular spasms of the face, arms, and legs), or rheumatic heart disease for over 30 years. This study shed light on the numerous complications of streptococcal pharyngitis ("strep throat") even before the cause was fully understood.[9]

Upon returning from Haiti, Richard Krause collaborated with Robert Edelman to initiate a natural history study involving 1,000 gay men.

However, Dick Kaslow (EIS 1971) recommended a larger sample size of at least 2,000 men for a more meaningful study. Consequently, NIAID and the NCI issued a request for applications to establish cooperative agreements for AIDS research. Eventually, Krause secured funding to study 5,000 men, marking a significant step in the battle against AIDS.

On September 30, 1983, cooperative agreement awards were granted to investigators at five sites: Baltimore, Chicago, Los Angeles, Pittsburgh, and San Francisco. Each site's mission was to identify 1,000 gay men without AIDS and track their health over at least three years.

In the following months, Dick Kaslow collaborated with these five teams to establish a common protocol for understanding the natural history of AIDS, identifying risk factors for infection, and creating a repository of biological specimens for future research.[10] However, the teams encountered a stumbling block when it came to defining participants and recruitment strategies. Warren Winkelstein, the principal investigator of the San Francisco cohort, insisted on recruiting not only self-described gay men but also single (non-married) men aged 25–54 within a specific area of San Francisco using a probability sampling strategy. Winkelstein proposed a door-to-door recruitment approach in the Castro district of San Francisco. Conversely, the other four sites advocated for recruiting self-described gay men through a convenience sampling strategy. This disagreement eventually led to the San Francisco site's removal from the MACS when the cooperative agreements were up for renewal in 1986.

What is the distinction between a probability sampling strategy and a convenience one, and why was Warren Winkelstein so adamant about it? A probability sampling strategy involves selecting a sample so that each member of the population has a known and non-zero chance of being included. During EIS training, a probability sampling strategy was used to recruit participants for the household study of violence (Chapter 2). This method is less biased and allows for valid conclusions to be drawn about the entire population under study.

In contrast, a convenience sample is one that is readily available. For example, the Chicago site proposed recruiting men attending an STD clinic, while Baltimore, Los Angeles, and Pittsburgh planned to advertise in gay newspapers and place posters in gay bars, bookstores, and bathhouses to attract participants. Such samples inherently contain bias because they include only individuals who happen to be out and about or engaged in a specific activity during the recruitment period. Winkelstein argued that his sampling strategy ensured the inclusion of "closeted" gay men and those who had same-sex encounters but did not identify as gay.[11]

Starting in April 1984, nearly 6,000 men voluntarily participated in semiannual interviews, physical exams, and laboratory tests. Each subject provided informed consent for the study, received assurances of confidentiality, and received a stipend for their involvement.[12]

Review of the MACS

When I joined NIAID in the summer of 1984, I had the opportunity to review the five applications and the cooperative protocol that had been developed by Dick Kaslow. This project was incredibly ambitious, and our hope was that the study would provide insights into the natural history of HIV infection, including its incubation period, changes in behavior over time, and the impact of treatment on the course of the disease. Kaslow shared with me the challenging process of creating a common protocol, establishing a unified recruitment process (at four of the five sites), designing a questionnaire, and planning laboratory evaluations.

After carefully reviewing the materials, I had several suggestions for the NIAID team, although not all of them were well received. I agreed with Warren Winkelstein that the San Francisco approach was the most scientifically valid one. However, I also recognized that going door-to-door to recruit gay men in Pittsburgh, Baltimore, or Chicago might not be practical. Additionally, I expressed concern about the questionnaire and questioned why Kaslow hadn't utilized the questionnaire developed by Harold Jaffe from our CDC study (Appendix B). My rationale was that using Jaffe's questionnaire would allow us to compare the results from both studies. Dick Kaslow explained to me that many of the MACS investigators were gay men, some openly so and others "closeted," and they had reservations about the CDC because the Jaffe study had exposed the promiscuity and illegal drug use within the gay community. As a result, the MACS investigators had decided not to collect data on sexual behavior, bathhouse participation, or information on illegal drug use in the same way as the CDC study had done. Instead, they chose to focus on behaviors in the two years prior to the interview. Kaslow argued that this approach would reduce recall bias among participants.

I also expressed concerns about the survey mode, which involved participants completing a pencil-and-paper exercise supervised by a research assistant, in contrast to the face-to-face interviews conducted by physicians, with the physician completing the forms, as we had done in Jaffe's study. Additionally, I shared information with Kaslow about our KS vs. PCP study and the discovery that nitrites were associated with Kaposi's sarcoma (Chapter 10). In hindsight, I regretted disclosing this information to him (see Chapter 16).

Regarding the results of the first wave of HIV testing in MACS by the end of 1984, there were variations among the different sites. Using Bob Gallo's experimental HTLV-III/LAV antibody test, the results were as follows:

- Los Angeles: 51 percent of 1,637 men tested positive.
- San Francisco: 49 percent of 799 gay men tested positive, while none of the 204 heterosexual men were positive.
- Chicago: 43 percent of 1,102 men tested positive.
- Baltimore/Washington, D.C.: 31 percent of 1,153 men tested positive.
- Pittsburgh/Tri State: 21 percent of 1,063 men tested positive.[13]

These results were staggering, particularly the fact that approximately half of the gay men in Los Angeles and San Francisco had already been infected with HIV by the end of 1984. It raised significant concerns about the impending impact of AIDS and how many individuals would succumb to the disease in the coming years.

HIV Testing Commercially Available

On March 2, 1985, the FDA licensed an HIV ELISA (enzyme-linked immunosorbent assay) blood test to Abbott Laboratories of Illinois for commercial use (Chapter 5). Six additional test kits were licensed by the end of the year. The sensitivity of the tests detected antibody-to-HIV range between 93 and 99 percent, and all above 99 percent in specificity. Characteristics of each subsequent test licensed by the FDA had to exceed its predecessors.[14]

The availability of the HIV antibody test transformed the AIDS effort. It allowed case finding, followed by sexual contact investigation and partner notification. The HIV antibody test had several excellent characteristics to justify its use. It had a high sensitivity and specificity and a reasonable cost. AIDS was a suitable disease for screening because it was a serious, progressive disease. Identifying asymptomatic HIV-infected sexually active persons and blood donors provided information that could prevent transmission to others. Predictive value positive (PVP) is one measure of test feasibility, expressed as a percentage. PVP is the number of individuals with a positive test result who actually have the disease divided by the number who test positive. Assuming a prevalence of 30 percent among gay men, the positive predictive value of a single test exceeded 95 percent. In other words, among gay men, 19 of 20 testing positive were indeed infected with the virus.

Although the screening test was embraced and implemented by the American blood banking industry (Chapter 6), the test was not acceptable to many gay men. Although screening seems simple to many, it is quite complex. There are hidden costs and risks. For example, screening can cause great anxiety in those who test positive and result in morbidity. In one study of gay men who learned their antibody status in the course of research, one in seven of those testing positive developed suicidal ideation. Some considered a positive test result a "death sentence." In 1985, we had no specific treatments for HIV, and indeed, over 90 percent of PCP patients died within two years of diagnosis of AIDS. Moreover, the gay community feared that tests would be inaccurate, results would be divulged inappropriately, and they would suffer further stigmatization and discrimination.[15]

On February 28, 1985, the National Gay Task Force and the Lambda Legal Defense and Education Fund filed a petition in federal court to stay the licensing of the test pending validation of the test's accuracy and a guarantee that the test would not be used to screen men for homosexuality. Already health officials had received requests from school officials to use the test to weed out gay teachers; country club managers wanted to use the test to identify HIV-infected food handlers. An emergency meeting was held between the lawyers and the FDA commissioner. In response, the test was clearly defined for use in blood banks and laboratories, and not as a screen for AIDS or for high-risk groups for AIDS.[16]

Many gay men were eager to know their antibody status and had plans to take the test as soon as it became available. However, there was a concern that some individuals might try to donate blood just to get their test results. To avoid this, measures were put in place to ensure that the test was readily available to those interested without the need for blood donation.

In April 1985, the CDC collaborated with 55 state and local health departments to establish alternative test sites. These sites offered pre- and post-test counseling and facilitated referrals for medical evaluation when necessary. Importantly, these services were provided free of charge. By the end of that year, a total of 874 test sites had conducted tests on 79,100 individuals. Among those tested, 13,684 individuals (approximately 17.3 percent) were repeatedly found to be positive on the antibody test.[17] This initiative not only made testing more convenient and accessible but also helped identify a substantial number of HIV-positive individuals who might otherwise have gone undiagnosed.

New PHS Recommendations to Prevent HIV Transmission

On March 14, 1986, the Public Health Service issued recommendations for the voluntary serologic testing of all individuals at an elevated risk of HIV infection when they sought healthcare services, particularly in settings such as sexually transmitted disease clinics, drug abuse clinics, and clinics for examining commercial sex workers. These recommendations aimed to facilitate the identification of asymptomatic individuals who tested positive for HIV. The primary goals were to provide them with medical evaluations and counseling to prevent further transmission of the virus. The CDC emphasized the importance of maintaining strict confidentiality and safeguarding records from unauthorized disclosure.[18]

The PHS outlined several crucial measures for individuals who tested positive for HIV:

1. Inform prospective sexual partners: Individuals should inform their prospective sexual partners about their HIV infection status so that the partners can take appropriate precautions.
    A. Abstaining from sexual activity with another person is one option that eliminates any risk of sexually transmitted HIV infection.
2. Take precautions during sexual activity: Individuals should take precautions to prevent contact between their blood, semen, urine, feces, or saliva and their sexual partners. Although the efficacy of condoms was still being studied, consistent condom use was recommended to reduce transmission by preventing exposure to semen and infected lymphocytes.
3. Notify previous sexual partners: Those who test positive for HIV should inform their previous sexual partners about their potential exposure to HIV and encourage them to seek testing and counseling.[19]

For individuals who tested negative for HIV antibodies, the recommendations were as follows:

1. Reduce the number of sexual partners: Individuals should aim to reduce the number of sexual partners. Maintaining a stable, mutually monogamous relationship with an uninfected person eliminates the risk of acquiring sexually transmitted HIV infection.
2. Take precautions with potentially infected partners: When engaging in sexual activity with anyone who might be infected, individuals should take appropriate precautions, as outlined above.[20]

These guidelines represented a critical step in the effort to combat the spread of HIV by promoting responsible behavior, protecting sexual partners, and ensuring that individuals received the necessary support and information to make informed decisions about their sexual health.

Gay Marriage

Many within the gay community were able to discern the underlying message in these recommendations. It was clear that "safe sex" could indeed exist, but it necessitated HIV testing, serosorting (selecting sexual partners based on their HIV status), and a commitment to monogamy. In other words, individuals were encouraged to get tested for HIV and share their results with their partners. If both partners tested HIV-negative and maintained monogamy, they could consider themselves "safe." If one or both partners tested positive, it was crucial to seek medical evaluation and treatment.

These recommendations emphasized the importance of HIV testing, open communication about HIV status, and the value of monogamous relationships as measures to reduce the risk of transmission. It underscored the need for responsible sexual behavior and the importance of regular testing for those who were sexually active.

Moreover, the movement for legal protection for same-sex marriages had been ongoing for decades, but it gained significant momentum following the publication of these recommendations. The concept of gay marriage took on a central role at the Second National March on Washington for Lesbian and Gay Rights on October 11, 1987. Among the seven primary demands presented during the march, the first one called for the legal recognition of lesbian and gay relationships. These recommendations and the evolving understanding of safe practices played a pivotal role in advancing the fight for legal recognition and rights for same-sex couples.

Ambivalence in Gay Community Regarding Testing

The introduction of HIV testing brought about complex ethical and public health considerations. While the test was a valuable tool for diagnosing and preventing the spread of a deadly disease, it also carried significant psychological and social implications. Here are some key points related to the challenges and responses to HIV testing during that time:

1. Conflicting advice and campaigns: Activists and organizations had different perspectives on HIV testing. Some advised gay men not to get tested due to the potential psychological ramifications of a positive result. In San Francisco, the AIDS Foundation launched a campaign listing the pros and cons of the test in the gay press, encouraging individuals to study and decide for themselves whether to take the test.

2. Confidentiality concerns: In many cities, maintaining confidentiality was a paramount issue. In California, the state assembly prohibited the release of antibody test results, even if ordered by subpoena. Written informed consent was required before testing, and pre- and post-test counseling were mandated. Doctors who administered the test without consent or disclosed a person's antibody status could face criminal penalties.
3. New York City's restrictions: In New York City, where a substantial percentage of AIDS case-patients were reported, gay activists strongly opposed the test due to fear of discrimination. The city's health commissioner, Dr. David Sencer, former director of the CDC, issued a public order restricting the test's use to blood banks and scientific research only. This decision was met with surprise and disappointment by many physicians who had hoped to use the test for diagnosing patients with immunologic disorders and counseling individuals about their infectious status.[21]

I could not fathom how a former head of the CDC did not understand the value in HIV testing for prevention of a deadly disease. I would learn later that NYC mayor Ed Koch had given Dr. David Sencer a direct order to restrict the use of the test.

4. Political and legal response: Some public health proponents and "conservative" politicians in various states believed that widespread mandatory testing could control the disease's spread within the gay community. Several states imposed mandatory HIV reporting, collecting names of HIV-positive individuals for contact tracing and partner notification. Colorado was the first state to implement mandatory HIV reporting in 1985, followed by other states like Minnesota, Wisconsin, South Carolina, Idaho, and Arizona.[22] However, some clinicians humorously reported fictitious names like "Ronald Reagan" and "Mickey Mouse" in protest.
5. Resistance to name reporting: Activists in many regions opposed the use of names for HIV reporting. Georgia, in cooperation with the CDC, became the first state to require HIV case reporting using unique identifiers instead of names. The Soundex system, a phonetic algorithm for indexing names, was employed to protect privacy. Despite these efforts, public health officials estimated that only about 60 percent of HIV-positive case-patients were reported.

These challenges reflected the complex and evolving nature of the HIV epidemic during that era. Balancing the need for public health measures with concerns about privacy, stigma, and discrimination was a significant issue in the response to the AIDS crisis.

AIDS Coalition to Unleash Power (ACT-UP)

As more and more men found out that they were HIV-positive, and then discovered that public health departments were collecting their names, anxiety boiled over into anger. Gay men were angry at the government for not doing more to protect gay men from AIDS and discrimination.

In 1987, Larry Kramer (1935–2020) became the catalyst for the creation of the AIDS Coalition to Unleash Power (ACT-UP). ACT-UP units formed first in New York City, then spread rapidly throughout the United States and Europe to protest the lack of resources provided for healthcare and research on AIDS. Their slogan was "SILENCE=DEATH," and they were anything but silent. They marched and protested at AIDS meetings, interrupted scientists during lectures, and invaded government offices to implement change in policies. Kramer and ACT-UP created changes at the New York City Health Department, the FDA, the National Institutes of Health, and the pharmaceutical industry. They forced the government to quicken the research evaluation and drug approval processes leading to the approval of the first effective antiretroviral agent, AZT, and other antiviral drugs that would prolong the lives of millions infected with HIV.

Larry Kramer was a playwright, author, and gay activist. He was born June 25, 1935, in Bridgeport, Connecticut, and graduated Yale University in 1957. In 1976 he published *Faggots*, a novel describing the shallow, promiscuous lifestyle of gay men on Fire Island, New York. In 1983 he and others founded the Gay Men's Health Crisis to provide services for gay men with AIDS in New York City; however, he left the group when his colleagues refused to follow his lead for more militant protests. In 1985 Kramer expressed his frustration by writing a play, *The Normal Heart*, which was produced at the Public Theater in New York City. *The Normal Heart* was listed as one of the hundred best plays of the 20th century by the Royal National Theatre of Great Britain. According to Kramer, the AIDS plague was allowed to happen because of the inaction of three "closeted" gay men: Edward Koch, mayor of New York from 1978 to 1989; Ronald Reagan, Jr., the son of the president; and Dr. Richard Krause, the director of the National Institute of Allergy and Infectious Diseases from 1975 to 1984.[23]

A Rational Approach to the HIV Test

Ronald Bayer emerged as a mediator amid the turmoil surrounding the introduction of the blood test for HIV. Holding a doctorate in political science from the University of Chicago, Bayer's professional journey led him to become an associate at the Hastings Center in New York, where he delved into the ethical dilemmas surrounding health policy. In an October 1986 article published in *Journal of the American Medical Association* (*JAMA*), he articulated fundamental principles and essential criteria for evaluating the HIV screening test.[24]

Bayer's insights acknowledged that the most significant chance of halting the spread of HIV relied on the voluntary cooperation of individuals at elevated risk. Their willingness to undergo testing and adapt their personal conduct for the greater good of the community played a pivotal role. According to Bayer, those at high risk of developing AIDS carried a moral duty to take all necessary measures to prevent harm to others, which included undergoing the antibody test. Given the dire medical consequences of HIV infection, those who tested positive bore the responsibility of knowing their antibody status, informing their sexual partners, and adjusting their behavior accordingly.

On the contrary, Bayer recognized that HIV had primarily affected groups already susceptible to social and economic discrimination. He underscored the potential harm the test posed to those who underwent it. In his assessment, the sole justifiable purpose for screening was to curb the spread of AIDS. Bayer firmly argued against using the test as a means of expressing disapproval of sexual orientation or drug use, deeming such actions a violation of principles of justice and respect for others. However, he did concede that if an effective therapy or vaccine were to be developed, screening might be justified as a means of protecting those at risk. Universal mandatory screening could only be considered ethical when a therapeutic intervention was available or when infection posed a risk to others through casual contact. In 1986, neither of these conditions had been met.[25]

Confidentiality emerged as a central concern in this context. There were fears that some individuals might be compelled to undergo the test for employment purposes or to secure life insurance. The most vehement opponents of the test worried about the establishment of medical concentration camps for HIV-positive gay men, a practice implemented in Cuba. While several state legislatures considered quarantine as an approach to AIDS prevention, none ultimately legalized it. The challenge in applying enforced isolation measures to HIV infection lay in the fact that traditionally quarantined diseases, such as smallpox, yellow fever, and cholera, had relatively short periods of infectivity for most patients, typically measured in days or weeks. In contrast, HIV infection resembled leprosy, with the potential to remain infectious for several years.[26]

Six-Month Follow-Up Evaluations in MACS

On Valentine's Day 1987, a group of NIH-funded researchers unveiled the results of their second evaluation of gay men in Baltimore, Chicago, Los Angeles, and Pittsburgh. Impressively, 90 percent of participants returned for this follow-up visit, leading to the identification of 95 new HIV infections among the 2,507 individuals who had initially tested negative. These new infections were distributed as follows: Los Angeles (5 percent of 685), Chicago (5 percent of 554), Baltimore/Washington (3 percent of 749), and Pittsburgh/Tri State area (3 percent of 519). Notably, none of the 220 men who reported only engaging in oral sex seroconverted, while 58 out of 548 men (11 percent) who reported receptive anal intercourse with two or more partners during the study period did seroconvert.[27]

Upon conducting a multivariate analysis, the researchers determined that receptive anal intercourse was the sole significant risk factor for HIV seroconversion. The risk ratio escalated from threefold for those practicing receptive anal intercourse with one partner to a staggering 18-fold with five or more partners. Consequently, the authors concluded that receptive anal intercourse was the primary mode of HIV transmission among gay men, emphasizing that the prevention focus should be on avoiding such behavior.[28]

However, the promotion of this message inadvertently led to a misleading belief: that if anal sex was the mode of transmission, then oral sex must be safe. The MACS investigators were careful to note that their study did not prove the safety of oral sex, but this caveat was not effectively communicated to the gay community.

Immediately, I expressed skepticism regarding these findings and voiced my concerns to the investigators. The concept of a sexually transmitted disease spreading exclusively through anal intercourse seemed implausible. By 1986, virologists had already isolated HIV from blood, semen, saliva, and vaginal secretions. No other sexually transmitted infection was known to be transmitted exclusively through a single mode of sexual contact. I suggested that the data be reanalyzed, considering factors such as the number of partners, study site, and other variables. I was particularly concerned about excluding the number of partners from the MACS statistical analysis, as it was a central finding in the Harold Jaffe study.[29] The researchers countered that numbers of partners were considered a confounding variable now that it was established that HIV caused AIDS. While I agreed with that point, I continued to argue that receptive anal intercourse might also be a confounding variable. Additionally, I questioned how receptive anal intercourse could explain the growing number of heterosexual men with AIDS in regions like Africa, the Caribbean, and the United States. I highlighted three individuals who were infected but reported only insertive anal intercourse and not receptive anal intercourse. The MACS researchers assured me that they were re-interviewing these participants, but they underscored the strong statistical significance of their existing findings, deeming further analysis unnecessary.[30]

I hoped that other studies would refute their findings. However, the San Francisco cohort and Warren Winkelstein, operating independently of the MACS, reviewed the initial wave of visits conducted from June 1984 to January 1985. Their analysis revealed some significant insights: among gay men who reported no male partners in the two years preceding their entry into the study, 18 percent tested positive for HIV. In contrast, of those who reported more than 50 male partners in two years, a striking 71 percent were seropositive. Of various sexual practices, only receptive anal intercourse exhibited a significantly elevated risk of HIV infection.[31] Harold Jaffe's reanalysis of national case-control study data supported the MACS findings.[32] These results were reproducible and consistent across studies.[33]

The gay community largely embraced the MACS's findings, with the focus of educational messages centering on the avoidance of receptive anal intercourse as the primary prevention strategy for HIV in gay communities. However, the apparent contradiction between the recommendations of different arms of the Public Health Service, with the CDC recommending HIV testing and treatment referral for all high-risk individuals while the NIH recommended avoiding only one specific sexual act, raised valid questions.

As time passed, it became evident that as receptive anal intercourse decreased among participants in gay cohorts, receptive oral sex and insertive anal sex accounted for more infections. Moreover, systematic misclassification bias had influenced earlier reports. New infections among gay men who engaged in both oral and anal sex with multiple partners were solely attributed to anal sex, although it was impossible to definitively determine which sexual act or partner transmitted HIV. Additionally, there were growing anecdotal reports of HIV seroconversions among individuals who practiced only receptive oral sex, spanning gay men, heterosexuals, and lesbians.[34] The conclusion drawn from these observations was clear: oral sex was not safe. Consequently, the NIH recommendations were deemed inadequate. Surprisingly, the authors of the initial report never retracted their paper or provided updated information to the gay community.[35]

Regarding the disclosure of HIV results, starting in late 1985, all MACS participants were informed by letter that HIV antibody tests were available upon request. However, by June 1987, fewer than 20 percent of participants in Chicago had requested and returned for an HIV disclosure visit.[36] The MACS investigators had possessed HIV results for all participants as early as 1984 but chose to release results only to those who specifically requested them. Furthermore, they made no effort to contact participants who tested positive on a visit and did not return for their semiannual visits. The rationale behind this approach was that they were studying behavior change in those who received test results compared to those who did not seek results.[37] Nevertheless, the nondisclosure of test results drew comparisons to the Tuskegee experiments conducted by the PHS, where Black men with diagnosed syphilis were followed from 1932 to 1972 without being informed of their test results and available treatments for syphilis were withheld, reflecting a concerning ethical parallel.

The Natural History of HIV Infection

Tony Fauci's Laboratory of Immunoregulation played a crucial role in defining the natural history of HIV infection by categorizing it into six stages based on clinical and laboratory data collected from patients at the NIH Clinical Center and average time intervals measured in blood transfusion recipients and gay men by the CDC[38]:

1. Viral transmission (primary infection): This marks the initial stage of HIV infection.
2. Acute retroviral syndrome: In this stage, which occurs two to three weeks after infection, the virus widely disseminates, and lymph nodes become seeded with the virus. Patients may experience flu-like symptoms such as body aches, diarrhea, headache, and nausea, which can last for two to three weeks.
3. Recovery and seroconversion: Antibodies to HIV become detectable in the bloodstream.
4. Asymptomatic chronic infection (latency period): This stage can last for a few months to as long as a decade or more.
5. Symptomatic HIV infection and AIDS: Patients experience constitutional symptoms like persistent fever, weight loss, and diarrhea, which can be followed by the development of cancers and opportunistic infections (AIDS).
6. Death: The final stage of the disease.

The latency period is the time from HIV infection to the diagnosis of cancers and opportunistic infections and was projected as 7.8–8.2 years in the CDC studies of blood transfusion recipients and gay men.[39]

However, there is variability in measured latency periods, ranging from less than one year in some of the earliest blood transfusion case-patients to over a decade in some patients. Several factors or cofactors may contribute to this variation and the complexity of AIDS:

- Host immune factors: The strength and effectiveness of an individual's immune response to the virus can influence the course of the disease. Some people may have stronger immune responses that delay the progression of HIV to AIDS. Rapid progression had been noted among infants and young children as well as elderly persons after receipt of blood and blood products.[40]
- Viral factors: Variability in the virulence of different HIV strains may affect the rate of disease progression.
- Co-infections: Other infections, such as cytomegalovirus and hepatitis C, can accelerate the progression of HIV to AIDS.
- Drugs: Drugs, such as steroids, opioids, and nitrite inhalants, may enhance the immunosuppression induced by HIV.
- Genetic factors: Genetic variations in both the host and the virus may play a role in determining the rate of disease progression.
- Access to healthcare: Socioeconomic factors and access to healthcare can impact the ability to receive antiretroviral therapy and other treatments that can slow the progression of HIV.

Regarding the MACS, its primary purpose, as envisioned by Richard Krause, was to determine the natural history of AIDS and the variation in the course of illness from one patient to the next. However, the study faced challenges due to attrition, with only 90 percent of participants returning for the first six-month visit, and this attrition rate persisted over time. The MACS continued until 2019 and its investigators published over 1,000 scientific papers on various aspects of HIV infection among gay men. However, they were unable to define the complete natural history of the disease. This limitation was partly due to the lack of tracking mechanisms to follow participants until death, which was necessary to comprehensively define the natural history of the disease. In the end, it's possible that Richard Krause, who passed away in 2015, might have been disappointed in the outcome of MACS in achieving its intended goals.

14

U.S. Army and Heterosexual Transmission

> *The psychiatrists made many attempts at formulating reasons for the excessive promiscuity of wartime. Long absence from home was probably the most convenient explanation, and eighteen months' service overseas was apparently the zero line with men who were otherwise stable and not habitually promiscuous. Age played little part, marriage was not a strong deterrent and fear decreased with absence from home, particularly among certain colonial and allied troops. The arm of the Service did not seem to matter; rather it was a question of geographical position and opportunity. Some reviews say that the risks decreased with rank, but there always seemed to be a very large proportion of senior non-commissioned officers in venereal diseases ward.*
> —Colonel Donald J. Campbell, U.S. Army, 1946[1]

In mid–June 1984, I accompanied Dr. William Jordan, our division director and advisor to the military, to a secret meeting at Walter Reed Army Medical Center in Washington, D.C. Major Robert Redfield, an army physician in infectious diseases, presented the medical histories of about 20 soldiers with AIDS or AIDS-related complex who had been evaluated at WRAMC. These patients included several self-acknowledged gay men, but also seven married men with children who denied any homosexual behavior or intravenous drug abuse.

Colonel Edmund Tramont, U.S. Army lead infectious diseases physician and a well-respected researcher on sexual transmitted infections among the military, told the army high command and the Military Advisory Board that he was not surprised that AIDS was occurring among our troops. Sexually transmitted infections plague armies worldwide. Most of the high command thought of AIDS as a gay disease, and suggested that all HIV-infected soldiers be boarded out of the military immediately.

I returned to the office and told Bob Edelman about the meeting. He and I started collecting reports in the medical literature suggesting heterosexual transmission of HIV infection and AIDS.

In the March 15, 1985, issue of the *Journal of the American Medical Association* (*JAMA*), Bob Redfield and colleagues described a cluster of seven active duty soldiers, married heterosexual men, with AIDS or AIDS-related complex (ARC). Redfield examined their wives and children and tested serum from each for HIV using an experimental enzyme-linked immunosorbent assay (ELISA) and Western blot test for detection of antibodies developed by Bob Gallo. All seven husbands were HIV-positive, five of the wives tested positive, as did one of 11 children (age range 14 months–13 years). Redfield concluded that heterosexual activity had the potential to play a significant role in transmission of HIV.[2]

Bob Edelman and I wrote a letter to *JAMA* in response to Bob Redfield's paper, citing data from Haiti and Africa that supported the importance of heterosexual transmission of HIV and highlighted the likelihood of female-to-male transmission. How were the husbands getting HIV infection? If female-to-male transmission of HIV was occurring, the virus must be spread by sexual activities other than receptive anal intercourse or exposure to semen. We also suggested that the rate of increase of AIDS case-patients attributed to heterosexual transmission by the CDC was similar to that among gay men and the other established risk groups.[3]

In October 1985, Bob Redfield published a second report in *JAMA*, following his initial study involving 41 AIDS/ARC patients. Most of these patients had self-reported engaging in high-risk behaviors. Surprisingly, 15 of them identified themselves as exclusively heterosexual and denied any injection drug use. Among them, there were 10 men and five women, comprising eight Blacks, four Hispanics, and three whites. Redfield's study revealed that six patients had engaged in heterosexual contact with partners who had developed AIDS or were at risk for it. The remaining nine patients had multiple heterosexual partners (more than 50) and had sexual encounters with prostitutes in Germany, including Black women from Cameroon and Zaire. Notably, none of the five women reported engaging in receptive anal intercourse. Redfield's findings challenged the prevailing belief that receptive anal intercourse was a requirement for HIV transmission, directly contradicting the positions held by the NIH and the MACS (as discussed in Chapter 13).[4]

The MACS investigators responded to Redfield's assertions. Dr. Frank Polk, the principal investigator at the MACS site in Baltimore, addressed the issue in a letter published in the December 13, 1985, issue of *JAMA*. While Polk acknowledged that female-to-male transmission of HIV was a crucial epidemiological question in AIDS research, he expressed skepticism regarding Redfield's findings. Polk argued that there was insufficient data to support female-to-male HIV transmission, aside from potentially low-frequency occurrences. He cautioned against taking Redfield's work at face value and even suggested that U.S. Army personnel might be dishonest about their sexual histories. It was important to note that revealing homosexuality or drug abuse by military personnel automatically led to their discharge from the service. Furthermore, Polk contested the data from Africa, which indicated an equal ratio of male-to-female AIDS case-patients, asserting that this did not necessarily prove equal transmission between females and males. He proposed that these statistics might be heavily influenced by the reuse of inadequately sterilized needles and syringes in the treatment of sexually transmitted diseases among promiscuous heterosexuals.[5]

Colonel Edmund Tramont and HIV Testing in the Military

During the ongoing scientific debate surrounding heterosexual transmission of HIV, Colonel Edmund "Ed" Tramont (1939–2023) emerged as a prominent figure advocating for the Department of Defense to address HIV in the military in a manner similar to how it dealt with other sexually transmitted diseases like syphilis and gonorrhea.

Colonel Tramont was born on August 5, 1939, in New Haven, Connecticut. He graduated from Rutgers University in 1962 and earned his medical degree from Boston University School of Medicine in 1966. In 1968, he was drafted into the army and began an internal medicine residency at Walter Reed Army Medical Center. One of his early patients happened to be General Dwight D. Eisenhower, the former president, who was suffering from cardiac disease. Dr. Tramont's responsibility was to closely monitor Eisenhower's condition day and night. Tramont served a remarkable 23 years in the U.S. Army, during which he held positions such as chief of infectious diseases at WRAMC from 1972 to 1981 and consultant in infectious diseases to the Surgeon General of the U.S. Army at the Pentagon from 1974 to 1991. Tramont was widely recognized as an authority on sexually transmitted infections in the military, and he was not surprised when AIDS emerged among military personnel who were often stationed far from their families and deployed to various parts of the world.

Dr. Tramont made a compelling case to the army high command and the Military Advisory Board, emphasizing the need for comprehensive education, mandatory screening programs, and active contact tracing to contain the virus within the military. HIV infection posed unique challenges for the military, impacting issues like military readiness, promotions, and retention. For instance, recruits receive a series of immunizations over a few days, but HIV-infected recruits may not respond effectively to these vaccines if their immune systems are compromised. Additionally, live virus vaccines could potentially spread uncontrollably in such immunodeficient individuals. Dr. Tramont highlighted a case involving one of Bob Redfield's initial AIDS patients, a soldier who developed disseminated vaccinia infection and subsequently died after receiving the smallpox vaccine in preparation for deployment to Africa.

Furthermore, Dr. Tramont raised concerns about safeguarding the blood supply for wounded soldiers in combat situations, where fresh plasma and blood were often obtained from nearby troops. These were just some of the many issues that Colonel Tramont addressed, and he also projected the potential healthcare costs to the military if HIV infection rates continued to rise among military personnel.[6]

The U.S. Army command took a comprehensive approach to address the HIV problem within the military, implementing several key measures:

1. Mandatory HIV testing for applicants: The army established a mandatory HIV testing program for all individuals applying to join the army. Those who tested positive would be excluded from recruitment.
2. Regular HIV testing for active duty soldiers: All active duty soldiers would undergo annual HIV testing. Those who tested positive would be referred for medical evaluation at Walter Reed. If diagnosed with HIV, these soldiers would receive comprehensive medical care and be assessed for discharge.
3. Discharge for unfit soldiers: Soldiers who tested positive and were deemed unfit for duty, based on their inability to perform their job at an acceptable level, would be discharged. They would receive lifelong medical benefits.
4. Continued service for fit soldiers: Soldiers who tested positive but were still physically capable of meeting the physical fitness requirements and performing their job duties would be allowed to remain on active duty. However, they would be restricted to duty within the continental 48 states and not deployed outside the United States.
5. Limited contact tracing: Contact tracing would be conducted but limited to spouses and children of the infected soldier.
6. Comprehensive care with privacy respect: Compassionate and comprehensive care would be provided to all HIV-infected

soldiers and their dependents, with a strong emphasis on respecting privacy issues.

In the initial round of testing among army applicants conducted between October 1985 and March 1986, 466 individuals tested positive, with a prevalence rate of 1.5 per 1,000 tested. Several factors were associated with infection, including age, race (particularly Black), male sex, and residence in urban areas with high AIDS rates. Fourteen counties in the United States had rates higher than five per 1,000, including New York (four counties), New Jersey (three), California (two), Maryland (specifically Baltimore and Montgomery counties), Colorado (one), Texas (one), and the District of Columbia.[7]

The first wave of mandatory testing among active duty army personnel in 1985 revealed a prevalence rate of 4.4 per thousand (0.44 percent), which was three times higher than the rate among military applicants. This higher rate was particularly evident among older soldiers (over age 30), Black and Hispanic soldiers, and unmarried enlisted men.[8]

Other branches of the military, including the United States Air Force, Marines, Navy, and the Public Health Service, also initiated testing in 1986 and found similar rates to the army. I was active duty U.S. Public Health Service at the time and had my first test in 1987.

My admiration for Dr. Edmund Tramont and the U.S. Army's handling of the emerging AIDS problem led me to join the infectious diseases staff at Walter Reed in 1989, where I cared for HIV-infected soldiers and their spouses for 17 years. Early identification of infection among military personnel allowed for preventive measures to reduce transmission to spouses and children, showcasing the importance of early diagnosis and intervention in HIV/AIDS management.

CDC AIDS Projections 1986–1991

In June 1986, the Public Health Service organized a meeting in West Virginia to revise their plan for AIDS prevention. At that point, there were 21,517 reported case-patients of AIDS in the United States, and it was estimated that 1–1.5 million Americans were infected with HIV. PHS projected that 20–30 percent of those infected would develop AIDS by 1991, and in that year alone, over 145,000 individuals with AIDS would require medical care, resulting in more than 50,000 deaths. Remarkably, these projections turned out to be quite accurate.[9]

However, Alexander Langmuir, the renowned epidemiologist and founder of the Epidemic Intelligence Service (EIS) and the CDC's chief epidemiologist from 1949 to 1970, expressed skepticism about the CDC's AIDS projections, considering them to be too high. Langmuir applied Farr's Law of Epidemics, dating back to 1840, to the reported annual incidence of AIDS case-patients in the United States from 1982 to 1987. He argued that the epidemic would peak in the U.S. in 1988 and then decline. Langmuir predicted that the total number of Americans with AIDS would reach about 200,000 by the year 2000. His argument was based on the assumption that inefficient female-to-male transmission of HIV would limit the epidemic, with only gay men and injecting drug users being most affected. The Reagan administration used Langmuir's work to justify limiting AIDS spending. However, AIDS case-patients continued to rise in the United States and worldwide throughout the 1980s and into the mid-1990s, ultimately contradicting Langmuir's predictions.[10]

Masters and Johnson: Heterosexual Crisis in America

Dr. William Masters and Virginia Johnson, renowned sex therapists, were the next to suggest an increasing heterosexual transmission of HIV. They conducted a two-stage, cross-sectional survey involving exclusively heterosexual men and women aged 21–40 in Atlanta, Los Angeles, New York City, and St. Louis. They reached out to around 10,000 individuals through word of mouth and distributed short questionnaires in various settings such as church groups, childbirth classes, singles bars, singles dances, and university campuses. Of those, 3,805 individuals completed screening questionnaires and provided contact information, with 2,042 being single, 1,326 married, and 437 cohabiting adults. Masters and Johnson selected two groups for further study.[11]

They defined "case-patients" as men or women who denied any homosexual activity or injection drug use and had had six or more heterosexual partners annually for the past five years. The comparison group consisted of individuals who claimed to have been in mutually monogamous relationships for the past five years. These subjects were invited to face-to-face interviews to confirm their sexual histories and undergo HIV antibody testing.

Masters and Johnson reported their findings from the first 50 men and 50 women in the four cities, totaling 800 individuals. Only one male out of the 400 control subjects tested positive. However, 14 (7 percent) women and 10 (5 percent) men in the more sexually active group tested positive. The highest rates were observed in NYC (9 percent), while the lowest were in St. Louis (3 percent). As a result, Masters and Johnson concluded that HIV was "now running rampant" in the heterosexual community. They called for routine HIV testing of all pregnant women, all individuals between the ages of 15 and 60 years hospitalized for any reason, convicted commercial sex workers, and marriage applicants.[12]

October 7, 1988, Journal of the American Medical Association

In the fall of 1985, Bob Edelman and I collaborated on a review of data related to AIDS among heterosexuals, with a specific focus on evidence for female-to-male transmission. We submitted this review to *JAMA* in December 1985. In our paper, we examined emerging data suggesting heterosexual transmission in various regions, including Africa, Haiti, and the United States. Several studies documented heterosexual promiscuity and sexual contact with female sex workers among Africans, Haitians, and Americans.[13]

In the States, the initial case-patients among heterosexuals were observed among injecting drug users, hemophiliacs, blood transfusion recipients, Haitian Americans, and female prostitutes. The subsequent groups affected were the spouses (both male and female sexual partners) and children of these high-risk patient groups. In our paper, we concluded unequivocally that heterosexual transmission of HIV occurs and can play a significant role in the spread of HIV infection and AIDS.

Our paper sparked controversy among the editors at *JAMA*. Typically, one receives a response from a journal within six to eight weeks, either accepting or rejecting the submission. However, we didn't hear back for over a year. In January 1987, *JAMA* provided us with four extensive reviews of our paper, ranging from suggestions that it be published immediately "as is" to claims that it was complete nonsense and should be rejected. We were given 30 days to respond, during which Bob Edelman and I revised the paper extensively and addressed each comment point by point. We received notice of acceptance just two weeks after resubmission.

Finally, on October 7, 1988, *JAMA* published our article titled "The epidemiology of AIDS among heterosexuals." The article garnered global attention, leading to its reprinting in the Southeast Asian version of *JAMA* and translations into Yugoslavian and Japanese. In the paper, we raised issues similar to those addressed by Masters and Johnson. We reviewed their work, as well as the Department of Defense's findings. Additionally, we discussed the case series of HIV infections within families of intravenous drug users, hemophiliacs, blood transfusion recipients, Haitian Americans, Caribbean Islanders, and Africans. We described HIV as a sexually transmitted infection capable of transmission between men, from men to women, from women to men, and even between women. Reports of transmission among lesbians had also been documented and were on the rise.[14]

We hoped that our review would convince those at the CDC, NIH and beyond, working on AIDS, of the inevitability of heterosexual transmission of HIV and AIDS in the United States and worldwide. We were confident that *JAMA* would publish our article by the spring of 1988. However, our paper faced further delays as it awaited a rebuttal by Dr. Hunter Handsfield, a member of the CDC's AIDS Advisory Board.

Dr. Handsfield, an infectious diseases expert at the University of Washington, Seattle, wrote a rebuttal to our article, which was published in the same issue of *JAMA*. He acknowledged that heterosexual transmission occurs but suggested that female-to-male transmission might be limited in industrialized nations. He cited a female-to-male ratio of 3.5 to 1 among heterosexual case-patients reported in the United States. He also mentioned reports from New York City indicating that only 0.05 percent of domestically acquired AIDS case-patients among adult males were attributed to heterosexual contact. Anatomical considerations led him to believe that transmission might be more efficient from men to women due to the retention of secretions in the vagina, as opposed to the penis.[15]

In response, Robert Edelman and I pointed out the challenging social consequences of HIV infection, primarily its apparent lengthy period of infectivity. Many individuals remained viremic for years after infection. With HIV's apparent presence in the heterosexual community, societies would need to grapple with difficult questions such as notifying sexual partners and assessing the suitability of infected individuals for marriage and natural parenthood.[16]

Premarital HIV Testing

During that period, obtaining a marriage license in 20 states required couples to take a blood test for syphilis and share the results with each other, and if positive, with their physician or the health department. Bob Edelman and I were among a small number of public health officials who suggested that states should also require HIV testing for individuals applying for marriage licenses. We believed that initiating proactive prevention programs among young couples could yield long-term benefits in slowing down HIV transmission.

Illinois and Louisiana were two states that implemented mandatory premarital HIV testing programs on January 1, 1988. However, these programs turned out to be unsuccessful. Louisiana repealed its testing program after just six months, and Illinois followed suit after 17 months. In Illinois, out of the 221,000 individuals who took marriage vows while the law was in effect, only 44 tested positive for HIV (2 per 10,000), at a cost of approximately $9 million. Additionally, both states experienced a 20 percent decrease in marriage license applications compared to previous years, with a corresponding increase in the number of applications in surrounding states where testing was not required.[17]

To assess the effectiveness of premarital HIV screening as an approach to AIDS prevention, the CDC conducted an evaluation of HIV antibody seroprevalence in marriage license applicants in selected areas across seven states (Alabama, California, Connecticut, Georgia, Mississippi, New Mexico, and Oklahoma). This was done by conducting blinded testing of blood samples routinely collected for syphilis serology. Among marriage applicants, there were 44 positive case-patients out of 24,561 tested (0.18 percent), which was nearly identical to the positivity rate among military applicants (0.15 percent). HIV positivity correlated with AIDS incidence and was higher among Blacks than whites. The CDC estimated an annual cost of $167 million if mandatory premarital screening were implemented, and it was believed to have a minimal impact on HIV prevention.[18]

HIV-1 Load Is Chief Predictor of Transmission

In the year 2000, we finally gained insight into the mechanics of HIV sexual transmission. Thomas Quinn and his team conducted a retrospective review of a community-based study involving 15,127 individuals in a rural district of Uganda. They followed 415 monogamous heterosexual couples in which one partner was HIV-positive and the other was HIV-negative at the start of the study. These couples were monitored for 2–3 years, with a focus on measuring behavioral and biological variables. Among these couples, the male partner was HIV-positive in 228 couples, and the female partner in 187 couples. During the study period, 90 spouses (22 percent) seroconverted, meaning they became HIV-positive. The rate of male-to-female transmission was found to be similar to female-to-male transmission. It was discovered that viral load, the quantity of HIV in the bloodstream, was the primary predictor of the risk for sexual transmission.[19]

In summary, sexually transmitted infections have long been a significant issue within the military. It comes as no surprise that our troops were among the earliest groups to acquire HIV through heterosexual transmission. This global health concern disproportionately affects various populations, including men who have sex with men, women engaged in sex work, users of illicit stimulant drugs, long-distance truck drivers, seafaring fishermen, international refugees, and deployed military personnel.[20]

15

HIV Therapy
HPA-23 to AZT

The U.S. government had taken a business-as-usual approach to AIDS treatment.... Under standard scientific procedures, the tests would be both controlled and double-blinded. Half the subjects would be given xxxx [insert any candidate drug] and the other half a placebo. To ensure that no one's expectations biased the results, neither doctor nor patient were allowed to know who was getting which. The protocol made scientific sense. The limitations on study participants ensured that untested drugs that might have serious side effects were not distributed willy-nilly to the population. Moreover, only through such controlled experiments could science really determine whether a drug actually did hold promise as an AIDS treatment.

The scientific principles, however, were difficult to explain to patients facing a death sentence.

—Randy Shilts, 1987[1]

In July 1984, now at NIAID, as I read through our AIDS portfolio, I was quite impressed with the number of grants and the quality of the science. I focused on the grants studying treatments for the opportunistic infections and the use of antiviral therapies.

I noted two serious problems. First, the majority of national experts and NIAID-funded researchers on *Pneumocystis carinii* pneumonia (PCP), candidiasis, cytomegalovirus, and other opportunistic infections were not in AIDS-affected regions, such as New York or California, but in Alabama, Pennsylvania, Tennessee, and Texas. This presented a challenge as many of the protocols provided experimental treatments to cancer patients and organ transplant recipients while specifically excluding AIDS patients. Meanwhile, physicians in New York City, San Francisco, and Los Angeles were desperately seeking help in caring for dying

AIDS patients. We needed to find a way to bring these various groups together.

I discussed the issue with Bob Edelman, and together, we devised a simple solution. We decided to contact all our investigators and urged them to expand their studies and include AIDS patients in their research. Initially, I was concerned that we might face resistance from some researchers, but to my surprise, our request was universally accepted. Moreover, we noticed that the outlying investigators, who were located in larger cities, were already starting to witness a surge in AIDS patients as the HIV infection continued to spread across the country.

However, the other serious problem was less amenable to rapid correction. None of the extramurally funded laboratories had yet grown HIV in their laboratories. I would find out later that our own NIAID intramural laboratories did not have access to the virus. At that time, only the Institut Pasteur, the National Cancer Institute, the Centers for Disease Control, and the University of California at San Francisco, an NCI-funded laboratory, had isolated HIV. The French were sharing their virus with anyone who requested it, but many laboratories were unable to grow it. The NCI was still very stingy with their virus.

Over the next few years, both NIAID-funded researchers and many non-funded clinicians worked on developing additional drugs to treat PCP, in addition to trimethoprim-sulfamethoxazole and intravenous pentamidine. These new drugs included aerosolized pentamidine, atovaquone, clindamycin/primaquine, dapsone, and trimetrexate.[2] However, it was discovered that none of these drugs could fully "cure" PCP; at best, they were equally effective or generally less effective than the standard treatments. Despite this limitation, they proved to be valuable options for patients who could not tolerate the standard therapies. For instance, around one-fourth of patients treated with trimethoprim-sulfamethoxazole experienced adverse events like leukopenia (low white blood cell counts), rash, and fever that were severe enough to require stopping the treatment and switching to an alternate agent.[3]

Given the high relapse rate among PCP patients who survived their initial episode, preventive measures were explored and found to be effective. The most successful prophylactic agent was found to be oral trimethoprim-sulfamethoxazole taken once daily, followed by once-monthly aerosolized pentamidine. Other agents, such as dapsone and atovaquone, were also recommended for PCP prophylaxis. Ultimately, it was advised that patients recovering from a PCP episode and those diagnosed with oral candidiasis could receive lifelong PCP prophylaxis. Temporary prophylaxis was suggested for individuals with HIV infection and persistent helper T-cell counts less than 200. While PCP prophylaxis did increase patient survival, the extension was only by a few months. It became evident that significant progress in AIDS survival would require the development of agents targeting HIV itself.[4]

In the summer of 1984, I initiated a retrospective review of therapy for *Toxoplasma* encephalitis (TE). To aid in study design and identifying potential participants, I sought the assistance of Dr. Jack Remington, a renowned expert on toxoplasmosis from Stanford University. After obtaining approval from the NIH research review board, I reached out to 157 clinicians via mail, inviting them to participate. Among them, 65 investigators had previously reported case-patients of TE to the CDC's AIDS surveillance database as of March 1984, while Dr. Remington identified 92 others as potential participants.[5]

In total, 68 biopsy-confirmed case-patients of *Toxoplasma* encephalitis were reported by investigators from 31 medical centers. Seven case-patients were excluded as they had received no therapy and were identified only during postmortem examination. All case-patients involved AIDS patients; no TE patients were reported among organ transplant recipients or cancer patients. The patients' median age was 36 years, ranging from 20 to 58 years, and they represented diverse risk groups, with 65 percent being gay men, 18 percent injecting drug users, 11 percent Haitian natives, and 6 percent from other risk categories. The patients were reported from 14 states, the District of Columbia, and Haiti, with New York State being the most common location (26 percent).[6]

Among the patients, 58 (95 percent) initially received pyrimethamine-sulfonamide combination therapy. By the time of the report, 49 (80 percent) of the patients had succumbed to the disease. The median time from the onset of therapy to death was 121 days (4 months). For the 20 percent still alive at the time of the report, the median time from onset of therapy to the date of the last known report was five months, with a range of one day to 17 months. Notably, this median survival time was similar to that observed in the PCP study. Patients who were "alert" at the start of therapy had significantly longer survival times compared to those described as "lethargic" or "stuporous." Among the patients discharged from the hospital, 17 experienced clinical relapse. Autopsies were conducted on 36 study patients, and *Toxoplasma* was found in brain tissue in 67 percent of them, despite antimicrobial therapy. These antimicrobials did not kill *Toxoplasma*, but held it in check at least temporarily.

Over 60 percent of the patients reported experiencing toxicity attributed to pyrimethamine-sulfonamide therapy, with many case-patients being attributed to pyrimethamine-induced folic acid depletion and bone marrow suppression. Common adverse events included leukopenia, rash, thrombocytopenia (low platelet count), and fever.

Four patients experienced Stevens-Johnson syndrome, a severe rash that required hospitalization.

Our conclusion was that improvements in survival would necessitate the development of new anti–*Toxoplasma* agents, strategies to reverse or prevent immunosuppression, or interventions to eliminate or block the effects of HIV.[7]

In the subsequent years, researchers found that prophylaxis was effective for most patients recovering from TE, but it only added a few weeks to survival. Lifelong trimethoprim-sulfamethoxazole, the same drug used for PCP prophylaxis, was recommended for patients diagnosed with TE and temporarily for all HIV-infected individuals with less than 100 CD4+ T cells. The addition of folinic acid to the regimen helped decrease medication-related bone marrow toxicity.[8]

We also discovered some new antimicrobials or new uses for medications approved for other infections that proved effective against other opportunistic infections associated with AIDS. Examples included clarithromycin, ethambutol, and rifabutin for *Mycobacterium avium-intracellulare*, acyclovir for herpes simplex virus, and ganciclovir for cytomegalovirus. While these agents reduced fever and alleviated some signs and symptoms of disease, they did not significantly extend survival times.

Even before we knew that HIV was the cause of AIDS, clinicians were experimenting with various antiviral and immunomodulating agents. However, agents like interferons, isoprinosine, peptide T, phosphonoformate, and ribavirin were tried but rapidly discarded. Real progress in AIDS treatment only occurred when we were able to find agents that directly targeted HIV.[9]

Antiretroviral Drugs

Dr. Willy Rozenbaum, an infectious diseases physician, played a crucial role in identifying the first AIDS patients in Paris. He provided clinical samples to virologists at the Institut Pasteur, which led to the discovery of lymphadenopathy-associated virus (LAV), later known as HIV (Chapter 5). Following the discovery of the virus, Rozenbaum approached Jean-Claude Chermann to inquire about treatments for retroviruses. Chermann suggested using a heavy metal called antimonium tungstate, also known as HPA-23, which had shown activity against a murine retrovirus in laboratory tests.

Willy Rozenbaum conducted initial treatment trials with intravenous HPA-23 on four patients, three with AIDS and one with an AIDS-related complex. He observed some temporary decrease in viral load and a slight increase in survival rates but did not observe any changes in CD4 T-cell counts.[10]

After these initial findings, Dominique Dormont decided to expand the treatment to more patients.[11] Some Americans traveled to France to participate in these French trials, including the well-known Hollywood actor Rock Hudson, who was diagnosed with Kaposi's sarcoma on his neck in June 1984. He was referred to Michael Gottlieb, UCLA, for treatment. Gottlieb attempted to obtain HPA-23 from the FDA in the United States but was informed that it was not available here. As a result, he referred Hudson to Willy Rozenbaum in France. Hudson received a short course of HPA-23 in the fall of 1984 and reported some success with the treatment.[12]

These early efforts represented significant steps in the search for AIDS treatments, as researchers and physicians around the world worked to understand the disease and explore potential therapies to combat the devastating impact of HIV.[13]

Sam Broder, an oncologist, played a significant role in advancing AIDS research by providing clinical samples from AIDS-related Kaposi's sarcoma patients he cared for at the NIH Clinical Center. He collaborated with Robert Gallo, who provided live virus to Hiroaki "Mitch" Mitsuya in Broder's lab. Mitsuya developed an anti–HIV screening assay known as ATH8, which utilized a cell line infected with human T-lymphotropic virus (HTLV-I). Through this assay, Mitsuya discovered that different HIV isolates grew best in specific types of tissue cultures, such as T cells or monocytes. Moreover, he found that certain potential therapies acted as inert chemicals and required activation (phosphorylation) within a cell to be effective. Furthermore, some drugs could be activated only in monocytes, while others worked exclusively in T cells. By skillfully manipulating this system, Mitsuya was able to identify the most promising combination of drug and cell type for testing for *in vitro* effect on HIV.[14]

One of the first drugs to show promise in Mitsuya's ATH8 assay system was suramin, a synthetic urea-based chemical developed in 1916. Suramin had been previously studied in animal models and used in Africa to treat onchocerciasis, a parasitic tropical disease also known as river blindness. Due to its prior approval for human testing by the FDA and an established dosing schedule in Africa, Sam Broder was eager to use suramin as a potential treatment for AIDS.[15]

On August 6, 1984, Bob Yarchoan, an immunologist working with Broder, administered the first dose of suramin (200 mg intravenously) to a patient with Kaposi's sarcoma at the NIH Clinical Center. Ten patients with AIDS or ARC were treated as outpatients, receiving an initial dose of 200 mg followed by six doses of one gram intravenously over five weeks. Remarkably, HIV levels decreased for each patient, and by the end of therapy, three patients had undetectable HIV levels. The side effects were generally mild to moderate in severity and included urinary abnormalities (9/10 patients), rash (7/10 patients), elevated liver enzymes (6/10 patients), and fever (5/10 patients). The authors of the study suggested that these results provided a rationale for further investigation of longer-term regimens of suramin or combination therapy with T-cell stimulating agents like interleukin-2. Unfortunately, first one patient, then a few others on long-term suramin developed adrenal necrosis, and the studies were terminated.[16]

Meanwhile, Rock Hudson returned to Hollywood after receiving HPA-23 treatment in Paris. Sadly, he experienced weight loss and cognitive decline, which fueled speculations about his health. In June 1985, he was diagnosed with AIDS-related lymphoma and went back to Paris for additional outpatient treatments with HPA-23.[17] On July 25, 1985, Hudson issued a press release confirming that he had AIDS and was in France for treatment. Tragically, he passed away on October 2, 1985, in Beverly Hills, California, at the age of 59.

Shortly after Hudson's death, Tony Fauci and James Hill, deputy director of NIAID, were summoned to the White House and criticized by President Reagan for what were perceived as insufficient efforts in treating HIV. At the meeting, Fauci presented the idea of establishing an AIDS Clinical Trials Group (ACTG). He proposed setting up ten clinical sites to evaluate antiretroviral drugs, with a total annual budget of $20 million.

Fauci sought advice from Bob Edelman on how to construct such a program, but he was dissatisfied with Edelman's response. Instead, he assigned John La Montagne, Ph.D., to create a separate division at NIAID solely focused on AIDS activities. Fauci then assembled a team, including me, to work with La Montagne in developing a joint NCI/NIAID program announcement to solicit applications by research teams across the United States to facilitate the development of AIDS treatments. This announcement, essentially a call for applications, was released on March 28, 1986.

In response to the announcement, 28 medical research centers submitted applications, and eventually, all of them were approved and funded to join the ACTG. This marked a significant step forward in the fight against HIV/AIDS, as the ACTG played a crucial role in conducting clinical trials to evaluate the safety and efficacy of antiretroviral drugs and other treatment approaches. The establishment of the ACTG was a pivotal moment in AIDS research and demonstrated a commitment to finding effective treatments for HIV/AIDS.

Among Dr. Fauci's numerous accomplishments in AIDS research, the ACTG stands out as perhaps the most significant and successful.

Food and Drug Administration (FDA) Drug Approval Process

The FDA is a crucial regulatory agency in the United States that is responsible for overseeing a wide range of products that have significant impacts on public health and consumer spending. It covers various items, including food products (excluding meat and poultry), human and animal drugs, blood and blood products, vaccines, medical devices, cosmetics, and animal feed. The FDA's role is to ensure the safety, efficacy, and quality of these products for the general population.[18]

The process of bringing a new drug to the market involves several phases:

Preclinical Testing: This phase involves testing the drug in laboratory settings, typically using test tubes and animal models. The goal is to establish the drug's activity against the targeted disease and its safety profile in animals. If the drug shows promising results and is reasonably safe, the FDA grants the sponsor an investigational new drug (IND) status, allowing them to proceed to human trials.

Phase 1: Initial studies in human volunteers are conducted to assess the drug's metabolism, pharmacologic actions, and safety. These studies usually involve a small number of participants, typically 10 to 20.

Phase 2: Larger studies are carried out to evaluate the drug's efficacy and safety in a larger patient population and determine an appropriate dosage. These studies usually involve 50 to 100 patients.

Phase 3: Principal studies are conducted to confirm the drug's efficacy, closely monitor its safety profile, and compare it to a placebo or commonly used treatments. These studies typically involve hundreds of patients and are generally conducted as randomized double-blinded protocols.

Once the Phase 3 studies are completed, the drug sponsor submits a new drug application (NDA) to the FDA for review. In 1985, the FDA required at least two studies demonstrating the drug's efficacy and safety before granting approval for market authorization. The FDA's review process itself could take up to three years to complete.

Phase 4: After the drug is approved and is being prescribed clinically, post-marketing studies, known as Phase 4 studies, are conducted to gather additional information about the drug. These studies help in discovering and evaluating unexpected or rare adverse reactions, drug-drug interactions, long-term benefits, and the optimal use of the drug in real-world settings.

The FDA's rigorous evaluation process ensures that drugs in clinical use are safe, effective, and of high quality, providing the public with access to medicines that have undergone thorough testing and scrutiny. The FDA also uses highly qualified advisory committees representing medical scientists, clinicians, statisticians, community members, and ethicists.[19]

AZT (Originally Azidothymidine, Now Known as Zidovudine)

AZT (azidothymidine) was discovered to have potent antiretroviral activity through research conducted by Wellcome Research Laboratories using a murine retroviral system. In February 1985, Mitch Mitsuya found similarly promising results with AZT in NCI's ATH8 assay system. Building on these findings, on July 3, 1985, Sam Broder and Bob Yarchoan administered the first intravenous doses of AZT to AIDS patients as part of an FDA-approved Phase 1 protocol. This study involved 23 volunteer patients at the NIH clinical center and 12 at Duke University Medical Center.[20]

During the study, AZT was found to be well absorbed when taken orally. Two-thirds of the patients showed increases in T-cell numbers, a positive outcome. However, the researchers also observed some serious adverse effects, including severe drops in red blood cell counts, headaches in about half of the patients, and tremors, confusion, and low white blood cell counts in one patient. Several patients developed bone marrow suppression and persistent low red blood cell counts after extended AZT therapy.[21]

In the fall of 1985, Burroughs Wellcome Company proceeded with a Phase 2 study of AZT, conducted as a double-blind, randomized, placebo-controlled trial. The study involved 282 patients with *Pneumocystis carinii* pneumonia (PCP) or advanced AIDS-related complex, and it took place in various U.S. cities. Patients were randomized to receive either 250 mg of AZT or a placebo every four hours for a total of 24 weeks.[22]

The study was terminated September 18, 1986, by an oversight committee due to the overwhelmingly positive response to AZT. Nineteen placebo recipients and one AZT recipient died during the study ($p < 0.01$). Newly diagnosed opportunistic infections were more common in the placebo group (45 subjects) compared to those receiving AZT (24 subjects).

AZT showed statistically significant benefits in terms of T-cell counts, skin anergy testing, and overall functional status (Karnofsky score).[23] When the study was halted, all patients who received the placebo were given the option to switch to AZT treatment.

Although AZT demonstrated significant efficacy, it also led to some serious adverse events, particularly bone marrow suppression. In 24 percent of AZT recipients, there was severe anemia with hemoglobin levels dropping below 7.5 grams per deciliter (normal range 13.2 to 16.6), compared to only 4 percent of placebo recipients ($p < 0.001$). Additionally, 21 percent of AZT recipients and 4 percent of placebo recipients required multiple red blood cell transfusions. Other side effects reported more frequently among AZT recipients included insomnia, nausea, neutropenia (low white blood cell counts), myalgia, and severe headaches.[24]

Word of these positive results spread rapidly within the NIH and the gay community. There was a high demand for AZT as everyone sought access to the promising drug. To address the scarcity of AZT and help provide it to patients across the United States, Tony Fauci and the FDA implemented a rarely used mechanism that allowed physicians who were not part of clinical trials to obtain AZT for their patients.[25]

Dr. Joan Drucker, an infectious diseases physician at Burroughs Wellcome Company, and I were tasked with implementing the delivery of AZT to clinicians. Physicians who wished to obtain the drug for their patients were required to provide necessary information to the NIAID to demonstrate that their patients met the entry criteria. I set up a board of three infectious diseases fellows at the Clinical Center to evaluate the applications on a daily basis. If an application was approved, I would inform Drucker's office in Durham, North Carolina, to release AZT to the patient's pharmacy. Physicians receiving the drug were responsible for providing follow-up data on the patients to Burroughs Wellcome, which would be collected by Dr. Drucker and submitted as supplementary material to the FDA.

In December 1986, Burroughs Wellcome submitted a new drug application (NDA) to market AZT, but there were no Phase 3 studies as required by the FDA for approval. This sparked debates within the FDA, as there were conflicting pressures. The FDA had its expectations for drug approval, but people were dying daily from AIDS, and AZT offered a glimmer of hope.

On March 19, 1987, just 20 months after the first administration of AZT to patients at the NIH, the FDA approved AZT for public sale by Burroughs Wellcome under the trade name Retrovir®. The recommended dosage was 200 mg taken five times daily.[26]

Sam Broder, Mitch Mitsuya, and Bob Yarchoan continued to make significant strides in the fight against HIV by identifying drugs that inhibited different loci of the reverse transcriptase enzyme. Dideoxycytidine (ddC) and dideoxyinosine (ddI) were the next two FDA-approved drugs in this category. These were rigorously tested within the newly established ACTG and compared directly to AZT, rather than using a placebo.

The real breakthrough came when combinations of these approved drugs were found to be more effective than individual drugs alone, leading to the development of treatment "cocktails." Eventually, markers like CD4 counts and viral load measurements became essential tools for evaluating the effectiveness of antiretroviral therapy. These trials marked a turning point in the treatment of HIV infection, significantly extending survival times by several years or even decades. These new combination therapies were termed highly active antiretroviral therapy (HAART).

However, it's crucial to acknowledge that these treatments have their drawbacks. They can be toxic and expensive, and once initiated, they typically must be continued for life. Furthermore, improper use can lead to the development of drug resistance, which underscores the importance of careful and responsible management of HIV treatment.

A New Strategy

The proposal by Anthony Fauci and Robert Redfield in 2019 introduced a new strategy to address the ongoing HIV/AIDS public health crisis. This initiative had four key pillars:

1. Early diagnosis: The goal was to diagnose all individuals with HIV as soon as possible after infection.
2. Effective treatment: Rapid and effective treatment was to be provided to achieve sustained viral suppression in those with HIV.
3. Prevention: Preventing at-risk individuals from acquiring HIV infection, including the use of pre-exposure prophylaxis (PREP).
4. Rapid response: Swift detection and response to emerging clusters of HIV infections to further reduce new transmissions, using the strategies outlined in the first three pillars.[27]

Pillar one, focusing on early diagnosis, posed challenges. Although the CDC had recommended routine HIV screening in healthcare settings since 2006, implementation was incomplete. A national survey conducted in 2016–2017 revealed that only 39 percent of respondents reported ever being tested for HIV.[28]

To address this, I suggest a novel screening approach, similar to the

Public Health Services measures for syphilis developed in the 1930s. This approach includes routine HIV testing at various healthcare encounters, such as clinic visits for sexually transmitted infections, complete physical examinations, emergency room visits related to illicit drug use, hospital admissions, and during pregnancy. Seropositive patients would be immediately referred to qualified healthcare providers for antiretroviral therapy and to the health department for investigation of the infection's source and subsequent sexual contacts.[29]

HIV/AIDS is suitable for routine screening due to its serious and treatable nature, long latency period, and the availability of effective treatment. Properly treated individuals living with HIV can expect a nearly normal lifespan. Pre- and post-exposure prophylaxis also offer additional strategies to reduce transmission. Identifying asymptomatic HIV-infected individuals can provide opportunities to share information to decrease transmission through various means, including sexual behavior, needle sharing, and blood donation.

Various medical diagnostic HIV tests are available with high sensitivity and specificity, making them suitable for routine screening. As of 2019, the recommended algorithm for diagnosing HIV infection starts with an HIV-1/2 antigen/antibody combination immunoassay, followed by confirmation with HIV-1/HIV-2 antibody differentiation immunoassay. Western blot testing is no longer recommended for confirmation.[30]

Transfer to the National Institute on Drug Abuse (NIDA)

While I was working with Joan Drucker on distributing AZT to clinicians before AZT was approved by the FDA, I received a call from Carl Leukefeld, D.S.W. (Doctor of Social Work), from the National Institute on Drug Abuse. He invited me to an interview at the Parklawn Building in Rockville, which was located just minutes from our home.

At the interview with Leukefeld and Roy Pickens, they told me that the Reagan administration was disappointed with their lack of progress dealing with AIDS and drug abuse. They wanted me to come help them develop a program on AIDS. It was quite flattering to hear that they had queried the resumes of all 5,500 commissioned officers of the Public Health Service and found that I was the only one with first-author publications in all three areas: AIDS, drug abuse, and infectious diseases.

I must admit, by that time, I was feeling disgruntled with my job at NIAID. I really enjoyed working with Bob Edelman and our weekly chats reviewing infectious diseases literature, as well as collaborating on a paper on the epidemiology of AIDS among heterosexuals. But John La Montagne had taken our office off-campus to the Kenwood area, significantly increasing my daily commute and preventing me from rounding at the Clinical Center. He also wanted me to oversee research projects instead of conducting them myself, and he even suggested withdrawing the Haverkos-Edelman paper on heterosexuals and AIDS, which was under review at the *Journal of the American Medical Association (JAMA)* (see Chapter 14). The final straw was when I was denied a position in his division to run the epidemiology section of the new AIDS program; instead, they hired a psychiatrist with multiple doctorate degrees.

Given these circumstances, I considered the offer from NIDA, realizing that it would isolate me from the infectious diseases world. I thought it might be a good opportunity to shorten my commute and learn about the epidemic of illicit drug abuse sweeping through the U.S. population and contributing so devastatingly to the transmission of HIV. I planned to stay for a year before seeking another job in infectious diseases.

I made the decision and transferred to the Clinical Medicine Branch at NIDA on December 1, 1986. As it turned out, my time at NIDA lasted over 11 years, during which I hope I made significant contributions to the fields of AIDS and drug abuse research.

16

What Causes Kaposi's Sarcoma?*

> *To begin, we need to define cause. We can define a cause of a specific disease event as an antecedent event, condition, or characteristic that was necessary for the occurrence of the disease at the moment it occurred, given that other conditions are fixed....*
>
> *For many people, the roots of early thinking persist and become manifest in attempts to find single causes as explanations for observed phenomena. But experience and reflection should easily persuade us that the cause of any effect must consist of a constellation of components that act in concert. A "sufficient cause," which means a complete causal mechanism, can be defined as a set of minimal conditions and events that invariably produce disease; "minimal" implies that all of the conditions or events are necessary. In disease etiology, the completion of a sufficient cause may be considered equivalent to the onset of disease.... For biologic effects, most or sometimes all of the components of a sufficient cause are unknown.*
> —Kenneth Rothman and Sander Greenland, 1998[1]

What is Kaposi's sarcoma (KS) and what role did this otherwise obscure cancer play in recognition of what would be named AIDS? What prompted its change from an indolent and rare sarcoma of elderly Mediterranean men to become an aggressive neoplasm killing substantial numbers of younger men? What causes KS?

I joined NIDA in December 1986. Within two weeks, an opportunity to reexplore the causes of Kaposi's sarcoma emerged. An urgent meeting

---

*Chapter 16 adapted from H.W. Haverkos, "Koch's postulates & Kaposi's sarcoma," *The Pharos* 82 (3) (Summer 2019): 17–23.

was called in response to a request from the U.S. Congress (Public Law 99–570, enacted on October 27, 1986). This bill's Section 4015 tasked Dr. Robert "Charles" Schuster, Ph.D., the director of NIDA, to conduct a study on alkyl nitrites (nitrite inhalants). The study aimed to determine: (1) how much and in what ways the public used alkyl nitrite products, (2) whether this usage aligned with the products' advertised purposes, and (3) the potential health risks and their nature associated with selling these products to the public. I volunteered to lead the organization of the study by assembling experts to create a comprehensive report for Congress.

As I worked on arrangements for the nitrite inhalant meeting, a significant article in the *New England Journal of Medicine*, published on January 8, 1987, had a profound impact on me. The study, led by Dr. Frank Polk from Johns Hopkins University School of Hygiene and Public Health and colleagues presented findings from the NIAID/NCI-funded Multicenter AIDS Cohort Study (MACS) (Chapter 13). This study followed a group of 1,835 HIV-positive men, with 59 of them developing AIDS within 18 months of follow-up, including 24 with Kaposi's sarcoma. Their analysis revealed that lower immunity, high levels of CMV infection, and a history of sexual contact with a person with AIDS were all independently linked to AIDS development. Interestingly, a separate analysis examining risk factors for Kaposi's sarcoma found no connection between nitrite usage and the disease. In fact, the 24 gay men with Kaposi's sarcoma reported using nitrites during sex less frequently than 120 matched controls.[2] The nitrite industry interpreted this study as evidence against my findings (Chapter 10) and even suggested that nitrite use could protect against Kaposi's sarcoma.

On March 31, 1987, NIDA sponsored a technical review titled "The Extent of Use and Health Hazards of Nitrite Inhalants." [Note: On this day, President Ronald Reagan and Premier Jacques Chirac signed an agreement to declare Bob Gallo and Luc Montagnier co-discoverers of the AIDS virus (Chapter 5)]. The technical review took place in Rockville, Maryland, and was attended by approximately 25 scientists. Key findings included various adverse effects associated with nitrite inhalation, such as skin and tracheobronchial irritations (especially around the nose and lips), burns resulting from accidental ignition, headaches, hypotension, cyanosis, methemoglobinemia, intoxication, and the development of habitual use patterns.[3]

Several presentations during the meeting delved into the pharmacologic mechanisms by which nitrites may be involved in the genesis of KS in individuals with AIDS, specifically examining carcinogenicity and immunosuppression. Additionally, I presented a review of our KS versus PCP study, and and found that nitrites emerged as the most significant variable in distinguishing between these two indicators of AIDS.[4]

16. What Causes Kaposi's Sarcoma?

I also examined the existing six epidemiologic studies that explored the relationship between nitrite use and KS in gay men. These studies yielded inconsistent results: three indicated a strong association between higher nitrite inhalant usage and KS, two did not confirm this association, and one, the MACS study, suggested that nitrite inhalant use had a protective effect against KS. I acknowledged the variability in these findings but also highlighted the challenges in interpreting questionnaire data, especially when dealing with small sample sizes, varying research methods, different study populations, and diverse survey questions.[5]

Let's examine one specific study among the mentioned studies—the MACS (Multicenter AIDS Cohort Study), which is described in much greater detail in Chapter 11. To recap, the study commenced in 1984 with the enrollment of 4,955 men who were subsequently followed up every six months. Of those, 1,835 were HIV-seropositive at the outset. During a median follow-up period of 15 months, 59 individuals developed AIDS, with 24 of them presenting with KS. Trained interviewers administered questionnaires to collect data.[6]

The MACS questionnaire specifically focused on nitrites and included eight items related to nitrite use within the past week, six months, and two years. Particular emphasis was placed on nitrite inhalant use during sexual activities in the previous six months and two years. It's worth noting that, unlike the CDC questionnaire, the MACS questionnaire did not consider reduced sexual and drug use during the prodromal period of disease, and it limited questions to nitrite inhalant usage within the two years prior, rather than over a lifetime.[7]

The results from the MACS study did not indicate any association between nitrite inhalant use and the development of KS. Instead, significant associations for KS were identified with factors such as decreased hemoglobin levels, decreased T-helper lymphocyte counts, and increased immunoglobulin levels. The authors of the study acknowledged that they inquired about nitrite use only within the two years preceding entry into the study and that they did not attempt to quantify this usage in their analysis. Consequently they suggested it was possible that they might have missed or obscured a meaningful association. They anticipated that future analyses, involving quantitative data on nitrite use from their study, would help resolve this issue.[8]

At the conclusion of the March 31, 1987, meeting, I requested that all ten presenters provide manuscripts of their findings, which were compiled into a NIDA monograph, specifically numbered as 83. This monograph was titled "Health Hazards of Nitrite Inhalants" and was printed in August 1988.[9]

During the meeting, I had the opportunity to meet Hank Wilson

(1947–2008), a dedicated LGBTQ rights activist from San Francisco and a long-term survivor of AIDS. In 1981, he initiated the Committee to Monitor Poppers, where he meticulously compiled extensive research on poppers. Wilson was a strong supporter of our research on nitrite inhalants and their associations with immunosuppression and KS. Over time, he became a friend and ally.

After the completion of NIDA Monograph 83, Hank Wilson took proactive steps by mailing a copy to all 535 members of the U.S. Congress. He also approached his own congressman, Mel Levine, a Democrat from California, to propose legislation aimed at banning poppers.

In response to reports of adverse events associated with the recreational use of nitrites, the U.S. Congress implemented a ban on the manufacture and retail sale of butyl nitrites, with exceptions for legitimate commercial purposes. This ban was enacted as part of the Anti-Drug Abuse Act (Public Law 100-690, Section 2404) on November 18, 1988. Notably, the law designated the Consumer Product Safety Commission, not the FDA, as the responsible authority for enforcing the ban.[10]

While I supported the ban on butyl nitrites, I was disappointed with the decision to exclude the FDA from the responsibility of enforcing the ban. When Congress sought input on the hazards of nitrites, the FDA argued that nitrite inhalants were not drugs and therefore should not be subject to their regulation. I found this argument to be questionable, given that amyl nitrite had been used for over a century to treat angina pectoris and for several decades as an antidote for cyanide poisoning.

However, I also understood the FDA's reluctance to get involved in another controversial area related to AIDS. The gay press, which heavily relied on advertisements for "poppers" (nitrites), portrayed the nitrite ban as an example of the government infringing on personal freedom. They published personal attacks on Hank Wilson and me for supporting the ban. Simultaneously, the FDA faced criticism for excluding all gay men from donating blood, approving the use of the drug AZT, which some considered toxic, and withholding access to other drugs of interest to gay activists, e.g., HPA-23, ribavirin, and interleukin-2.

In fact, on October 11, 1988, one month before the ban was signed by President Reagan, thousands of gay men stormed and occupied the FDA headquarters in the Parklawn Building in Rockville, Maryland, as a powerful demonstration of their concerns and frustrations regarding FDA policies and actions related to AIDS.

Following the ban, the rates of nitrite inhalant use among participants in the MACS study dropped significantly, from 66 percent in 1985 to 35 percent in 1989. It's important to note that this decline could also be attributed to the progression and increased rates of illness among this group.[11]

16. What Causes Kaposi's Sarcoma?

Age-adjusted Rates of Kaposi's sarcoma by Gender, 1973-2001

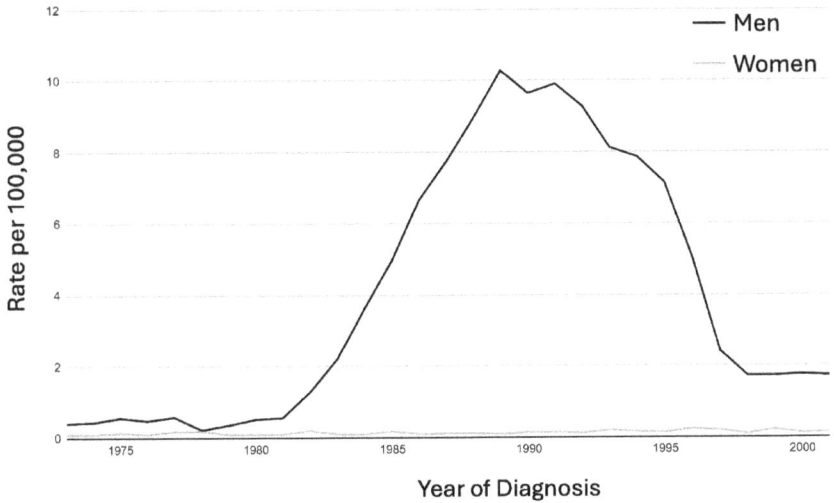

Source: SEER incidence and age-adjusted rates of Kaposi's sarcoma, nine registries, 1973-2001.
Reference: Haverkos HW. Viruses, chemicals and co-carcinogenesis. Oncogene 2004; 23:6492, Figure 1.

Incidence and age-adjusted rates of Kaposi's sarcoma, nine registries of SEER (Surveillance, Epidemiology and End-Results), 1973-2001 (National Cancer Institute, DCCPS, Surveillance Research Program, Cancer Statistics Branch. The data was released in April 2003, based on November 2002 submission. [Haverkos, H.W. "Viruses, chemicals and co-carcinogenesis." *Oncogene* 2004; 23: 6492-9.]).

Rates of KS among men reached a peak of 10.1 case-patients per 100,000 in 1989 and subsequently declined as shown in the "Age-adjusted Rates of Kaposi's sarcoma by Gender, 1973-2001" graph.[12] Of course, it's crucial to recognize that changes in KS incidence cannot be solely attributed to the nitrite ban, as the timing of the decline is influenced by the emergence of AZT and, later, the introduction of other antiretroviral therapies as part of treatment "cocktails."

To evade the clear intentions of the law, nitrite manufacturers resorted to marketing alternative alkyl congeners, such as isopropyl nitrite, by disguising them as "new and improved" room odorizers and "video head cleaners." This marketing approach often carried sexual undertones. In response, Congress made significant efforts to close this loophole by enacting Public Law 101-647, Section 3202, on November 29, 1990.[13]

Despite facing regulatory hurdles, the nitrite industry persisted in

Isopropyl Nitrite
$C_3H_7NO_2$

Cyclohexyl Nitrite
$C_6H_{11}NO_2$

Left: Chemical structure of isopropyl nitrite (C3H7NO2). *Right:* Chemical structure of cyclohexyl nitrite (C6H11NO2).

its quest to develop legal forms of inhalants, frequently promoting them as "safer" alternatives. They swiftly introduced cyclohexyl nitrite, characterized by a ring of carbons (instead of branched chains). This particular form of nitrite was deemed legal (as it did not fall under the category of alkyl nitrites) by the Consumer Product Safety Commission in 1992.[14]

In response to a decline in profits in the United States attributed to regulatory changes, nitrite manufacturers strategically rebranded their products. New names such as Bang, TNT, Buzz, Purple Haze, Liquid Gold, and RAVE were adopted, with a marketing emphasis on labeling them as "Room Odorisors" (please note the intentional misspelling of "Odorizers") or simply as "Aroma." Simultaneously, the nitrite industry redirected its focus toward aggressive marketing in regions such as the Caribbean, Europe, and Asia, where these products remained legally accessible.

The more popular brands within this market feature isopropyl nitrite as the primary ingredient. These products were manufactured in the United Kingdom, Australia, and other countries that had not implemented bans on nitrite inhalants.

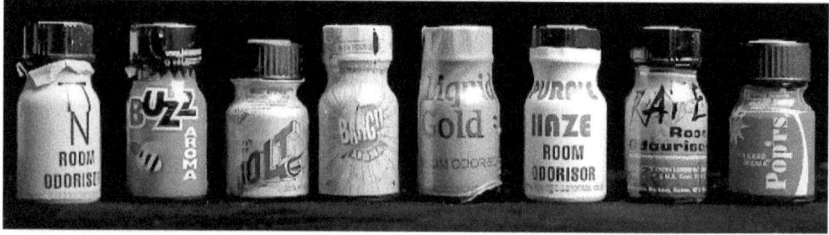

This image displays a range of "poppers" or nitrite inhalants currently available in the United Kingdom. Isopropyl nitrite is the main ingredient across the featured brands (UK Home Office, 2005, Wikipedia).

16. What Causes Kaposi's Sarcoma?

While I believed that I had unraveled the mystery surrounding AIDS-related KS, my colleagues at the CDC and NIH were less convinced. They continued to reference the Frank Polk study as evidence that nitrites were not a contributing factor to KS.[15]

However, in the early 1990s, the MACS updated its research on the relationship between nitrite inhalants and KS. By January 1993, 826 men had developed AIDS, with 316 of them also developing KS. Their baseline interview information was carefully analyzed, revealing several significant findings. The KS patients were predominantly from Los Angeles; reported higher usage of "recreational" drugs, particularly nitrite inhalants and hashish; engaged in more sexual activity based on various specific behaviors; and reported more instances of gonorrhea, hepatitis, herpesvirus infections, genital and anal warts, and scabies. A model combining these factors, including sexual activity, nitrite inhalant use, and having sexual partners from the West Coast, predicted the occurrence of KS. Nitrite inhalant use was reported by 284 out of 314 KS patients (90.5 percent) and 421 out of 508 non–KS AIDS patients (82.9 percent) in the two years prior to the baseline interview, with an odds ratio of 1.96, and confidence intervals of 1.27–3.04. The use of nitrites was one of several variables found to be significant in multivariate analysis.[16]

Following this updated report from the MACS supporting the role of nitrites in the development of AIDS-related KS, I approached Mr. Richard Millstein, the acting director of the National Institute on Drug Abuse, with a request to convene a second meeting to reevaluate the role of nitrites in the context of AIDS-related KS. NIDA sponsored a "Technical Review: Nitrite Inhalants" on May 23–24, 1994, in Gaithersburg, Maryland. Approximately 150 individuals attended, including scientists, gay activists, and members of the press. Participants included Robert Gallo, Harold Jaffe, Peter Duesberg, and Hank Wilson.[17]

The agenda included discussion of several key questions:

1. What is the epidemiology of nitrite use?
2. Do nitrites lead to increased risky sexual behavior and HIV transmission?
3. Do nitrites suppress the immune system?
4. Do nitrites act as a cofactor in Kaposi's sarcoma (KS)?
5. What further research is required to determine whether nitrite inhalants promote HIV risk behaviors and play a role in the natural history of HIV infection?

A lively discussion among the participants yielded four key recommendations:

1. Avoid the use of nitrite inhalants: It was advised that the public should steer clear of nitrite inhalants due to their adverse effects on health.
2. Foster further research: More research was deemed necessary to gain a deeper understanding of the role that nitrite inhalants play in the development of HIV disease. This would help clarify their impact on health.
3. Address media coverage and advertising: The meeting attendees recognized that media coverage and advertising, particularly in the gay press, did not align with current scientific knowledge regarding nitrites. As a result, there was a need for additional educational efforts to bridge this gap and ensure accurate information was disseminated.
4. Enhance enforcement: The Consumer Product Safety Commission was encouraged to take a more proactive role in enforcing the bans on the sale of alkyl nitrite inhalants. This would help limit public access to these substances.[18]

These recommendations reflected a concerted effort to address the concerns surrounding nitrite inhalant use and its potential implications for HIV disease, as well as the need for accurate information and enforcement of bans to protect public health.

I was elated by the outcomes of the meeting and believed that we were poised to make significant strides in unraveling the mysteries behind Kaposi's sarcoma. In 1994, I collaborated with Hank Wilson and other colleagues on a paper that explored the historical and epidemiological aspects of nitrite inhalant usage in the United States, as well as their potential contributions to AIDS.[19]

December 1, 1994, marked another day of challenge for me. Researchers Yuan Chang, Patrick Moore, and their team at Columbia University in New York unveiled a novel human herpesvirus known as KSHV (Kaposi's sarcoma herpesvirus) or HHV-8 (human herpesvirus type 8) through a technique called representational difference analysis. This method is used in biological research to identify genetic sequence disparities within viral DNA samples. Yuan Chang and Patrick Moore, who were a husband-wife duo, detected this virus in over 90 percent of Kaposi's sarcoma lesions, including those case-patients not linked to HIV—such as classical, endemic (African) and iatrogenic forms of the disease. Their findings were published in the December 1, 1994, issue of the journal *Science*.[20]

Harold Jaffe and Jim Curran celebrated their prediction and the discovery of a new sexually transmitted agent for Kaposi's sarcoma, a development they believed refuted the notion that nitrite inhalants were a causative factor. They viewed nitrite inhalants as merely an additional confounding variable. This turn of events left me as though I were back at square one in my research.

History of the Five Variants of Kaposi's Sarcoma

Let's explore the historical development of the five currently recognized epidemiologic variation settings of Kaposi's sarcoma:

Variant 1—Classic Kaposi's Sarcoma (Multiple Idiopathic Pigmented Hemangiosarcoma)

In 1866, a pivotal discovery in the realm of medicine was made by a Scottish medical student named T. Lauder Brunton (1844–1916). Brunton documented the vasodilatory effects resulting from inhaling amyl nitrite vapor. This discovery proved to be revolutionary as he introduced the novel use of amyl nitrite in the medical treatment of angina pectoris. Patients suffering from this condition experienced swift relief from chest pain, with discomfort often subsiding in less than a minute.[21]

Brunton's groundbreaking work quickly gained recognition among the medical community, establishing amyl nitrite as a potent solution for angina pectoris. Following his graduation from the University of Edinburgh in 1868, Brunton continued to hone his expertise through mentorship from esteemed physiologists at renowned European institutions. Notably, he spent a significant period of time at the University of Vienna, a location and era when Moritz Kaposi was initially treating patients afflicted by a novel dermatologic disorder.[22]

In 1872, Kaposi (1837–1902), of the University of Vienna, published a report that detailed five case-patients of an enigmatic condition known as idiopathic multiple pigmented sarcoma of the skin. The first case he documented involved a 68-year-old married master smith from Brodes in Lower Austria, identified as L.K. This patient had been admitted to the dermatological department on July 25, 1868, grappling with excruciating hand tension and severe foot swelling, which severely impaired his ability to stand and practice his trade. Among the striking observations was a palm-sized pigmented, dark gray, depressed area on his right instep, surrounded by firm brown-red to bright-red nodules. Similar nodules were scattered across his legs, hands, upper arms, chin, cheek, and upper lip, each varying in size, shape, and texture. Biopsies conducted on two of these nodules revealed microscopic evidence of a small cell sarcoma with inclusions, signs of minor hemorrhages, and extracellular yellow-brown to black pigment. Despite a two-month stay at the hospital, the nodules displayed minimal change, with only a few new lesions appearing on his thighs and upper arms. Filled with longing to be reunited with his loved ones, L.K. departed the hospital on September 22, marking the 60th day of his hospitalization.[23]

The second case of Kaposi's sarcoma involved a 66-year-old married distiller from Cracow. He was admitted to a medical facility on April 5, 1869, after enduring a 14-month battle with the disease. His condition was marked by distinctive coarse, nodular, violet-red infiltrations on his skin that were sensitive to touch. These troubling symptoms were notably present on his feet, upper extremities, and both eyelids.

Tragically, his health took a dire turn on May 12 when he developed severe bloody diarrhea and fever. Despite medical attention, he succumbed to the illness on May 21. A postmortem examination uncovered the pervasive nature of the disease, with extensive lesions detected throughout his gastrointestinal tract.[24]

What would review of those medical records indicate about preexisting medical conditions, i.e., heart disease, prior medications, travel history, sexual history, and more? If preserved blood samples were available for those patients, one could measure immune function, and test for antibodies to HHV-8 and HIV. If even tissue (biopsy) fragments or histopathology slides were available to science, one could today perform molecular marker studies or searches for HHV-8 genome fragments (e.g., via polymerase chain reaction).

Over one hundred years later, data regarding KS in the United States were accessible through the National Cancer Institute (NCI) and various case reports. The NCI's Surveillance, Epidemiology, and End Results (SEER) program conducted surveys in ten regions across the country, including the states of Connecticut, Hawaii, Iowa, New Mexico, and Utah and the cities of Atlanta, Detroit, New Orleans, San Francisco, and Seattle. These surveys aimed to track the incidence and outcomes of various cancers. The SEER program covered slightly over 10 percent of the entire U.S. population and offered a reasonably representative sample of the nation. Between 1973 and 1977, NCI reported approximately 30 case-patients of KS each year, with a male-to-female ratio of three to one.[25]

In 1981, researchers at Memorial Sloan Kettering Cancer Center in New York City shared their findings from treating 92 KS patients spanning the years from 1949 to 1975. Among these patients, 76 percent were men, and their average age was 63 years. Notably, over one-third of these KS patients also experienced at least one other primary malignancy during the study period. Many of these additional cancers were related to the lymphoreticular system, encompassing conditions like lymphosarcoma, reticular cell sarcoma, Hodgkin's disease, leukemia, other forms of lymphomas, and multiple myeloma.[26]

Bijan Safai, a dermatologist, and Robert Good, an immunologist, underscored that KS serves as an intriguing model for studying virus-associated malignancies. The unique geographical distribution and clustering of KS case-patients suggested potential involvement of genetic, environmental, and infectious factors.[27]

Variant 2—Endemic Kaposi's Sarcoma (Africa)

In 1914, a second form of Kaposi's sarcoma gained recognition in Africa, primarily affecting Black males between the ages of 25 and 40. The male-to-female ratio was remarkably 17 to one, and the clinical presentation varied widely. At one end of the spectrum were benign, nodular lesions that were confined to the extremities, while at the other end were florid, disseminated lesions. Survival after presentation ranged from three to ten years. Within this African form, a lymphadenopathic subvariant affected children at an average age of three years, with a male-to-female ratio of three to one.[28]

Italian medical scientist Gaetano Giraldo and his colleagues made significant observations in Uganda in the 1960s, 1970s and beyond. They used electron microscopy to identify herpes-type particles in five out of eight tissue culture cell lines obtained from KS patients.[29] During this period, five different human herpesviruses were already recognized: herpes simplex type 1 and 2, Epstein-Barr virus, varicella-zoster virus, and cytomegalovirus (CMV). Giraldo noted that nucleic acid segments from these KS tumors bore a resemblance to CMV.[30]

With the advent of the HIV antibody test, Jay Levy, Giraldo, and other researchers conducted tests on blood samples collected from 74 men and one woman with KS, including patients from Algeria, Cameroon, Senegal, Tunisia, Uganda, and Zaire during the years 1971–1974. The results were significant—all individuals tested negative for HIV.[31]

In 1994, a significant breakthrough in our understanding of the etiology of KS came to light with Chang and Moore's identification of a new human herpesvirus, HHV-8 (Human Herpesvirus 8). Furthermore, they detected this virus in sera from more than 90 percent of KS patients, irrespective of whether they had HIV infections.[32]

HHV-8 was found to be transmitted through various means, including sexual activity, kissing, and contact with saliva—similar to the transmission routes of other herpesviruses. The prevalence of HHV-8 antibodies was observed to increase with age, exhibit significant geographical variability, and depend on the specific detection assay employed.[33]

This discovery raises an intriguing question: Could HHV-8 be the herpesvirus that Gaetano Giraldo observed in KS tissues under electron microscopy in 1972, initially identifying it as cytomegalovirus (CMV)[34]? Upon reviewing Giraldo's papers from the 1970s and 1980s, it was noted that he reported high CMV antibody titers in KS patients but also high rates in control patients. This begs the question of whether these serologic results could potentially represent cross-reacting antibodies to HHV-8 or even co-infection.

The identification of HHV-8 as a key player in KS etiology opens up new avenues for understanding the complex interactions between viral infections and the development of this disease. Further research and exploration are necessary to unravel the intricacies of these viruses and their roles in Kaposi's sarcoma.

During this time, Dr. John Ziegler at University of California, San Francisco conducted important epidemiological studies involving both HIV-seropositive and HIV-seronegative KS patients in Uganda. His research led to a proposal that KS might result from the activation of latent HHV-8 by a combination of immune suppression and inflammation, ultimately triggering an oncogenic, or cancer-causing, lytic state in endothelial cells.

Dr. Ziegler's investigations extended to the unique environmental conditions in Uganda, particularly the practice of walking barefoot among volcanic soils. In this setting, chemicals such as iron oxides and aluminosilicates, possibly aided by abrasions from quartz particles, were believed to cause trauma and inflammation on the extremities. These environmental factors were thought to predispose individuals infected with HHV-8 to developing KS on their limbs.[35]

Dr. Ziegler's work highlighted the intricate interplay between viral infections, environmental factors, and the development of KS, shedding light on the multifaceted nature of this disease.

Variant 3—Iatrogenic Kaposi's Sarcoma

In the 1970s, oncologists observed an increase in the occurrence of KS among patients with compromised immune systems. These included individuals who were on graft-versus-host immunosuppressive therapy after renal transplant surgeries, patients on long-term corticosteroid treatments, and those whose immune systems were suppressed due to various therapeutic treatments for cancer. Notably, the male-to-female ratio for this iatrogenic form of KS was 2.3:1. Some case-patients even showed signs of improvement or resolution when immunosuppressive medications were discontinued.[36]

Fast-forward to 2003. During medical rounds at Walter Reed Army

Medical Center, a dermatology colleague shared three case reports of KS patients. Interestingly, these patients had developed KS lesions after initiating therapy with captopril or lisinopril, which are angiotensin-converting enzyme (ACE) inhibitors. What stood out was that when these medications were discontinued, the KS lesions either improved or completely disappeared.[37] It's worth noting that ACE inhibitors and nitrite inhalants both affect blood vessels and are used to lower blood pressure.

Variant 4—Epidemic (AIDS-related) Kaposi's Sarcoma

In the spring of 1981, Dr. Alvin Friedman-Kien and his colleagues met at a national dermatology meeting in California. They reported 26 case-patients of Kaposi's sarcoma to the CDC. Prior to 1980, there were roughly 300 new case-patients of KS annually in the United States, primarily among men aged 60 or older and renal transplant recipients. In elderly patients, KS typically manifested as persistent skin lesions and seldom led to fatalities. However, these 26 case-patients, all gay men, had skin lesions of KS confirmed by biopsy, but their disease followed a more aggressive course, spreading to the lungs, stomach, and intestines.[38]

In October 1981, the CDC conducted a national case-control study in Atlanta, Los Angeles, New York City, and San Francisco (Chapter 2). The study included 50 gay men with KS and/or *Pneumocystis* pneumonia, along with 120 controls identified at sexually transmitted diseases clinics or by private practitioners. Case-patients and controls were matched for age, race, and residence. The most significant variables identified in this study were the number of sexual partners and engaging in sexual activities at bathhouses. These findings suggested that a new sexually transmitted agent was the cause of the outbreak.[39]

In 1983, French investigators identified a new retrovirus as the cause of AIDS.[40] This virus was eventually named the human immunodeficiency virus (HIV).

Meanwhile, a national case-comparison study was conducted, combining interview and laboratory results from three studies conducted by the CDC. This study revealed that the most significant variable distinguishing gay men with KS or both KS and PCP from those with PCP alone was the lifetime use of nitrite inhalants.[41]

Variant 5—Kaposi's Sarcoma in Men Who Have Sex with Men but Without Evidence of HIV Infection

In 1985, the HIV antibody test became available, and researchers discovered that most gay men with KS were HIV-positive, though not all. The first report of an HIV-negative gay man with KS was reported in 1986.[42] In a separate report, Alvin Friedman-Kien and his colleagues at New York University documented six HIV-negative gay men with KS ranging in age from 32 to 62 years; five of the six reported using nitrite inhalants.[43] Additional instances of HIV-negative gay men with KS had been documented by others including Ethel Cesarman in New York.[44]

I believe this is a most important variant and should generate a number of research questions. For example, if immunosuppression is an important factor for the development of KS, what causes immunosuppression among HIV-negative gay men with KS? Could the immunosuppression result from various infectious agents and drugs of abuse employed by promiscuous gay men independent of HIV? Are there gay men with opportunistic infections who are not infected with HIV? Do these HIV-negative case-patients support the concept that cofactors alone could cause immunosuppression and AIDS-like diseases?

Table 1 provides an overview of the changing patterns of KS variants over time, encompassing various populations and clinical characteristics.[45]

Table 1

Variant, Year of First Report	Affected Population	Clinical Presentation	Immunocompromised
Classic or sporadic, 1872	Elderly men of Eastern European, Middle Eastern or Mediterranean origin	Typically localized to lower extremities. Mucosal and visceral disease are rare.	No
Endemic (African), 1914	Young Black males (15–40 years) and children in Africa—HIV-negative	Aggressive cutaneous lesions in adults, lymphadenopathic form in children	No
Iatrogenic, 1960s	Immunosuppressed individuals (e.g., post organ transplant)	Localized or widespread involvement	Yes
Epidemic (AIDS-related), 1981	Initially gay men in New York and California	Most common in head, face, neck, gastrointestinal tract, and lungs	Yes
Fifth form (HIV-negative), 1986	Gay men globally	Mainly cutaneous, with infrequent mucosal and visceral involvement	No

Hypothesis: Multifactorial Causes of Kaposi's Sarcoma

Over four decades of research into the causation of KS, I have formulated a multifactorial hypothesis regarding the five distinct variants of this disease as presented in Table 2.

Table 2. Multifactorial Causes of KS[46]

KS Variant	Herpesvirus	Factors Affecting Immune System Functions	Vasoactive Agents
Classic	HHV-8	Immunosenescence, concurrent primary cancers	Unknown (possibly amyl nitrite)
Endemic (African)	HHV-8	Environment factors (parasites, diet, herbs), drugs (antimalarials)	Aluminosilicates/ iron oxides (taken up by lymphatics)
Iatrogenic	HHV-8	Steroids, other immunosuppressants	ACE inhibitors
Epidemic (AIDS-related)	HHV-8	T-cell defect due to HIV infection	Nitrite inhalants
Fifth form	HHV-8	Unknown (possibly CMV and drug abuse)	Nitrite inhalants

ACE, angiotensin-converting enzyme; HHV, Human herpesvirus.

British investigators conducted an extensive study of 676 Kaposi's sarcoma (KS) patients who were referred to an HIV cancer center in Chelsea between 2000 and 2021. They analyzed demographic, clinical, pathological, virological, and immunological parameters and categorized the patients by KS variant, as detailed in Table 3.[47]

Table 3. Characteristics of KS Patients by Variant[48]

	Classic KS	Endemic KS	Iatrogenic KS	HIV+ KS	MSM KS	Total
Total	23	19	21	572	41	676
Sex						
Male	18	14	18	531	41	622 (92%)
Female	5	5	3	39	0	52 (7%)
Other	0	0	0	2	0	2 (1%)
Mean age	74	59	55	41	52	43
Range	39–88	15–78	22–73	16–75	31–84	16–88
Disease						
Skin only	21	15	11	429	39	515 (76%)
Advanced	2	4	10	143	2	161 (24%)
HHV						
Available	15	18	16	435	39	523 (77%)
Positive	7 (47%)	9 (50%)	7 (44%)	217 (50%)	11 (28%)	251 (48%)

	Classic KS	Endemic KS	Iatrogenic KS	HIV+ KS	MSM KS	Total
CD4 count						
Available	12	17	15	492	40	576 (85%)
Mean	637	688	543	261	814	317
CD8 count						
Available	12	17	15	505	40	578 (85%)
Mean	448	470	1214	884	439	839
CD4/CD8 ratio	1.4	1.5	0.4	0.3	1.0	0.4

Normal values: CD4 500–1200 cells/microliter; CD8 150–1000 cells/microliter; CD4/CD8 ratio > 1.0.

Based on these findings, Mark Openshaw and colleagues proposed reclassifying KS variants into two categories, considering the presence or absence of immunosuppression, particularly abnormal CD4/CD8 ratios.[49] While this proposal has merit, I advocate for a more comprehensive evaluation of the entire immune system before declaring patients immunocompetent. Additionally, gathering more information about potential cofactors in KS pathogenesis, such as the use of ACE inhibitors and nitrite inhalants, remains crucial.

To explore the multifactorial causes of KS further, I recommend that investigators expand their research on KS and collect data on potential cofactors in KS etiology, such as concurrent cancers, immunosuppressive medications, ACE inhibitors, and nitrite inhalants. For those interested in revisiting the etiology of KS, establishing active KS surveillance and conducting case-comparison studies of the various KS forms would be beneficial.

Steps for Establishing Active Surveillance for KS

1. Identify a project manager.
    Find a dedicated project manager, such as a dermatology fellow, a young attending dermatologist, or an epidemiologist who is enthusiastic about KS research and committed to publishing results.
2. Develop a case definition.
    Create a clear case definition for KS, including a specific time frame of reference. This will ensure consistency in identifying and categorizing case-patients.
3. Establish surveillance systems.

Active surveillance:

- Identify and engage well-connected dermatologists, such as those associated with medical schools.
- Develop a protocol and a standardized report form.
- Contact these dermatologists via phone, email, or mail, inviting them to participate.

Passive surveillance:

- Promote passive reporting by distributing flyers at national dermatology meetings and publishing notices in dermatology journals.
- Encourage dermatology colleagues to voluntarily report KS case-patients they encounter.

4. Create a comprehensive Case Report Form (CRF).

- Design a detailed case report form (CRF) to gather essential data, including age, race/ethnicity, gender, sexual orientation, country of birth, current residence, immunologic status, concurrent cancers, HIV status, HHV-8 status, ACE inhibitor use, and nitrite inhalant use.
- Recognize that many respondents will not have answers to every question. However, including these questions in the CRF will raise awareness among clinicians about potential connections and encourage them to gather such information from future patients.
- Provide guidance on how to inquire about factors like nitrite inhalants, which can be unfamiliar to some clinicians due to changing product contents and labeling.

5. Perform descriptive epidemiology.

- Analyze data to create a descriptive epidemiological profile by organizing information by time, place, and person.
- Identify trends, patterns, and correlations within the data.
- Consider further epidemiologic studies to explore similarities and differences among various forms of KS.

Conclusion

The findings suggest that Kaposi's sarcoma (KS) results from a complex interplay of factors, with HHV-8 infection at its core. However, the specific factors contributing to KS development will vary across regions and populations.

In North America and Europe, AIDS-related KS appears to be the result of intricate interactions between HHV-8, HIV, and nitrite inhalant abuse, emphasizing the need for a comprehensive understanding and development of prevention strategies.

In contrast, in Africa, HHV-8 infection may be reactivated by environmental factors found in the soil, such as aluminosilicates and iron oxides. Parasitic infections, dietary factors, the use of antimalarials, and coexisting HIV infection may also exacerbate the disease. Additionally, anecdotal evidence suggests that ACE inhibitors may play a role in activating HHV-8 among classical KS patients, renal transplant recipients, and other immunosuppressed individuals carrying the virus.

For investigators focusing on KS in gay men, particularly the fifth form, it is crucial to consider the potential impact of nitrite inhalant abuse. This consideration is especially important given the evolving nature of "poppers," with new formulations including isopropyl and cyclohexyl nitrites and their deceptive marketing as room odorizers and "aromas."

Given these intricate interactions and multifaceted factors, it is time to move beyond Koch's postulates that attribute HHV-8 as the sole causative agent of KS. Instead, embracing Kenneth Rothman's theory of sufficient causation will provide a more comprehensive framework for understanding the disease. This approach acknowledges that HHV-8 may be necessary, but it is not sufficient to cause KS, and multiple contributing factors should be considered.

17

Paradigm Shift
From Koch's Postulates to Rothman's Sufficient Causal Theory

> *The research worker is a solver of puzzles, not a tester of paradigms.... Like the chess player ... he tries out various alternate moves in the search for a solution. These trial attempts, whether by the chess player or by the scientist, are trials only of themselves, not of the rules of the game. They are possible only so long as the paradigm is taken for granted. Therefore, paradigm-testing occurs only after persistent failure to solve a noteworthy puzzle has given rise to crisis. And even then it occurs only after the sense of crisis has evoked an alternate candidate for paradigm.*
> —Thomas S. Kuhn, 1962[1]

In January 1998, I transitioned from NIDA to join the FDA's Center for Drug Evaluation and Research, specifically the division of antiviral drug products, as a medical reviewer. My role included contributing to the approval of drugs targeting herpesviruses and HIV. I concentrated on antiretroviral drugs like efavirenz and nevirapine, both crucial inhibitors of HIV's reverse transcriptase enzyme.

In 2006, I retired from the Public Health Service and took an associate professor position at the Uniformed Services University of the Health Sciences (USU) in Bethesda, Maryland. There I taught various courses, with a notable focus on "Classic Studies in Epidemiology," exploring the history of medicine and disease causation paradigms.

Paradigm 1. Koch's Postulates
—Single Infectious Agent, Single Disease

In the 19th century, visionaries like John Snow, Ignaz Semmelweis, and Louis Pasteur advanced the germ theory of disease causation. Jacob

Henle and Robert Koch established crucial criteria for proving a microbe's role in disease:

1. The microorganism must be abundant in all afflicted organisms.
2. It should be isolated from the diseased host and cultivated in pure culture.
3. Introducing the microorganism into a healthy organism should cause disease.
4. The microorganism must be re-isolated from the newly diseased host, matching the initially inoculated agent.

Anthrax

Robert Koch (1843–1910) employed his postulates to definitively establish the causative agents of diseases like anthrax, cholera, diphtheria, and tuberculosis. Let's delve into his proof of spore-forming bacteria as the cause of anthrax.

Koch's method involved a meticulous step-by-step process to distinguish causation from mere association. To confirm the link, he removed parasites from the host, isolated them from any potential disease-inducing tissues, and introduced these isolated parasites into a healthy animal, reproducing the disease's unique characteristics.

For instance, in anthrax, Koch observed colorless, non-motile rod-like structures in the blood of infected animals. Initially considered lifeless crystalline formations, these structures were later seen to grow, produce spores, and regenerate into rods, suggesting a connection to lower plants. Injecting small blood samples containing these rods into healthy animals consistently induced anthrax, although it couldn't conclusively prove the rods as the sole disease agents due to the presence of other blood components.

To definitively establish anthrax bacilli as the sole cause, Koch isolated them from the blood through serial cultivation. After several passages, the pure bacilli, when injected into healthy animals, unequivocally induced fatal anthrax, mirroring the disease's natural occurrence. This groundbreaking work solidified the connection between anthrax bacilli and the disease itself.[2]

Cholera

In 1854, a deadly cholera epidemic swept through London's Soho district, claiming 530 lives in just ten days. Driven by curiosity and armed with a death list from the registrar, John Snow (1813–1858) began a meticulous investigation. His findings revealed a stark pattern: most deaths clustered around the Broad Street water pump. Those closer to other pumps still preferred Broad Street water, except the workhouse residents, who remained largely unscathed. Equally curious was that no Broad Street brewery workers fell ill, as they favored malt liquor over the pump water.

Suspecting the Broad Street pump, Snow's initial examination found limited impurities, leading to uncertainty. But as he delved deeper, fluctuations in visible organic matter emerged, including small white particles. Microscopic analysis confirmed the presence of disorganized particles, likely from decomposed matter, and oval animalcules, signaling organic contamination. Mr. Eley, a Broad Street resident, noted the water's foul odor and taste after storage, aligning with sewage contamination. Presenting these findings to the St. James parish board led to the pump's handle removal on September 8, halting the outbreak.[3]

In 1854, Filippo Pacini identified the cholera bacterium, describing it as a disease causing fluid and electrolyte loss. His work, however, went unnoticed.[4]

In 1884, Robert Koch pinpointed the comma-shaped cholera bacillus. Although he successfully cultured *Vibrio cholera*, his attempts to induce infection in animals fell short of his postulates. Max von Pettenkofer's self-inoculation experiment, where he and others ingested the bacterium, fulfilled Koch's criteria.[5]

Using similar methods, Koch proved bacterial causes for diphtheria and tuberculosis. The "single agent, single disease" concept shaped infectious disease and microbiology sciences, leading to disease prevention and control. Antibiotics and vaccines further reduced infectious disease incidence and mortality.

Does HIV Satisfy Koch's Postulates for AIDS?

In my view, HIV does not fully align with Koch's postulates when it comes to causing AIDS. HIV is a necessary component but is not adequate on its own to induce AIDS, as defined by the presence of Kaposi's sarcoma and/or opportunistic infections.

One of the initial challenges in applying Koch's postulates to viruses, including HIV, is their inability to grow in pure culture. Unlike many bacteria that can be cultivated in pure culture through serial passage, most viruses are reliant on host cells and cannot be isolated independently.

However, if we consider the transfer of cell-dependent HIV, we can partially meet the third and fourth Koch's postulates, as illustrated by the case of two patients identified by Michael Gottlieb in 1984 (Chapter 5). In this instance, a 24-year-old gay man who later developed PCP donated blood to a 38-year-old female blood transfusion recipient, who subsequently developed PCP one year later.[6]

In this case, both the donor and the recipient exhibited PCP as their AIDS manifestation. However, I am not aware of any blood donor-recipient pairs in which both individuals developed KS. This observation raises the question of whether there are additional factors at play that explain the various manifestations of AIDS. I firmly believe that HIV is responsible for the immunosuppression observed in AIDS, but it alone does not suffice to cause AIDS as evidenced by the presence of PCP, toxoplasmosis, or KS as distinct manifestations.

Transitional Period in Public Health

From the early 1900s to the mid–20th century, public health underwent a significant transformation. Initially, communicable diseases like pneumonia, tuberculosis, and gastrointestinal infections were the leading causes of death in the United States, constituting a substantial portion of mortality (Appendix C).

Mortality trends fluctuated, with infectious disease–related deaths declining from 1900 to 1917 but surging during the 1918–1919 influenza

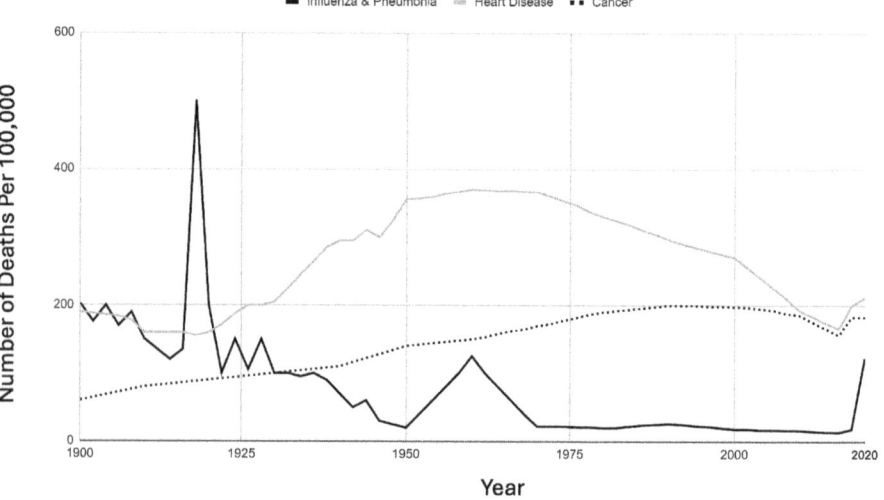

Mortality attributed to influenza/pneumonia, heart disease, and cancer (number of deaths per 100,000) USA, 1900–2020. Data for the year 2020 also includes COVID-19 deaths in addition to influenza/pneumonia (Centers for Disease Control and Prevention).

pandemic. After World War I, there was a sustained reduction in infectious disease-related mortality (Figure 1).

Medical breakthroughs in the 1940s, including antibiotics like penicillin and sulfa drugs, along with vaccines, further reduced morbidity and mortality from infectious agents. This led to increased life expectancy, rising from 48.2 years in 1900 to 67.2 years in 1950.

By 1950, noncommunicable diseases like heart diseases, cancer, and cerebrovascular diseases became the predominant causes of death, posing new challenges for public health. These conditions required different approaches to understanding causation.

Robert Koch's postulates, used for infectious diseases, proved inadequate for noncommunicable diseases like myocardial infarction, stroke, cancer, diabetes mellitus, and schizophrenia. Consequently, new theories and methodologies were developed to investigate and address these complex diseases, marking a crucial shift in public health priorities toward chronic disease understanding and prevention.

Paradigm 2. Sir A. Bradford Hill Criteria— Single Noninfectious Cause, Multiple Diseases

In 1965, Sir Bradford Hill (1897–1991) suggested nine criteria to distinguish association from causation, focusing his evaluation on cigarette smoking and lung cancer.[7]

1. Strength of association
2. Consistency
3. Specificity
4. Temporality
5. Biological gradient
6. Plausibility
7. Coherence
8. Experiment
9. Analogy

Smoking Tobacco and Lung Cancer

In the 1920s, concerns arose regarding cigarette smoking and its potential connection to cancer. Thomas Edison, the famous American inventor, was one of the early voices suggesting this link. Some of Edison's employees, exposed to high levels of benzene while working on rubber production in Florida, developed leukemia. Edison's defense argued that many of these men were heavy cigarette smokers, leading to his legal victory. However, subsequent research confirmed the link between benzene exposure and leukemia, dispelling doubts about its harmful effects. This historical episode highlights the complex relationship between smoking, occupational hazards, and evolving health knowledge in the early 20th century.

In the early 1900s, as lung cancer rates rose, two hypotheses emerged. Miasma (bad air) was considered due to increased air pollution with the rise of automobiles. Concurrently, cigarette smoking surged, especially after soldiers were given cigarettes during World War I.

To investigate the smoking–lung cancer link, Richard Doll (1912–2005) and Sir A. Bradford Hill (1897–1991) conducted key studies. The first began in 1947, comparing the smoking habits of 1,357 male and 108 female lung cancer patients with age- and sex-matched hospitalized controls. Astonishingly, 99.5 percent of male case-patients and 95.5 percent of controls smoked, revealing an overall smoking rate of over 95 percent. The odds of smoking among case-patients were 9.1 times as high as the odds of smoking among controls.

Examining daily cigarette consumption before illness onset, we find a dose-response pattern for males and females. The more cigarettes smoked daily, the higher the odds of lung cancer, demonstrating a clear link.[8]

Table 2. Amount of Cigarettes Smoked Daily Before Onset of Lung Cancer Case-patients and Matched Controls, Men, 1948–1952[9]

Daily Number of Cigarettes	Number of Case-patients	Number of Controls	Odds Ratio
0	7	61	Referent
1–14	565	706	7.0
15–24	445	406	9.5
25+	340	182	16.3
All smokers	1,350	1,296	9.1
Total	1,357	1,357	

Table 3. Amount of Cigarettes Smoked Daily Before Onset of Lung Cancer Case-patients and Matched Controls, Women, 1948–1952[10]

Daily Number of Cigarettes	Number of Case-patients	Number of Controls	Odds Ratio
0	40	59	Referent
1–14	44	40	1.6
15–24	12	8	2.2
25+	12	1	17.7

Daily Number of Cigarettes	Number of Case-patients	Number of Controls	Odds Ratio
All smokers	68	49	2.0
Total	108	108	

Richard Doll and Bradford Hill's second study focused on 59,600 physicians listed in a national medical registry in England and Wales as of October 1951. The questionnaire they received inquired about their smoking habits, including the quantity, method, and when they started and stopped smoking. Those who had not smoked at least one cigarette a day for over a year were classified as nonsmokers.[11]

About 68 percent of the physicians responded to the questionnaires, a response rate considered good, but not ideal. A response rate exceeding 80 percent was expected.

From November 1951 to October 1961, lung cancer occurrences were documented through death certificates and medical records. Among the 4,597 deaths in the cohort, 153 male physicians had confirmed lung cancer diagnoses. Data on the number of cigarettes smoked were available for 136 of them.[12]

Table 4. Number and Rate (per 1,000 person-years) of Lung Cancer Deaths by Number of Cigarettes Smoked Per Day, 1951–1961[13]

Daily Number of Cigarettes Smoked	Deaths from Lung Cancer	Person-years at Risk	Mortality Rate per 1000 Person-years	Rate Ratio	Rate Difference Per 1000 Person-years
0	3	42,800	0.07	Referent	Referent
1–14	22	38,600	0.57	8.1	0.50
15–24	54	38,900	1.39	19.8	1.32
25+	57	25,100	2.27	32.4	2.20
All smokers	133	102,600	1.30	18.6	1.23
Total	136	145,400	0.94	13.4	0.87

The population attributable risk percent, indicating the proportion of deaths attributed to smoking, stands at 92.5 percent. In simpler terms, 92.5 percent of all lung cancer deaths among male physicians in Great Britain are directly linked to cigarette smoking. This study significantly reinforces the association between smoking and lung cancer.[14]

Determining causation for noninfectious diseases involves careful evaluation, and in 1965, Sir Bradford Hill presented nine criteria to distinguish association from causation, focusing on the relationship between cigarette smoking and lung cancer.[15]

1. Strength of Association: The death rate from lung cancer in cigarette smokers is 9–10 times higher than in nonsmokers, with heavy smokers facing rates 20–30 times higher.
2. Consistency: The Surgeon General of the U.S. Public Health Service identified the smoking-lung cancer association in 29 retrospective and seven prospective studies.[16]
3. Specificity: While lung cancer death rates are higher in smokers, the association is not specific; smokers also exhibit higher death rates for various other diseases like cardiovascular disease, gastric bleeding, tuberculosis, and different cancers.
4. Temporality: Cigarette smoking typically precedes lung cancer development by several decades in most case-patients.
5. Biological Gradient: Lung cancer death rates increase linearly with the number of cigarettes smoked daily.
6. Plausibility: While biological plausibility is helpful, it shouldn't be a strict requirement, as it depends on the available biological knowledge.
7. Coherence: The temporal rise in both cigarette smoking and lung cancer over the last few decades, along with sex-specific mortality patterns and the effects on the lungs, align with general knowledge.
8. Experiment: Those who quit smoking have lower lung cancer death rates compared to those who continue to smoke, supporting a causal link.
9. Analogy: Examples like scrotal cancer in chimney sweeps exposed to soot or birth defects in those exposed to thalidomide illustrate the analogy criterion.[17]

Bradford Hill's criteria have been widely used to establish causation in various contexts, including occupational exposures and lifestyle factors like alcohol consumption, for a range of chronic diseases. They offer valuable guidance when investigating the complex relationships between single causes and multiple diseases, as outlined in the 1965 paper.[18]

Paradigm 3. Kenneth Rothman—Sufficient-Component Causation Theory—Multifactorial Cause of Chronic (Noncommunicable) Diseases

In 1976, Kenneth Rothman introduced the sufficient-component causal model, aiming to bridge theoretical causation concepts with epidemiological practice. In this model, a sufficient cause comprises all necessary factors to inevitably induce disease. Component causes contribute to completing a sufficient cause, and a necessary cause is a component cause present in every sufficient cause. Synergy denotes factors with a combined effect greater than their individual impacts.[19]

Rothman's idea that multiple risk factors, not a single agent, drive chronic diseases was exemplified by the Framingham Study of heart disease. Since 1920, heart disease has consistently ranked as the leading cause of death among Americans, surpassing infectious diseases (see Figure 1).

FDR and Coronary Heart Disease

Franklin Delano Roosevelt (FDR), the unique figure in U.S. history who was elected as president four times, abruptly died in 1945 during his fourth term, bringing attention to the inadequate understanding of cardiovascular disease prevailing at the time. This significant incident served as a catalyst for the inception of the Framingham Heart Study, a groundbreaking research initiative aimed at unraveling the mysteries surrounding heart-related conditions and contributing to advancements in cardiovascular health knowledge.[20]

During his 1932 campaign, FDR's blood pressure measured 140/100 mm Hg (mercury). From 1935 to 1941, his blood pressure escalated from 136/78 to 188/105 mm Hg. His physician asserted that the president's health was sound, attributing his elevated blood pressure to his age.

In March 1944, FDR was admitted to Bethesda Naval Hospital due to breathlessness, sweating, and abdominal distension. A cardiologist observed signs of heart trouble, including cyanosis and a chest X-ray indicating an enlarged heart. The diagnosis was hypertension, hypertensive heart disease, and heart failure. Treatment involved digitalis and salt reduction but proved ineffective, with his blood pressure surging to 240/130 mm Hg a month later.

In February 1945, during the Yalta Conference, Lord Charles Moran, Winston Churchill's physician, noted FDR's deteriorating condition, suspecting arterial hardening and giving him only a few months to live. On April 12, 1945, at age 63, FDR succumbed to cerebral hemorrhage with a blood pressure reading of 300/190 mm Hg.[21]

In response, President Harry Truman signed the National Heart Act on June 16, 1948. This act recognized heart and circulatory diseases, including high blood pressure, as grave threats to the nation's health. It allocated a $500,000 grant for a 20-year epidemiological study on heart disease, marking a pivotal moment in the pursuit of cardiovascular health knowledge in the United States.[22]

The Framingham Study

Framingham, a self-contained town 20 miles west of Boston with a population of 28,000 (10,000 aged 30–59), became the focal point for the groundbreaking Framingham Heart Study. The aim was to enroll 5,000 individuals without coronary heart disease (CHD) at the outset and follow them every two years for two decades. Local health officials identified a committee of community leaders, offering them a clinic examination to understand enrollment procedures. This committee then reached out to 6,507 randomly selected residents for clinic visits, with two-thirds responding. In addition, 740 volunteers were actively sought. This formed the Framingham Study Group, totaling 5,127 participants free of CHD (2,845 women and 2,282 men).

Each participant underwent an extensive medical history review, lifestyle assessment, and thorough physical examination by at least two physicians. Various laboratory tests were performed, including chest X-rays, electrocardiograms, and blood sample analyses. The data were shared with participants' personal physicians. Those initially free of CHD were reexamined every two years for two decades, even if they relocated, with comparable examinations arranged. In case-patients of death, efforts were made to determine the cause, particularly related to cardiac disease, often involving autopsies.

The New York Heart Association criteria were used to identify CHD outcomes, encompassing myocardial infarction, angina pectoris, coronary occlusion, myocardial fibrosis, and possible myocardial infarction, as determined by clinical evidence and ECG changes.[23]

After the initial follow-up cycle, 65 men and 32 women developed new CHD, with 18 men and 2 women succumbing to it. Myocardial infarction was the predominant diagnosis among men (30 case-patients), while angina pectoris was more common among women (24 case-patients).[24]

For men aged 45–62, factors associated with new CHD included high blood pressure (above 160/95 mm Hg), high cholesterol (over 260 mg percent), left ventricular hypertrophy on ECG, and a weight gain of 30 percent or more since age 25.[25]

In 1961, William Kannel introduced the term "risk factor" and emphasized that there is no single essential or sufficient cause for cardiovascular disease (CVD). Instead, CVD risk factors encompass increased age, hypertension, hyperlipidemia, cigarette smoking, and diabetes mellitus.[26]

Statistical Methods: Multivariate Analysis

Jeanne Truett, a statistician at the National Heart Institute, devised a multivariate analysis to explore the impact of numerous variables on CHD risk in the Framingham study. This approach, similar to the one used in AIDS research among gay men, examined seven risk factors initially measured during exams:

1. Age (years)
2. Serum cholesterol (mg/100ml)
3. Systolic blood pressure (mm Hg)
4. Relative weight (100 × actual weight divided by median for sex-height group)
5. Hemoglobin (g/100 ml)
6. Cigarettes per day (coded as 0 = never smoked, 1 = less than a pack per day, 2 = one pack per day, 3 = more than a pack per day)
7. ECG (electrocardiogram, coded as 0 = normal, 1 = definite or possible left ventricular hypertrophy, definite nonspecific abnormality, and intraventricular block).

At the 12-year follow-up, the most influential risk factors for CHD, aside from age, included high cholesterol, increased cigarette smoking, ECG abnormalities, and hypertension. Relative weight also played a role but to a lesser extent.[27]

Table 5. Linear Discriminant Function Coefficients (Standard Units) of Risk Factors for CHD at 12 Years Follow-up[28]

Risk Factors	Coronary Heart Disease Men	Coronary Heart Disease Women
Age	0.5934 (1)	0.6259 (1)
Cholesterol	0.4444 (2)	0.2844 (4)
Cigarettes smoked	0.4192 (3)	0.0625 (6)
Systolic blood pressure	0.3334 (4)	0.5556 (2)
ECG abnormality	0.2626 (5)	0.3048 (3)
Relative Weight	0.1890 (6)	0.0975 (5)
Hemoglobin	-0.1050	0.0392 (7)

(x) Rank order
 - = Insufficient data

Over time, the Framingham research team expanded their analysis by incorporating additional variables such as diabetes mellitus and proteinuria (Table 7).[29] These coefficients gauge the strength of the relationships between risk factors and cardiovascular events. Larger values indicate more robust associations, while some factors like heart rate and proteinuria failed to attain statistical significance at p < 0.05.

Table 6. Coefficients for Regression of Specified Cardiovascular Events on Cardiovascular Risk Factors for Men and Women, Ages 45–74, in the Framingham Study, Over 20-year Follow-up[30]

Risk Factors	Cardiovascular Disease Men	Cardiovascular Disease Women
Hypertension	0.414 (1)	0.509 (1)
Serum Cholesterol	0.236 (2)	0.255 (2)
ECG-LVH	0.222 (3)	0.219 (3)
Cigarettes	0.198 (4)	0.029 *
Diabetes	0.160 (5)	0.192 (5)
Relative Weight	0.156 (6)	0.219 (3)
Heart Rate	0.144 (7)	0.058 *
Proteinuria	0.090 (8)	0.062 *
Vital Capacity	-0.0179	-0.330

These numbers represent the strength of the relationships between the risk factor and cardiovascular events. The higher the number, the stronger the relationship.
(x) = rank order
*Not statistically significant at p < 0.05.
- = Insufficient data

In essence, this meticulous examination of risk factors in the Framingham study highlighted the complex interplay of variables contributing to CHD development. It emphasized the significance of age, high cholesterol, smoking habits, ECG abnormalities, and hypertension as critical factors. As research evolved, the inclusion of additional variables further enriched our understanding of cardiovascular health, paving the way for more effective preventive strategies and treatments.[31]

Armed with knowledge about the risk factors for cardiovascular disease, researchers embarked on a mission to alter behaviors, formulate medications to lower blood pressure and cholesterol levels, and pioneer innovative surgical techniques to address blocked coronary arteries.

From 1980 through 2000, the age-adjusted death rates for coronary heart disease witnessed a remarkable reduction, plummeting from 540 to 270 deaths per 100,000 population for men and from 260 to 130 deaths for women. This significant decline can be attributed to a combination of factors. Approximately 47 percent of this decrease was credited to medical or

17. Paradigm Shift

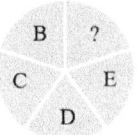

Sufficient Cause 1
72 year-old Female

Sufficient Cause 2
65 year-old Male

Sufficient Cause 3
55 year-old Male

A = Hypertension; B = High Cholesterol; C = Cigarette Smoking; D = Diabetes
E = Electrocardiogram - Left Ventricular Hypertrophy; ? = Unidentified Factors

Causal pies to demonstrate multifactorial causes of cardiovascular disease (Colleen Brauer/Harry Haverkos).

surgical treatments, including resuscitation in both community and hospital settings; the utilization of medical treatments such as aspirin, heparin, beta-blockers, ACE inhibitors, and statins; and surgical interventions like angioplasty and coronary artery bypass grafting (CABG). Nearly 44 percent of the decrease was linked to modifications in risk factors, which involved reductions in total cholesterol levels and systolic blood pressure, a decline in smoking prevalence, and more physical activity. However, it's worth noting that these achievements were somewhat offset by rising rates of obesity and diabetes.[32]

In a broader context, the overall life expectancy in the United States surged from 67.2 years in 1950 to an impressive 77.0 years by 2020. A significant portion of this increased longevity can be attributed to advancements in the prevention and treatment of coronary heart diseases. The groundbreaking Framingham study played a pivotal role in revealing the multifactorial nature of heart disease and identifying key areas for intervention within the disease process.

As we look to the future, strategies for preventing coronary heart disease must adopt a comprehensive approach. This approach should aim to maximize the reach of effective treatments while actively promoting population-based prevention through the reduction of risk factors.[33]

New Paradigm to Consider—Multifactorial Causes of Infectious Diseases—a Modification of Rothman's Sufficient-component Causal Theory

The question of what causes AIDS is a complex and multifaceted one, and there have been various hypotheses proposed over time. The four hypotheses mentioned by Harold Jaffe (Chapter 2) are as follows:

A. Cytomegalovirus
B. An environmental toxin, most likely nitrite inhalants
C. Immune overload due to multiple infections and immunosuppressant drugs
D. A new virus

I propose an additional answer:

E. All of the above

Cytomegalovirus as a component cause of immune suppression and AIDS?

In 1981, Cytomegalovirus (CMV) was considered a potential cause of AIDS. In a national case-control study:

1. Antibodies to CMV were detected in 100 percent of AIDS case-patients and 98 percent of controls.
2. Cytomegalovirus complement fixation titers were significantly higher in case-patients compared to controls.
3. CMV was found in 25 percent of case-patients and 9 percent of controls in cultures of urine and throat swabs ($p < 0.05$).
4. DNA restriction endonuclease studies, used to "fingerprint" each CMV isolate, were conducted on 20 samples isolated in cell culture (10 from patients and 10 from controls). Each of the 20 isolates had distinct restriction endonuclease patterns with no matches.[34]

In the study comparing Kaposi's sarcoma (KS) and *Pneumocystis* pneumonia (PCP) patients:

1. Serologic evidence for CMV infection was found in 100 percent of both KS and PCP patients.
2. CMV was cultured in 50 percent of PCP patients and 21 percent of KS patients.[35]

While there was no evidence of a unique or "new" CMV strain suggesting it as a necessary cause of AIDS, there was enough evidence to suggest that CMV played a role in AIDS as a component cause. This involvement occurred through its impact on the immune system and its potential to cause life-threatening opportunistic infections among AIDS patients.[36]

Nitrite Inhalants as a Component Cause of Immunosuppression, KS and AIDS

Let's begin by revisiting the results of two key studies: the original case-control study (Chapter 4) and the KS vs. PCP study (Chapter 10).

Table 7. Significant Variables Associated with AIDS in 50 Gay Men, Selected by Linear Logistic Regression Analysis

Variable	Rank* Grouped Factor	Rank* Ungrouped Factor	Rank* Individual Variables
Number of male sexual partners per year	1	1	1
Proportion of sex partners from bathhouses in past year	1	3	–
Syphilis previously	2	–	2
Non–B hepatitis previously	2	–	5
Italian, Jewish, or Eastern European ancestry	3	3	2
Drugs for enteric parasites	3	–	2
Sperm exposure and rectal trauma score	3	3	–
Feces exposure score	3	–	4
Number of different "street" drugs used	4	4	–
Lifetime nitrite use	4	–	–
Age at initiating regular sex with men	–	2	2
Ever married	–	2	5

*Highest rank variables are most strongly associated with illness. Dash indicates that the variable was not selected.[37]

The final epidemiological results revealed that the variables most strongly associated with AIDS were those related to the number of male sexual partners and meeting those partners in bathhouses, indicating a potential sexually transmitted agent. However, nitrite inhalant use was also statistically significantly associated with AIDS on multivariate analysis.[38]

Let's look again the multivariate results of the KS vs. PCP study (Chapter 10):

Table 8. Significant Variables Associated with KS Versus PCP Among 87 Gay Men, as Selected by Linear Logistic Regression Analysis and Ranked by Level of Statistical Significance[39]

KS vs. PCP	Both vs. PCP	Both vs. KS
Nitrite inhalant use	Nitrite inhalant use	No variables selected
Receptive anal intercourse	Income	
Income		
Bathhouse partners		
Marijuana use		
Unlabeled nitrite use		

We interpreted these results as saying that nitrite inhalant use was a causative agent for KS in combination with HIV. Let's look at the Bradford Hill criteria to determine a potential role for nitrite inhalants and KS.

1. Strength of Association: Gay men with KS inhaled about twice as many nitrites compared to those with opportunistic infections, as observed in several studies.[40]
2. Consistency: Among 12 studies comparing gay men with KS and those with opportunistic infections, four found a strong association between extensive nitrite use and KS, one found a weak association, six found no association, and one initially suggested a protective effect of nitrites for KS but later reversed this finding. This variation in outcomes reflects differences in study design, sample size, timing, quality of interviews, and laboratory studies. More research is needed for clarification.[41]
3. Specificity: Nitrite inhalants are uniquely linked to Kaposi's sarcoma, with no other known associations with cancer.
4. Temporality: The discovery of the relief of angina pectoris with amyl nitrite dates back to 1866 when a Scottish medical student made this breakthrough. Interestingly, two years later, Dr. T. Lauder Brunton was a visiting physician at the University of Vienna, where he coincidentally shared the wards with Dr. Moritz Kaposi. Dr. Kaposi was tending to and diagnosing the first patients afflicted with a multi-pigmented hemangiosarcoma.[42] Fast forward to the 1980s, a notable surge in Kaposi's sarcoma case-patients occurred among gay men who were frequent users of "poppers" or nitrite inhalants.[43]
5. Biological Gradient: Studies linking nitrite use to KS show a biological gradient where the rate of KS among gay men increases with greater use of nitrite inhalants.
6. Plausibility: Nitrites have been shown to be carcinogenic in

laboratory tests (Ames test) and affect blood vessels, which are the site of hemangiosarcoma. The occurrence of AIDS-related KS on body areas heavily exposed to nitrite vapors, such as the face, head, and nose, further supports this plausibility.
7. Coherence: Among patients with AIDS, gay men are more likely to use nitrite inhalants compared to intravenous drug users, Haitians, and hemophiliacs, and they have the highest rates of KS.
8. Experiment: The decline in nitrite inhalant use following their prohibition in 1989, as observed in the MACS, coincided with a decline in the rates of KS.
9. Analogy: Other nitrogen-containing compounds, such as nitrosamines, are known to cause cancer.

Moreover, it's worth noting that nitrites are also recognized for their capacity to induce immunosuppression. In a study conducted by the intramural component of the National Institute on Drug Abuse (NIDA), 18 male volunteers were exposed to three inhalations of amyl nitrite for either three or 18 consecutive days. Blood samples were collected immediately after the final inhalation and then at intervals of 1, 4, and 7 days afterward. The analysis of these samples revealed a modest decrease in T-lymphocyte counts and a reduction in natural killer cell activity, both of which gradually returned to baseline levels several days after the last inhalation.[44] This immunosuppressive effect has also been observed in animal studies by other researchers.[45]

By applying the Bradford Hill criteria, it becomes evident that nitrite inhalant use may play a significant role in the development of KS.

Multifactorial Causes of Immunosuppression in AIDS and Carcinogenicity in KS

The utilization of multivariate analysis in the national case-control study was particularly impressive, as it offered a systematic approach to evaluate a wide range of variables distinguishing case-patients from controls among gay men. Instead of seeking the most significant single variable, I now believe there is an alternative interpretation of these results. The data strongly suggest a multifactorial cause for the immunosuppression that characterizes AIDS.

This implies that a combination of factors, such as infectious agents (like syphilis and hepatitis C viral infections), environmental toxins (including antibiotics for GI infections, nitrite inhalants, and "street drugs"), and genetic factors (such as Eastern European, Italian, and Jewish ancestry), collectively strain the immune system. Alternatively, they may intensify the immunosuppressive effect of HIV infection. Subsequently, the introduction of other infectious agents such as *Pneumocystis carinii*, *Toxoplasma gondii*, and Human herpesvirus type 8 (HHV-8) manifests clinically as opportunistic infections and cancers (refer to Table 3).[46]

Similarly, one can interpret the multivariate results of the KS vs. PCP study as indicating that KS results from immunosuppression caused by HIV and carcinogenicity induced by other factors, including nitrite inhalants, additional infectious agents, and possibly marijuana use. The association of increased income with the development of KS raises intriguing possibilities, such as the ability to purchase more drugs and have increased opportunities for travel, which can enhance the pool of sexual partners and exposure to various infectious agents.[47]

These alternative interpretations highlight the complexity of the disease and recognize that multiple factors may contribute to the development and progression of AIDS. This underscores the importance of considering a comprehensive range of variables and not solely focusing on a single causal factor, such as HIV.

Two New Viruses Associated with KS and AIDS

Back in 1983, French investigators made a significant discovery. They identified a new retrovirus, later named HIV, which was later confirmed as a direct cause of AIDS by three American research groups.[48] While HIV is responsible for the immunosuppression observed in AIDS, it doesn't solely determine the specific disease manifestations like KS, PCP, or CNS toxoplasmosis. In simpler terms, according to Rothman's perspective, HIV is a necessary but not a sufficient factor for causing AIDS. HIV plays a crucial role as a component cause in the development of KS.

Fast forward to 1994, when researchers at Columbia University in New York made another groundbreaking discovery. They identified a new herpesvirus, known as Kaposi's sarcoma herpesvirus (KSHV) or Human herpesvirus type 8 (HHV-8).[49] This virus was found in all forms of Kaposi's sarcoma and is transmitted, like other herpesviruses, through mucosal-mucosal contact, such as kissing and sexual behavior. However, how HHV-8 causes KS is a conundrum.[50] HHV-8 is a necessary factor for the development of KS and is a contributing factor or component cause of AIDS.

In summary, I am of the opinion that we have made significant strides in unraveling the intricate puzzle of AIDS. The next crucial step

17. Paradigm Shift

is to develop strategies for deconstructing each component of this puzzle, thereby enabling us to both prevent and treat individuals afflicted by this devastating disease. Moreover, the knowledge we've gained from this research serves as a valuable blueprint that we can employ in our efforts to decipher the mysteries surrounding other infectious diseases, cancers, autoimmune disorders, and various other medical conditions.

18

Multifactorial Causes of Infectious and Chronic Diseases

> *The etiology of cancers appears to be complex and multifactorial. Peyton Rous and others demonstrated the process of co-carcinogenesis by exposing rabbits to a virus and tars. Epidemiologists have proposed virus-chemical interactions to cause several cancers. For example, one might propose that the etiology of cervical cancer results from a complex interplay between oncogenic viruses and cervical tar exposures through tar-based vaginal douching, cigarette smoking, and/or long-term cooking in poorly ventilated kitchens. Hepatocellular carcinoma may result from the joint effects of viruses and hepatotoxic chemical carcinogens. Kaposi's sarcoma might happen following reciprocal actions of human herpesvirus-8 infection, immunosuppression, and chemical exposures, such as nitrite radicals and alumino-silicates. Use of Koch's postulates will not help one prove or disprove a multifactorial causation of disease; new criteria are needed. Delineating the web of causation may lead to additional strategies for prevention and treatment of several cancers.*
>
> —Harry Haverkos, 2004[1]

In April 1989, I approached Dr. Kellogg Hunt, a pulmonary specialist and chief of internal medicine at Walter Reed Army Medical Center, about joining their infectious diseases staff. He referred me to Ed Tramont (Chapter 14), and I began caring for HIV-infected soldiers one morning a week for the next 17 years.

In August 1989, Roy Pickens, Ph.D., my boss at NIDA, was called to the Addiction Research Center in Baltimore to address an ethical issue involving the improper administration of cocaine to research subjects without informed consent. Pickens asked me to manage the division of clinical research and act as AIDS coordinator during his absence, roles I would fulfill for over five years.

Amid this busy period, two family emergencies led me to investigate the causes of cervical cancer and type 1 diabetes mellitus.

Squamous Cell Cervical Cancer

In June 1991, my 66-year-old mother was diagnosed with squamous cell cervical cancer, the size of a tennis ball, presenting with vaginal bleeding. Despite undergoing surgery and radiation therapy, she succumbed to metastatic disease in December 1994. What causes cervical cancer?

My mother's cervical cancer journey had a lengthy and remorseful history. Born in Ohio in 1924, she and her twin sister married on the same day in 1948. At 37, after their final Papanicolaou (Pap) tests, my aunt tested positive and underwent a hysterectomy. Although my mother tested negative, she never returned for further screening. Diagnosed with invasive cervical cancer at 66, she passed away at 70, while her twin lived to 93. The lack of awareness about my mother's medical history hindered my encouragement for regular exams.

Cervical cancer ranks as the fourth most common life-threatening cancer among women globally, following breast, colon, and lung cancers. However, it is the leading cause of cancer mortality among women in sub–Saharan Africa and Central America. Papanicolaou cervical screening, introduced in the 1950s, has contributed to mortality declines in the United States and other developed nations.

In 1842, an Italian surgeon noted elevated uterine cancer rates among married and widowed women compared to Catholic nuns and virgins.[2] Subsequently, epidemiologists linked sexual behaviors, such as age at first intercourse, commercial sex work, and giving birth, to cervical cancer deaths, suggesting a sexually transmitted agent.

In the 1970s and 1980s, German physician Harald zur Hausen identified human papillomavirus types 16 and 18 (HPV-16 and HPV-18) in cervical cancers. Although HPV didn't fulfill Koch's postulates, zur Hausen proposed that synergistic actions with initiators like herpes simplex type 2 or factors like cigarette smoking could induce cancer.[3]

Cigarette Smoke as a Cofactor for Cervical Cancer

Dr. Warren Winkelstein, M.D. (Chapter 13) established a connection between cigarette smoke and cervical cancer. Utilizing data from the

1973 Surveillance, Epidemiology, and End Results (SEER) study, he noted a direct correlation (Pearson's coefficient of +0.60) between the incidence rates of cervical cancer and male lung cancer across nine U.S. communities. These included metropolitan Atlanta, Birmingham, Dallas–Ft. Worth, Detroit, Minneapolis–St. Paul, Pittsburgh, San Francisco–Oakland, and the states of Colorado and Iowa.[4]

In the 1960s, the surgeon general confirmed the causal link between cigarette smoking and lung cancer. Winkelstein, intrigued, investigated the potential connection to cervical cancer. Analyzing rates of cigarette smoking among women with cervical cancer and controls from 33 studies, 26 supported his hypothesis. Critiquing seven negative studies, he identified biases and highlighted the fulfillment of Bradford Hill criteria, including a dose-response relationship and temporal association. Winkelstein concluded that cervical cancer should be recognized as tobacco smoking-related.[5]

In 1995, I transitioned to NIDA's intramural program in Baltimore. There, I collaborated with Wallace Pickworth, Ph.D., a tobacco researcher, to update Winkelstein's studies. We examined 72 epidemiologic studies worldwide, revealing a crude odds ratio of 2.13 for current smokers.[6] Our ecologic study found a direct correlation between cervical cancer and male lung cancer in U.S. states but an unexpected negative result globally.[7]

In 2002, the International Agency for Research on Cancer affirmed the association between smoking and invasive cervical cancer, citing over 150 studies. Tobacco smoke, with about 6,000 compounds including carcinogens like benzyl pyrenes and nitrosamines, was implicated. Researchers challenging HPV-infected cell lines with benzo[a]pyrene demonstrated biological plausibility.[8]

In essence, Winkelstein's pioneering work laid the foundation for recognizing smoking as a risk factor for cervical cancer, further supported by laboratory studies linking tobacco smoke compounds to HPV-induced DNA damage.[9]

Smoking and Squamous Cell Cervical Carcinomas Versus Adenocarcinomas

A notable observation is that while cigarette smoking may correlate with squamous cell cancer, it is not implicated in the development of adenocarcinomas, underscoring the dissimilarity in risk factors for these two forms of uterine cervical cancers. A meta-analysis of 12 case-control studies, involving 8,097 women with invasive squamous cell carcinomas, 1,374 women with invasive adenocarcinomas, and 26,445 control women, revealed that a higher lifetime number of sexual partners, earlier age of first sexual experience, increased number of births, and extended use of oral contraceptives were associated with both histological types of cancer.[10]

However, the analysis showed a distinctive pattern concerning cigarette smoking. Current smoking was linked to an increased risk of squamous cell cancer (odds ratio = 1.47, 95 percent CI 1.15–1.88) but not adenocarcinomas (OR = 0.82, 0.60–1.11).[11]

Examining HPV-DNA presence, the meta-analysis found that 94 percent of squamous cell cancers, 85 percent of adenocarcinomas, and 16 percent of controls exhibited HPV-DNA of any genotype. Notably, HPV-16 and/or HPV-18 were prevalent in 74 percent of squamous cell cancers, 78 percent of adenocarcinomas, and 8 percent of controls. This suggests a strong association of HPV with both types of uterine cervical cancers. However, the data implies that tar-based factors may be linked to squamous cell cancers but not adenocarcinomas of the cervix.[12]

The Crucial Link—Wood-Burning Stoves

World Health Organization investigators conducted a study comparing lifestyle factors in 99 Honduran women with cervical cancer and 199 matched controls. HPV infection showed a strong association with cervical cancer (OR = 7.66, 95 percent CI 3.88–15.1). Among HPV-positive women, significant relationships were found for age at first intercourse, education, and unexpectedly, exposure to woodsmoke. Women with 25–34 years of woodsmoke exposure had an OR of 3.67 (95 percent CI 1.48, 9.09), and for those with over 35 years, the OR was 6.35 (2.10, 19.29). Case-patients had more frequent and prolonged woodsmoke exposure than controls (Chi-squared = 14.66, p = 0.00001), indicating a dose-response. No differences in cigarette smoking were observed.[13]

If cigarette smoke is a cervical cancer cofactor, why not woodsmoke? Indoor air pollution from woodsmoke contains a similar chemical spectrum as cigarette smoking. Approximately three billion people, half the global population, rely on wood, coal, crop residues, or dung for cooking and heating. In a second ecologic study, solid fuel use was directly correlated with cervical cancer rates worldwide (Pearson correlation coefficient = 0.498, p < 0.001).[14] Regions with high cervical cancer rates, like Africa and Central/South America, also have high rates of solid fuel use. The shift from solid fuels to natural gas and electricity in developed nations may explain Brinton's observation of declining cervical cancer rates with increasing cigarette smoking.

- Cervical cancer death rates also declined with widespread Pap smear use. George Papanicolaou (1883–1962) introduced a screening strategy in 1941, implemented in the United States and Europe in the 1950s. U.S. Preventive Services Task Force guidelines recommend screening women aged 21–65 every three years with cytology. Pap testing may be discontinued in women over 65 with adequate prior screening and no other high-risk factors for cervical cancer.

Tar-based Vaginal Douching

Vaginal douching, an ancient practice involving the introduction of liquids or gases into the vagina, has utilized various substances over the years, including bleach, perfumes, soaps, vinegars, water, and yogurt. In the early 1900s, chemists discovered that resins from coal-tar distillation possessed antiseptic properties, leading to the emergence of tar-based douches.

In 1931, a New York City clinician observed a higher usage of commercially available vaginal douche products (such as Lysol®) among women with cervical cancer in his practice. Describing these products as coal-tar derivatives, he noted their experimental use in inducing cancers in animals.[15] Epidemiologists in Massachusetts and California later confirmed associations between cervical cancer and products containing

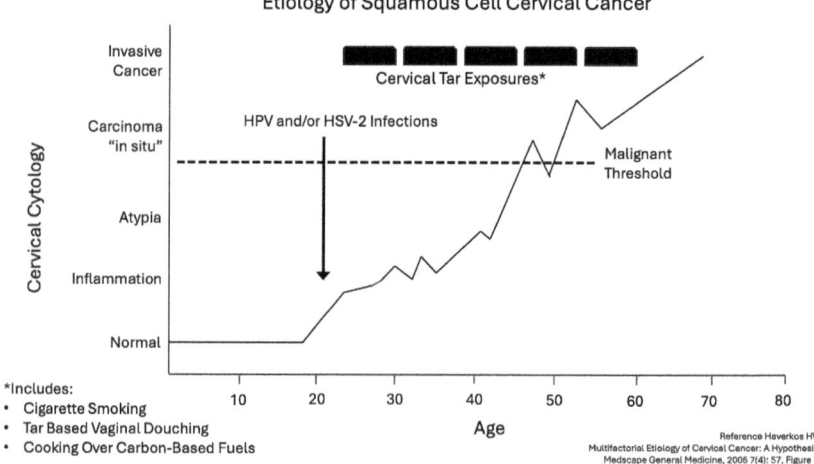

"Etiology of squamous cell cervical cancer: an interactive hypothesis" (Haverkos et al., *Biomedicine & Pharmacotherapy* 2000; 54:57).

carbolic acid, creolin, or sulfonaphthol, leading to the voluntary discontinuation of these products in the United States by 1970, though their distribution continued globally.[16] Notably, these studies did not account for HPV infection status, raising questions about whether tar-based douching serves as a cofactor or a confounder.

We proposed an alternative hypothesis: co-carcinogenesis,[17] outlined in Figure 1. Acknowledging that HPV did not satisfy Koch's postulates for cervical cancer, we explored alternative causes. Our review included sexually transmitted infections (such as HPV, herpes simplex virus-2, and human immunodeficiency virus), noninfectious factors (like cigarette smoking and oral contraceptives), and tar-based vaginal douche products. Nutrition was also considered as a potential protective factor.[18]

Rous Rabbit Model

Peyton Rous (1879–1970) and his colleagues conducted experiments on rabbits to study the development of squamous cell cancers. They exposed rabbit ears to tars and then injected Shope papillomavirus into the rabbits. Interestingly, they observed that the formation of cancers occurred more rapidly when the rabbits were first exposed to the virus and then to methylcholanthrene. This led them to conclude that papillomavirus and tar have a synergistic effect in the development of cancer.[19]

Rous's challenge studies suggest that cancer wasn't induced by either factor alone. Instead, cancer emerged only when both the virus and chemical factors interacted.

HPV Vaccine Breakthrough

In June 1995, the World Health Organization (WHO) gathered 36 scientists in Lyon, France, to scrutinize over 1500 papers on papillomaviruses and cancers. Their consensus was that proteins from HPV types 16 and 18 could cause cervical cancer by disrupting cellular regulatory pathways.[20]

Papillomaviruses, double-stranded DNA viruses, infect mucous membranes and skin in a species-specific manner, inducing cellular growths. With over 200 identified human papillomavirus types, the discovery rate continues to rise. More than 90 percent of women with invasive cervical cancer harbor one or more HPV types, notably HPV-16 (found in about 50 percent of all CC) and HPV-18 (15–20 percent). Around 20 other HPV types are linked to cervical cancer, earning them the label "oncogenic."[21]

In 1997, a pharmaceutical company initiated a clinical development program for a recombinant HPV virus-like particle vaccine to prevent cervical cancer. By 2002, a randomized, placebo-controlled trial commenced, involving 12,167 women aged 15 to 26 across 13 countries. The vaccine targeted four HPV types to prevent high-grade cervical lesions associated with HPV-16 and HPV-18. The three-year study demonstrated a remarkable 98 percent efficacy in the per-protocol susceptible population. The FDA approved the vaccine in May 2006.[22] This marked a groundbreaking milestone in cervical cancer prevention, offering hope and protection against the most prevalent oncogenic HPV types.

In summary, significant strides have been made in comprehending the origins of cervical cancer. The HPV vaccine stands as a beacon of hope for preventing this lethal disease. Nevertheless, there remains room for further efforts to mitigate the impact of smoking, douching, and cooking over wood-burning stoves as co-carcinogens. An essential question lingers: what are the cofactors that precipitate adenocarcinoma of the cervix?

Type 1 Diabetes Mellitus

In June 1995, our 16-year-old son, Daniel, was diagnosed with type 1 diabetes mellitus during his annual sports physical. Glucose was detected in his urine, and he had been experiencing fatigue and nocturia while participating in various sports for several months. His blood sugar measured 235 mg/dl, and his hemoglobin A_{1C} was 9.7 percent. The question arises: What causes type 1 diabetes mellitus?

None of my three siblings or Lynne's three siblings had diabetes. However, I did have two male cousins among my 34 first cousins (13 males and 21 females) who had type 1 diabetes, one diagnosed at age 15 and the other at 39. Lynne had one male cousin diagnosed at age 26 out of her 18 first cousins (8 males and 10 females).

Our son was admitted to Walter Reed Army Medical Center, where he started insulin therapy and received education on diabetes self-care. Despite the challenges, he went on to play college soccer at the University of Richmond, got married, and became a father. Daniel has three boys, one of whom was adopted. Thanks to remarkable advancements in medical technology for diabetes care and our son's diligent self-care, he has become a successful entrepreneur, playing highly competitive sports into his 40s.

Type 1 diabetes mellitus is the most common life-threatening endocrine disorder of children and young adults. In a 2007 multicenter American study, the incidence of type 1 diabetes mellitus was approximately 2 per 10,000 among youth less than 20 years of age; no gender differences were noted.[23]

Enteroviruses and Type 1 Diabetes Mellitus

In 1926, S. Franklin Adams reported a seasonal variation and a higher incidence of acute diabetes in northern U.S. states compared to southern states, suggesting an infectious etiology.[24] The search for an infectious etiology of type 1 diabetes focused on enteroviruses.[25]

Enteroviruses are a common cause of childhood "flu-like" illnesses during late summer/early fall. In 1979, J.W. Yoon reported a 10-year-old previously healthy boy who presented to the National Naval Medical Center (now the Walter Reed National Military Medical Center) in Bethesda, Maryland, in diabetic ketoacidosis, and he died one week later. Coxsackie B4 virus, now identified as human enterovirus B4, was grown from his pancreas at autopsy. Inoculation of that virus into mice produced high blood sugars and pancreatic necrosis.[26]

Cofactors for Type 1 Diabetes Mellitus

A genetic component in the etiology of type 1 diabetes is suggested by the notable familial clustering of the disease. Genes located on chromosome 6, responsible for specific proteins, have been associated with an increased risk of type 1 diabetes. Children carrying both the highest-risk haplotypes on chromosome 6 face a 5 percent risk of developing the disease by the age of 15. However, the intricate interaction between high-risk alleles on chromosome 6 and those on other chromosomes, influencing the onset of the disease, remains unclear.[27]

The heightened occurrence of type 1 diabetes at higher latitudes implies a potential role for vitamin D deficiency in its etiology. Finland, boasting one of the world's highest rates of type 1 diabetes mellitus, conducted a study in 1966 involving 10,366 children born in two Finnish cities. The study recommended 2000 international units of vitamin D3 per day. By 1998 revealing that by 1998, 81 children were diagnosed with type 1 diabetes mellitus at a median age of 14. The incidence rate was significantly lower for those using vitamin supplements regularly, suggesting a potential protective effect (relative risk, 0.22: 95 percent confidence intervals 0.05–0.89).[28]

Several investigators propose that "enhanced" nutrition may trigger type 1 diabetes mellitus. The Swedish Childhood Diabetes study, dedicated to studying risk factors, investigated nutrients and food additives. Comparing the dietary histories of 339 children with type 1 diabetes mellitus and 528 controls matched for age, sex, and residence, the study found a direct relationship between the intake of foods rich in complex carbohydrates, meats, nitrates, nitrites, and nitrosamines in the diet.[29] Additionally, various studies suggest a correlation between higher socioeconomic status and increased rates of type 1 diabetes in Finland, Estonia, and the United States.[30]

Linking Enteroviral Infection, Vitamin D Deficiency, and Type 1 Diabetes Mellitus

In the context of a viral infection during a period of vitamin D deficiency in a well-fed child, we propose a mechanism for the induction of autoimmune disease. This hypothesis centers on the idea that vitamin D deficiency may compromise the immune system, leading to an abnormality that causes the immune system to mistakenly recognize enterovirus proteins as pancreatic tissues. This phenomenon is referred to as molecular mimicry, where the immune system, in a state of imbalance due to vitamin D deficiency, falsely identifies viral proteins as similar to the body's own tissues.[31]

Furthermore, we suggest that a metabolite of dietary nitrosamines, specifically a streptozotocin-like nitrosourea, might contribute to pancreatic destruction. Streptozotocin is a compound known for its diabetogenic properties, and its structural similarity to certain nitrosamines raises the possibility that dietary sources of nitrosamines could result in a similar destructive effect on the pancreas.[32]

In summary, the proposed mechanism involves a dual impact: vitamin D deficiency compromising the immune system's ability to distinguish between self and non-self, leading to molecular mimicry, and the potential diabetogenic effect of a nitrosamine metabolite contributing to pancreatic destruction. This integrated hypothesis provides a framework for understanding how a viral infection, coupled with vitamin D deficiency and dietary factors, could collectively contribute to the development of autoimmune diseases such as type 1 diabetes mellitus. Further research and exploration of these interconnections may yield valuable insights into preventive and therapeutic strategies for autoimmune diseases.[33]

Hypotheses—Etiology of Selected Diseases

During my tenure teaching epidemiology courses at the Uniformed Services University of the Health Sciences from 2006 to 2021, I opted for a unique approach—students were tasked with writing papers instead of taking traditional tests. I encouraged them to select a disease with an unknown cause and formulate hypotheses for its causation. I have supplemented the following table with my own and colleagues' investigations into various diseases featuring one or more infectious agents.

Table 1. Hypotheses on the Etiology of Selected Diseases[34]

Featured Infectious Agent(s)	Disease	Cofactor(s)
Adenovirus	Obesity	Diet, lack of exercise, processed foods, vitamin excess
CMV	Coronary artery disease/stroke	Genetics, diabetes, diet, high cholesterol, hypertension, lack of exercise, obesity
Coronavirus	COVID-19	Asthma, COPD, diabetes, HIV infection, older age, pulmonary hypertension, sickle cell disease
EBV	Burkitt's lymphoma	Malaria, dietary nitrosamines
EBV	Multiple sclerosis	Vitamin D deficiency, other viruses
EBV	Nasopharyngeal cancer	HLA genotype
EBV	Non-Hodgkin's lymphoma	Pesticides, PCBs, hair dyes
Enteroviruses	Type 1 diabetes mellitus	Genetics, dietary nitrosamines, vitamin D deficiency
HBV and HCV	Hepatocellular carcinoma	Alcohol, aflatoxin, *Schistosoma japonicum*
HHV-8	AIDS-related Kaposi's sarcoma	HIV, nitrite inhalants, ACE inhibitors
HHV-8	Other forms of KS	Aluminosilicates, diet, immunosuppressants, amyl nitrite, ACE inhibitors, nitrite inhalants, secondary cancers
HIV	AIDS	Antimicrobial agents, CMV, drugs of abuse, genetics, gonorrhea, HHV-8, "opportunistic" organisms, other immunosuppressants, syphilis
HPV-5, 8, 17	Skin cancers	Genetics, sunlight, radiation
HPV-16, 18, et al.	Cervical cancer—adenocarcinoma	Alcohol, HSV-2, oral contraceptives

Featured Infectious Agent(s)	Disease	Cofactor(s)
HPV-16, 18, et al.	Cervical cancer—squamous cell	Coal/dung/wood cooking. HSV-2, tar-based vaginal douching, tobacco/marijuana smoking
HPV-16, 18, et al.	Oral cancer—Adenocarcinoma	Alcohol, HSV-1
HPV-16, 18, et al.	Oral cancer—squamous cell	Betel use, HSV-1, marijuana, tobacco
Influenza B/VZV	Reye's syndrome	Enzyme deficiencies, salicylates
SV40	Mesothelioma	Asbestos, tobacco
Helicobacter pylori	Stomach cancer	Alcohol, dietary nitrosamines, genetics, smoked fish, spicy foods
Mycobacterium tuberculosis	Reactive tuberculosis	Alcohol, diabetes, end-stage renal disease, HIV, immunosuppressants, malabsorption, silicosis, substance abuse
Staphylococcal, Streptococcal toxins	Toxic shock syndrome	Highly absorbent tampons, surgery
Toxoplasma gondii	Schizophrenia	Bartonella species, decreased fish consumption (omega acids), vitamin D deficiency
None	Apocrine adenocarcinoma	Radiation, textile dyes, alcohol
None	Autism	In utero exposures, processed foods, vaccines
None	Breast cancer	Alcohol, estrogen therapy, increased breast density, genetics
None	Colon cancer	Alcohol, genetics, well-cooked red meat consumption
None	Lung cancer	Asbestos, marijuana, pneumonia, silicosis, tobacco, tuberculosis

Apocrine Adenocarcinoma

In December 2001, at the age of 50, I observed a reddened area in my right armpit, initially mistaking it for a single hair folliculitis. Over the next three months, it grew to the size of a pea, though it remained non-painful and non-itchy. Seeking medical attention, I consulted my internist at Walter Reed Army Medical Center, who then referred me to dermatology. In May 2002, a dermatologist conducted a biopsy, identifying the lesion as an apocrine (sweat gland) adenocarcinoma. Subsequently, I was promptly referred to the chief of oncology, who conducted

18. Multifactorial Causes of Infectious and Chronic Diseases 233

a comprehensive medical history and physical examination, ordering tests to rule out primary breast, colon, and prostate cancers.

In August, the chief of oncologic surgery at Walter Reed performed a debridement of the tumor and sentinel node biopsies, revealing that four out of 21 lymph nodes were positive for cancer. Following this diagnosis, radiation and chemotherapy were recommended.

Throughout my life, I had enjoyed outdoor sports, particularly tennis and golf, and spent considerable time in the sun. In my youth, I underwent radiation treatments for persistent acne at the University of Cincinnati Medical Center. Additionally, at ages 39 and 44, I had basal cell cancers treated on my chest and right temple, respectively. After these incidents, I became meticulous about sunscreen application and wore dark shirts during tennis matches, believing they offered better sun protection. However, after prolonged summer matches, I noticed blue/black dyes in my armpits during showers.

Driven by a desire to understand my condition, I delved into medical literature at the NIH and FDA libraries, finding approximately 50 reported case-patients of apocrine adenocarcinomas. Based on my research, I hypothesized that my cancer was triggered by the radiation received during my youth, compounded by dyes seeping into my armpit in the summer.[35]

Armed with this knowledge, I opted against chemotherapy and radiation, choosing instead to manage my condition by postponing all diagnostic radiation exams and adopting preventive measures such as using roll-on deodorant and wearing white sports/undershirts to avoid contact with dark dyes. While I cannot definitively prove the connection between radiation/chemical dyes and apocrine adenocarcinoma, I have remained cancer-free for over 20 years and am content with the decisions I made.

In summary, recognizing the complexity of diseases—whether infectious or chronic, like cancers, autoimmune disorders, and mental health issues—is crucial. These conditions often arise from a mix of factors, including infectious agents, genetics, and environmental elements. Embracing this multifactorial perspective necessitates a shift in our approach, urging us to investigate and understand the diverse causes that contribute to these health challenges.

Epilogue

The AIDS pandemic continues to affect people worldwide. According to the World Health Organization, HIV infection has claimed the lives of approximately 40 million individuals to date, with an estimated 39 million people currently living with the virus. New infections persist globally, and in some regions, the numbers are even rising. In 2022, roughly 630,000 people lost their lives due to HIV-related causes, and 1.3 million individuals contracted HIV.[1]

While the prevailing message remains that HIV leads to AIDS, significant advancements have been made in HIV treatment. The FDA has granted approval for over 30 antiretroviral drugs, spanning various classes such as reverse transcriptase-, protease-, and integrase-inhibitors. Combination therapies have demonstrated their ability to reduce viral loads, increase CD4 counts, and extend survival rates. Additionally, both pre- and post-exposure prophylactic regimens have been tested and shown to be around 50 percent effective as of 2013.[2]

Despite these substantial breakthroughs, there are still concerns regarding HIV medications. They can be both toxic and costly, necessitating lifelong treatment. Misuse may also result in drug resistance. While not always explicitly acknowledged, coexisting factors are implied by the use of antimicrobial drugs to prevent life-threatening opportunistic infections, such as *Pneumocystis* pneumonia, toxoplasmic encephalitis, and mycobacterial infections.

In the face of the challenges that lie ahead, one striking and welcome fact emerges in the battle against HIV/AIDS: individuals receiving antiretroviral treatments now experience life expectancies approaching those of individuals without HIV.

On the other hand, Kaposi's sarcoma, which is considered one of the precursor diseases of AIDS, remains less understood. Initially, when HIV was discovered, it was believed to be the cause of Kaposi's sarcoma. However, once a blood test became available, HIV could not be detected in the vast majority of Kaposi's sarcoma case-patients that occurred before 1980.

Epilogue

It wasn't until 1994 that HHV-8 (human herpesvirus 8) was found in all forms of Kaposi's sarcoma and presumed to be its sole cause. Nevertheless, a simple explanation for the origins of Kaposi's sarcoma has proven to be incomplete.[3] This disease results from a complex interplay between HHV-8 infection, immunosuppression, and vasoactive agents.

It's also crucial to recognize that chronic diseases, including coronary artery disease, stroke, cancer, autoimmune diseases, and mental health disorders, often have multifactorial causes that involve infectious agents in conjunction with genetic and environmental factors. For instance, coronary artery disease presents a complex web of risk factors, such as cigarette smoking, genetics, hypertension, infectious agents, obesity, and lack of exercise.[4] Reye's syndrome appears to result from a multifaceted combination of salicylates, varicella-zoster virus/influenza B viruses, and genetic metabolic errors.[5] Building on our experience investigating the causation of Kaposi's sarcoma, we have developed multifactorial hypotheses for the etiologies of diseases like cervical cancer, hepatocellular carcinoma, multiple sclerosis, schizophrenia, and type 1 diabetes mellitus.[6]

In conclusion, I advocate for a much-needed shift in the paradigm through which we perceive and understand infectious diseases. I challenge the entrenched belief that HIV is the exclusive cause of AIDS, as defined by Robert Koch's postulates. Instead, I embrace Kenneth Rothman's comprehensive component causal model, asserting that AIDS, like many chronic ailments, arises from a complex interplay of various factors. By championing this perspective, I aim to foster a profound and sophisticated understanding of infectious diseases, steering us away from the simplistic and outdated viewpoint of the 19th century. I firmly believe that by acknowledging the intricate complexities of the contemporary landscape, we can pave the way for a more comprehensive and effective approach to tackling AIDS, Kaposi's sarcoma, and other infectious diseases.

Appendix A: Report Form— AIDS Surveillance

Knowing the number of case-patients alone is not sufficient to understand an epidemic. To define its descriptive aspects, it is essential to gather detailed information about each affected patient.

First, collect key details such as age, gender, sexual orientation, place of residence, onset dates, and diagnostic criteria. Next, document relevant signs, symptoms, and laboratory results. Finally, obtain the reporting physician's contact information to facilitate follow-up inquiries or potential recruitment for future epidemiologic studies, such as case-control or cohort studies.

To streamline data collection, the form should be designed for efficiency, incorporating check-box formats to facilitate quick responses during phone calls with busy clinicians.[1]

Our initial form collected the following information:

Case identification number (to be assigned sequentially)

Date of call and name of person taking call

Patient name (first, middle, last)

Age

Status (alive, dead)

Date of Birth (month, day, and year)

Date of Death (month, day, and year)

Sex (male, female)

Sexual preference (male, female, both, unknown)

Marital status (married, never married, divorced, widowed, separated, unknown)

Race [White, not Hispanic; Black, not Hispanic; Hispanic; Asian or Pacific Islander; American Indian or Alaska Native; Other country (specify); Not stated]

Residence (City, Borough, State)

If hospitalized, name and location of hospital (Name, City, State)

Illness: [Date of Diagnosis (month, year) Method of Diagnosis (Biopsy, Culture, Other specimen)]
    Kaposi's sarcoma
    Pneumocystis
    CMV Infection
    Progressive Herpes Simplex (duration)
    Toxoplasmosis (CNS)
    Cryptococcosis (CNS)
    GI candidiasis
    Other Opportunistic Infection (specify)
    Other medical condition

Signs and Symptoms: [Date of Onset (month, year)]
    Skin lesions only if related to opportunistic infection (specify location)
    Lymphadenopathy more than 3 months duration (specify location)
    Fever
    Dyspnea
    Weight loss
    Diarrhea
    Oral thrush
    Other (specify)

Does (did) patient have any serious underlying condition (e.g., malignancy, organ transplant, immunosuppressive therapy? (Yes, No, Unknown)

If steroids: dose, duration, last dose

1. Reporting Source: (Name, Title-Specialty, Phone, Address)

2. Primary Physician (Name, Title-Specialty, Phone, Address)

Immunologic test results: (Absolute lymphocytes (WBC X % lymphs)

Additional Notes (optional):

Report form July 1981 developed by Harry W. Haverkos

Report Form—AIDS Surveillance

Other pertinent information added February–August 1982 by Richard Selik, M.D.:

Race: Haitian

IV drug use? [Yes, No, Unknown (If yes, specify)]

Blood transfusions past 5 years? [Yes, No, Unknown (If yes, specify dates)]

Any other blood products? (Yes, no, unknown)

Patient ever in prison? (Yes, no, unknown)

Patient ever receive Hepatitis B vaccine? (Yes, no, unknown)

Appendix B: Questionnaire— AIDS Case-control Study

Once you have identified the hypotheses to be tested, you must determine the necessary data to collect. If the disease is transmitted through person-to-person contact, such as sexual transmission, gather details on the frequency, duration, and nature of personal interactions. If the mode of transmission is uncertain, a broader set of questions covering all possible risks should be included.

Data collection tools, such as questionnaires, should go beyond risk factors. They should also capture identifying details, clinical information, and descriptive characteristics. Identifying information allows for follow-ups, while clinical data ensures that individuals meet the case definition. Additional clinical details, such as the severity of illness, hospitalizations, and long-term effects, can provide valuable insights. Descriptive factors related to time, place, and person help characterize the affected population, compare case-patients with controls, and generate new hypotheses about disease causes.

If a newly developed questionnaire is being used for the first time, it must be pretested. This process helps refine survey procedures by assessing the ability to locate respondents, their willingness to participate, the time required for interviews, and other logistical factors.[1]

Questionnaire—CDC Case-control Study

Identification
(for CDC use)

ID No.
Birthdate (month, day, year)
Zip code

Interview Information

Interviewer

Interview facility [Hospital, VD clinic, Home, Private physician's office, Other (specify)]

Date of interview (month, day, year)

Time started (: am or pm)

Time completed (: am or pm)

Time of interview (in minutes)

For case-patients only: Has case been interviewed before as part of a study (yes, no)

Present Illness Data
(ask only for case-patients)

1. Which of the following illnesses have you had? (Kaposi's sarcoma, Pneumocystis pneumonia, Both)
2. When, would you say, did your illness begin? (month, year) (if both illnesses are present, when did the earlier of the two begin?)
3. From the time your illness began, until now, which of the following symptoms have you had?

    Symptom [Yes, No, Don't know, Date first noted (month, year)]
    - Skin abnormalities (describe)
    - Shortness of breath
    - Fever for more than a week
    - Diarrhea for more than a week
    - Swollen glands for more than a week
    - Cough for more than a week
    - Unintentional weight loss (number of pounds)
    - Cold sores (painful blisters in mouth)
    - Shingles (painful blisters on skin)
    - Thrush (white patches in mouth)
    - Others (describe)

    (Compare the earliest of these symptom dates to the date the patient felt the illness began. If dates are the same, record below as "onset date." If dates are different, discuss difference with patient and come to an agreement regarding "onset date.")

4. Onset date (FOR CASE-PATIENTS RECORD DATE DERIVED FROM PREVIOUS SECTION. FOR CONTROLS RECORD DATE

OF THE MATCH CASE. THIS DATE WILL BE USED IN THE REST OF THE QUESTIONNAIRE.) Month, Year

Sociodemographic Data

5. In what city and state were you born?
6. How old were you on (onset date)? (years)
7. Into which of the following categories would you place yourself? (CHECK ONE)
    White, not Hispanic
    Black, not Hispanic
    Hispanic
    Asian/Pacific Islander
    American Indian or Alaska Native
    Not stated
8. How many years of school had you completed by (onset date)? Years
9. I am going to read you a list of income categories. Considering the year before (onset date), into which of these categories would you place your personal income before taxes. (CHECK ONE)
    Less than $10,000
    $10,000 to $20,000
    $20,000 to $30,000
    More than $30,000
10. What was your marital status on (onset date)? (CHECK ONE)
    Married
    Separated or divorced
    Widowed
    Never married
11. If ever married: How many times have you been married?
    How many total months have you been married?

Past Medical History

12. Let's talk about your medical history up until (onset date). Before (onset date) did you ever have any kind of surgery? Yes, No

    IF YES, ASK: Starting with your most recent operation and working backwards, what kind of surgery did you have and when did you have it? Type of surgery Year

13. Before (onset date), had a doctor ever told you that you had any of the following infections. (READ EACH INFECTION. IF RESPONSE IS YES, RECORD OF INFECTIONS AND DATE OF LAST INFECTION.)

Infection   Yes, No, Don't know, How many times? Year of last infection

Gonorrhea (clap)
Syphilis
Nongonnococcal urethritis (discharge from the penis not caused by gonorrhea)
Nongonnococcal proctitis (discharge from the rectum not caused by gonorrhea)
Genital Herpes simplex (IF YES, ASK: Was it on the penis? Was it on or in your rectum?
Venereal warts: (IF YES, ASK: Were they on the penis? Were they on or in your rectum?
Pubic lice ("crabs")
Scabies ("itch mites")
Any other sexually transmitted infection (specify)

14. Still thinking back to before (onset date), did you ever have diarrhea the was so bad that you had to go to the doctor for treatment? CHECK ONE: Yes, No

IF YES, ASK: Did the doctor tell you that your diarrhea was caused by (READ EACH ITEM SLOWLY). IF YES TO AN ITEM, ASK: How many times did you have diarrhea caused by (ITEM). When was the last time you had diarrhea caused by (ITEM)?

Cause of diarrhea   Check if yes   How many times? Year of last infection

Salmonella
Shigella
Camplyobacter
Yersinia
Amebiasis
Giardiasis
Strongyloidiasis
Some other cause the doctor told you about (specify)

15. Before (onset date), did a doctor ever tell you that you had hepatitis?

(CHECK ONE) Yes, No: IF YES, SAY: I am going to read you a list of different causes of hepatitis. Did the doctor mention any of these as the cause of your hepatitis? Were you sick with hepatitis (jaundice, poor appetite) or was the hepatitis diagnosed by a blood test at a time you felt well? When was the diagnosis made?

Cause of hepatitis   Check if cause   Check if sick   Check if not sick   Year

Hepatitis A ("infectious")
Hepatitis B ("serum")
Cytomegalovirus
EB virus ("mono")
Some other cause the doctor told you about? Specify

16. Did you ever receive hepatitis B vaccine? (CHECK ONE) Yes, No. (EXCLUDE GAMMA GLOBULIN INJECTION)

   IF YES, ASK: Where and when did you receive it? Place year

17. Again, before (onset date), were you ever told by a doctor that you had mononucleosis? (CHECK ONE) Yes, No

   IF YES, ASK: What year was that?

   Did the doctor do a blood test for mono? (CHECK ONE) Yes, No, Don't know

18. And what about cancer? Before (onset date), were you ever told by a doctor that you had cancer? (CHECK ONE) Yes, No

   IF YES, ASK: What kind of cancer was it and when did the doctor tell you about it?

   Type of cancer, Year

19. Did you ever receive any x-ray treatment for a medical condition, such as acne or an enlarged thymus gland before (onset date?) (CHECK ONE) Yes, No

   IF YES, ASK: What was the condition? What year was the treatment given?

20. Did you ever have a serious infection, such as pneumonia, that required hospitalization before (onset date)? (CHECK ONE) Yes, No

   IF YES, ASK: What kind of infection was it and when were you hospitalized?

   Type of Infection, Year

21. Finally, have you ever had any medical problems besides the ones we discussed that required hospitalization before (onset date)? (CHECK ONE) Yes, No

   IF YES, ASK: What were those problems and when were you hospitalized? Illness, Year

Recent Illness Data
(ASK ONLY FOR CONTROLS)

SAY TO ALL CONTROLS: So far, we have talked about your medical history up until (onset date). The next few questions are about your health from (onset date) to (today's date).

Questionnaire—AIDS Case-control Study

22. From (onset date) to (today's date), have you had any of the following symptoms?

    Symptom   Yes, No, Don't know   Date Noted (month, year)
    Skin abnormalities (describe)
    Shortness of breath
    Fever for more than a week
    Diarrhea for more than a week
    Swollen glands for more than a week
    Cough for more than a week
    Unintentional weight loss (number of pounds)
    Cold sores (painful blisters in mouth)
    Shingles (painful blisters on skin)
    Thrush (white patches in mouth)

23. ASK CONTROLS: What was the reason for your most recent visit to the sexually transmitted diseases clinic or to your doctor?

Occupational History

24. Let's talk about the different kinds of employment you've had and the type of work you have done. Start with your job as of (onset date) and work backwards over the past 10 years. Include time spent in the military and going to school and mention periods of unemployment.

    Occupation   Type of business/description of work   Years

Hobby History

25. Let's talk about any hobbies you might have spent time on regularly during the 10 years before (onset date). I am interested in hobbies which involve exposures to substances such as painting, rather than hobbies like sports or music. Hobby, Years

Exposure History

26. Have any of your activities at home or at work before (onset date) EVER resulted in you being exposed to any of the following: (READ EACH ITEM)

    ITEM   Yes   No   Don't know   Years of exposure (from, to)
    A. Industrial chemicals (e.g. solvents) specify
    B. Agricultural chemicals (e.g. pesticides) specify
    C. Defoliants (e.g. Agent Orange) specify

D. Other chemicals (e.g. photographic) specify
E. Radioactive materials (specify)

Travel History

27. Where were you living during (onset date)? City, state
28. Before then, how long had you lived continuously in this metropolitan area? Months

    IF RESIDENCE IN THIS AREA WAS LESS THAN 120 MONTHS, SAY: What other cities did you live in? During which years did you live in them? Start with the most recent and work backwards over the last ten years. City, state, years
29. During the 10 years before (onset date), did you spend any time travelling in foreign countries? (CHECK ONE) Yes, No

    IF YES, ASK: In what countries did you travel? Start with your most recent trip and work backwards. Include the year of the trip. (LIST COUNTRIES VISITED DURING A SINGLE TRIP ON EACH LINE.) Country, Year

Pets

30. In the 10 years before (onset date), did you keep or live in a household with any pets? (CHECK ONE) Yes, No

    IF YES, ASK: What kind of pets? When did you live with them? Did any have any unusual illnesses? Did they die of such illnesses?
    Pet, Years of ownership, Unusual illness? (yes, no)
    Specify illness, Did illness cause death? (yes, no)

Alcohol Use

31. Did you ever take least an occasional alcoholic drink before (onset date)?

    IF YES, ASK: On the average how many days in a week would you have a drink? Days

    If we consider on an average day, about how many drinks would you have? Consider a can of beer, a glass of wine, or a mixed drink to be equal to one drink? Drinks

    How many years would you say you have drunk alcoholic beverages? Years

    When was the last year up until (onset date)? Year

Cigarette Use

32. Have you ever smoked cigarettes at least occasionally before (onset date)?
    (CHECK ONE) Yes, No

    IF YES, ASK: On the average how many cigarettes do you smoke in a day? number

    How many years would you say you have smoked cigarettes? years
    When was the last year up until (onset date)? Years

Medications

33. During the 10 years before (onset date), did you take any of the prescription medications I am going to mention? If you did take any of them, I would like to know how many times you took the medication and why you took it.
    Medication   Yes, No, Don't know, No. of times taken, Reason(s) taken
    Penicillin (shots)
    Ampicillin (pills)
    Tetracycline (tablets)
    Flagyl (for amebiasis)
    Diiodoquin (for amebiasis)
    Humatin (for giardiasis)
    Atabrine (for giardiasis)
    Kwell (for lice or scabies)
    Cortisone (exclude topical)
    Prednisone

34. Other than the medications I have mentioned, can you recall any other prescription medications that you have taken during the 10 years before (onset date)?
    (CHECK ONE) Yes, No   IF YES, ENTER THESE MEDICATIONS BELOW

    Medication, Reason(s) taken

    The illnesses which we are studying might be related to drug use. Therefore, I would like to ask you about your use of certain drugs before (onset date). Some of these questions may not be applicable to you. First we will talk about "street drugs," then about inhalant stimulants.

    "Street" drugs

35. I am going to read you a list of some street drugs. If you have used any of them, I would like to know how you used them (e.g. smoking, by mouth), how often you used them and when you used them.

Drug   Yes, No, Don't know, Smoke, Nasal, Oral, IV,
        No. of times per month, Years used

Marijuana
Cocaine
Heroin
Amphetamines ("speed")
Barbiturates ("downers")
LSD ("acid")
Quaaludes
PCP ("angel dust")
Any others I didn't mention (specify)

Inhalants

36. Had you used any type of inhalant sexual stimulants or "poppers" (amyl or butyl nitrite) before (onset date)? (CHECK ONE) Yes, No   IF YES, ASK:

    A. When did you first use "poppers"? (year)
    B. When did you last use "poppers" before (onset date)? (year)
    C. During the period that you used "poppers," how many months, altogether did you use them? (months)
    D. If we take an average month of use, during how many days (or nights) would you use them? (days and nights)
    E. If we take an average day (or night) of use, how many "sniffs" might you take? (sniffs)
    F. When you use "poppers" about what percent of the use is in:
        Bathhouses (%)
        Discos (%)
        Other (specify) (%)
    G. Of the "poppers" that you have used, about what percent have been
        Ampules (%)
        Labelled bottles (%)
        Unlabelled bottles (%)
    H. If you use labelled bottles, which brands have you used (CHECK IF USED)
        1. Locker Room
        2. Bolt
        3. Rush
        4. Hardware

Questionnaire—AIDS Case-control Study

   5. Bullet
   6. Disco-Roma
   7. Head
   8. Hit
   9. Highball
   10. Pig Poppers
   11. Quicksilver
   12. Kryptonite
   13. Other (specify)
  I. If you use unlabelled bottles, where do you usually buy them?
     Name of store, City
37. Have you ever inhaled ethyl chloride before (onset date)?
    (CHECK ONE) Yes, No
    (Ethyl chloride is a substance that comes in a bottle and is usually sprayed on a handkerchief, then inhaled.)
    IF YES, ASK:
    A. When did you first use ethyl chloride? Year
    B. When did you last use ethyl chloride before (onset date)? Year
    C. During the period you have used ethyl chloride, how many months altogether, have you used it? Months
    D. If we take an average month of use, during how many days (or nights) would you use it? days
    E. If we take an average day (or night) of use, how many "sniffs" might you take? Sniffs
    F. When you use ethyl chloride, about what percent of the use in:
        Bathhouses (%)
        Discos (%)
        Other (specify) (%)

Sexual Behavior

The illnesses which we are studying may be related to sexual behaviors. Therefore, I would like to ask you some questions about your initial sexual experiences, then focus on your sexual practices during the year before (onset date). Some of the questions may not be applicable to you.

A. Initial Sexual Experiences. If we define sexual intercourse as the entrance of your penis into another person's mouth, anus or vagina, or the entrances of a penis into your mouth or anus, …
38. How old were you when you first had sexual intercourse with:
    (a) A male (man or boy) __ years or never (check here)

(b) If sexual contact with a male: How old were you when you first began having regular (at least once a month) sexual intercourse with males? ___years or never (check here)

39. And how old were you when you first had sexual intercourse with:
    (a) A female (woman or girl) ___ years or never (check here)
    (b) If sexual contacts with a female: How old were you when you first began having regular (at least once a month) sexual intercourse with females? ___ years or never (check here)

B. Sexual Experiences in the Year before Onset Date.

40. Going back one full year (365 days) from (onset date), how many different people have you had sexual intercourse with? ___ people

41. Of these ___ different people, how many were:
    (a) Males ___ men or boys
    (b) Females ___ women or girls
    If no male partners, check here and go to question 45.

42. If male sexual partners in the past year:
    Of your ___ male partners, about what percent did you meet or have sex with in:
    (a) Bath houses (%)
    (b) Gay bars and discos (%)
    (c) Book stores and movie houses (%)
    (d) Public parks and restrooms (%)

43. If male sexual partners in the past year:
    Frequency
    Of your ___ male partners, about what percent did you have sex with:
    (a) Only once (one night, not again) (%)
    (b) Intermittently (2-10 different nights) (%)
    (c) Frequently (more than 10 different nights) (%)

44. Considering all the episodes of sexual contact with male partners during the past year, about what percent of these episodes have involved the following activities (one "episode" may involve multiple activities):
    Activity, % male partners
    (a) Partner put his penis in your mouth (%)
    (b) You put your penis in your partner's mouth (%)
    (c) Partner put his penis in your rectum (%)
    (d) You put your penis in your partner's rectum (%)
    (e) Partner put his tongue in your rectum (%)
    (f) You put your tongue in your partner's rectum (%)

Questionnaire—AIDS Case-control Study

(g) Partner put his hand or fist in your rectum (%)
(h) You put your hand or fist in your partner's rectum (%)

45. If female sexual partners in the last year:
    Of your ___ female sexual partners, about what percent did you meet in bars, discos, or other public places? (%)

46. Of your ___ female partners, about what percent did you have sex with:
    Frequency
    (a) Only once (one night, not again) (%)
    (b) Intermittently (2–10 different nights) (%)
    (c) Frequently (more than 10 different nights) (%)

47. If female partners in the last year:
    Considering all the episodes of sexual contact with female partners during the past year, about what percent of these episodes have involved the following activities (one "episode" may involve multiple activities):
    Activity, % female partners
    (a) You put your penis in partner's vagina (%)
    (b) You put your penis in partner's mouth (%)
    (c) You put your penis in partner's rectum (%)
    (d) You put your hand or fist in partner's rectum (%)
    (e) You put your tongue in partner's rectum (%)
    (f) Partner put her hand or fist in your rectum (%)
    (g) Partner put her tongue in your rectum (%)

48. Would you consider your sexual activities during this year to be <u>typical</u> of your sexual activities during the preceding 5 years? Yes, No
    (a) If not typical: In what ways was this year significantly different?
    _____

    (b) If not typical: In a typical year, Please tell me the answer to these four questions:
        (1) Number of different male sexual partners
        (2) Number of different female sexual partners
        (3) Percent of different male partners who were "one night" partners
        (4) Percent of different female partners who were "one night" partners

49. Finally, could we talk about your lifetime sexual experiences up until (onset date). During (onset date) you were ___ years old. (subtract answer to question 38a or 39a, whichever is longer), about how many different people have you had sexual intercourse with?
    You may find it easiest to take a typical year and multiply.
    _____ lifetime partners

50. Of these different lifetime partners, how many were
    (a) male partners ____
    (b) female partners ____
51. Is there any other aspect of your sexual experience that we should talk about?
    (RECORD VERBATIM)

Family History

Just a few more questions about the background and medical history of your family.

52. Where was your father born? Country
53. What (is) (was) his ethnic background? Ethnicity
54. Where was your mother born? Country
55. What (is) (was) her ethnic background? Ethnicity
56. Is your family background Jewish? (CHECK ONE) Yes, No
57. Considering your grandparents, parents, your brothers and sisters, if any, and your children, if any, have any of these family members had cancer (CHECK ONE) Yes, No
    IF YES, ASK: Which family member(s) was that? What type of cancer did (he) (she) have?
        Family Relationship   Type of Cancer
58. Have any of your friends had cancer since January 1979? (CHECK ONE) Yes, No
    IF YES, ASK: What was your relationship with this friend? What type of cancer did he have?
    Relationship? Roommate, Sexual Partner, Type of Cancer
59. Have any of your friends been hospitalized because of infections since January 1979? (CHECK ONE) Yes, No
    IF YES, ASK: What was your relationship with this friend? What type of infection did he have?
    Relationship? Roommate, Sexual Partner, Type of Infection
60. Have any of your friends had unexplained weight loss and/or fever since January 1979?
    IF YES, ASK: What was your relationship with this friend? Try to describe his illness.
    Relationship? Roommate, Sexual Partner, Description of Illness

Transcribed by Harry W. Haverkos 2/16/2025

Appendix C: Leading Causes of Death in the United States Since 1900

Table 1. Leading Causes of Death in the U.S. Since 1900 (number of deaths per 100,000)

1900 (1,719.1)*	1950 (963.8)*	2000 (872.0)*	2020 (835.4)*
1. Pneumonia + Flu (202.7)	1. Heart Diseases (355.5)	1. Heart Diseases (257.9)	1. Heart Diseases (168.2)
2. Tuberculosis (194.4)	2. Cancer (139.8)	2. Cancer (201.0)	2. Cancer (144.1)
3. Diarrhea (142.7)	3. Stroke (104.0)	3. Stroke (60.8)	3. COVID-19 (85.0)
4. Heart Diseases (137.4)	4. Accidents (60.6)	4. CLRD# (44.3)	4. Accidents‡ (57.5)
5. Stroke (106.9)	5. Infancy Diseases (40.5)	5. Accidents (35.5)	5. Stroke (38.8)
6. Kidney Disease (88.6)	6. Pneumonia + Flu (31.3)	6. Diabetes Mellitus (25.2)	6. CLRD† (36.4)
7. Accidents (72.3)	7. Tuberculosis (22.5)	7. Pneumonia + Flu (23.7)	7. Alzheimer's dx (32.4)
8. Cancer (66.4)	8. Arteriosclerosis (20.4)	8. Alzheimer's dx (18.0)	8. Diabetes (24.8)
9. Senility (50.2)	9. Kidney Disease (16.4)	9. Kidney Disease (13.5)	9. Pneumonia + Flu (13.0)
10. Diphtheria (40.3)	10. Diabetes Mellitus (16.2)	10. Septicemia (11.4)	10. Kidney Disease (12.7)

*Death rate from all causes.
  †CLRD reported as chronic lower respiratory diseases, including chronic obstructive pulmonary disease.
  ‡Accidents (unintentional injuries only), 2020
  Modified from various National Vital Statistics Reports, CDC

Chapter Notes

Preface

1. Kurian GT (editor). *A Historical Guide to the U.S. Government.* Oxford University Press; 1998.
2. Thacker SB, et al. Epidemic Intelligence Service of the Centers for Disease Control and Prevention: 50 years of training and service in applied epidemiology. *Am J Epidemiol.* 2001; 154 (11): 985–92; Pendergrast M. *Inside the Outbreaks: The Elite Medical Detectives of the Epidemic Intelligence Service.* Houghton Mifflin Harcourt; 2010.

Chapter 1

1. CDC. *Pneumocystis* pneumonia—Los Angeles. *MMWR.* 1981 Jun 5; 30: 250–2.
2. Pazin G, et al. Prevention of reactivated herpes simplex infections by human leukocyte interferon after operation on the trigeminal root. *N Engl J Med.* 1979; 301: 225–230.
3. Haverkos HW, et al. Follow-up of interferon treatment of herpes simplex. *N Engl J Med.* 1979; 225–230.
4. Haverkos HW, et al. Diagnosis of pneumonitis in immunocompromised patients by open lung biopsy. *Cancer.* 1983; 52(6), 1093–1097.

Chapter 2

1. Pendergrast. *Inside the Outbreaks.* xi.
2. CDC. *Pneumocystis* pneumonia. 1981.
3. Walzer P, et al. Pneumocystis carinii pneumonia in the United States: epidemiologic, diagnostic, and clinical features. *Ann Intern Med.* 1974; 80:80–93.
4. CDC. Kaposi's sarcoma and *Pneumocystis* pneumonia among homosexual men—New York City and California. *MMWR.* 1981 Jul 3; 30 (25): 305–08.
5. Haverkos HW, Curran JW. The current outbreak of Kaposi's sarcoma and opportunistic infections. *CA. Cancer J Clin.* 1982; 32(6): 330–9.
6. CDC. *Pneumocystis* pneumonia. 1981; Gottlieb MS, et al. *Pneumocystis carinii* pneumonia and mucosal candidiasis in previously healthy homosexual men: evidence of a new acquired cellular immunodeficiency. *N Engl J Med.* 1981; 305 (24): 1425–31.
7. Haverkos. Current outbreak. 1982.
8. Auerbach DN, et al. Cluster of cases of AIDS. Patients linked by sexual contact. *Am J Med.* 1984; 76 (3): 487–92.

Chapter 3

1. Shilts, R. *And the Band Played On.* St. Martin's Press; 1987, 171.
2. CDC. *Pneumocystis* pneumonia. 1981.
3. CDC. Kaposi's sarcoma and Pneumocystis pneumonia among homosexual men—New York City and California. *MMWR.* 1981 Jul 3; 30 (25): 305–8.
4. CDC. Follow-up on Kaposi's sarcoma and *Pneumocystis* pneumonia. *MMWR.* 1981 Aug 28; 30 (33): 409–10.
5. Masur H, et al. An outbreak of community-acquired PCP: initial manifestation of cellular immune dysfunction. *N Engl J Med.* 1981 Dec 10; 301 (24): 1431–8.
6. Masur H, et al. Opportunistic infection in previously healthy women: initial

manifestations of a community-acquired cellular immunodeficiency. *Ann Intern Med.* 1982 Oct; 97 (4): 533-339.
  7. Haverkos. Current outbreak. 1982.
  8. *Ibid.*
  9. CDC. Epidemiologic Notes and Reports: Persistent, generalized lymphadenopathy among homosexual men. *MMWR.* 1982 May 21; 31 (19): 249-51; CDC. Diffuse, undifferentiated non-Hodgkin lymphoma among homosexual males—United States. *MMWR.* 1982 Jun 4; 31 (21): 277-79.
  10. CDC. AIDS in Prison inmates—New York, New Jersey. *MMWR.* 1983 Jan 7; 31 (52): 700-1.
  11. Guinan ME, et al. Heterosexual and homosexual patients with AIDS: a comparison of surveillance, interview, and laboratory data. *Ann Intern Med.* 1984 Feb; 100 (2): 213-18.
  12. Haverkos HW, et al. Disease manifestation among homosexual men with AIDS: a possible role of nitrites in Kaposi's sarcoma. *Sex Transm Dis.* 1985; Oct-Dec; 12 (4): 203-8.
  13. Miller B, et al. The syndrome of unexplained generalized lymphadenopathy in young men in New York City. Is it related to the acquired immune deficiency syndrome? *JAMA.* 1984 Jan 13; 251 (2): 242-6. PMID 6690782.
  14. CDC. Opportunistic infections and Kaposi's sarcoma among Haitians in the United States. *MMWR.* 1982 Jul 9; 31 (26): 353-4, 360-1.
  15. CDC. Epidemiologic notes and reports: *Pneumocystis carinii* pneumonia among persons with hemophilia A. *MMWR.* 1982 Jul 16; 31 927): 365-367.
  16. *Ibid.*
  17. CDC. Update on AIDS among patients with hemophilia A. *MMWR.* 1982 Dec 10; 31 (48): 644-6, 652.
  18. CDC. Current trends update on AIDS—United States. *MMWR.* 1982 Sep 24; 31 (37): 507-508, 513-514.
  19. Guinan, et al. Heterosexual and homosexual patients with AIDS in the United States: a comparison of surveillance, interview, and laboratory data.
  20. *Ibid.*
  21. Jaffe HW, et al. AIDS in the United States: the first 1,000 cases. *J Infect Dis.* 1983 Aug 1; 148 (2):3 39-345.
  22. *Ibid.*

  23. CDC. Epidemiologic notes and reports: possible transfusion-associated AIDS—California. *MMWR.* 1982 Dec 10; 31 (48): 652-54.
  24. CDC. Unexplained immunodeficiency and opportunistic infections in infants—New York, New Jersey, California. *MMWR.* 1982 Dec 17; 31 (49): 665-667.
  25. Oleske J, et al. Immune deficiency syndrome in children. *JAMA.* 1983 May 6; 249 (17): 2345-2349.
  26. CDC. Current trends update: AIDS—USA. *MMWR.* 1984 Jan 6; 32 (52): 688-691 (Pediatric AIDS definition).
  27. *Ibid.*
  28. Online CDC Year-end Reports. Dec 31, 1984.

Chapter 4

  1. Shilts. *And the Band Played On.* 243.
  2. Jaffe HW, et al. National case-control study of KS and PCP in homosexual men. I. Epidemiologic results. *Annals of Internal Medicine.* 1983; 99:145-151.
  3. *Ibid.*
  4. Modified table 4 from Jaffe. Epidemiologic results. 1983.
  5. Jeffe. Epidemiologic results. 1983.
  6. Rogers MF, et al. National case-control study of KS and PCP in homosexual men. II. Laboratory results. *Annals of Internal Medicine.* 1983; 99:151-158.
  7. *Ibid.*
  8. *Ibid.*
  9. Francis DP, et al. Infection of chimpanzees with LAV. *Lancet.* 1984; ii: 1276-7.
  10. Rogers. Laboratory results. 1983.
  11. Jaffe. Epidemiologic results. 1983.
  12. Modified from tables and text from Jaffe. Epidemiologic results. 1983.
  13. Modified table 3 from Jeffe. Epidemiologic results. 1983.
  14. Jeffe. Epidemiologic results. 1983.
  15. *Ibid.*
  16. CDC. Current Trends Prevention of AIDS: Report of Inter-Agency Recommendations. *MMWR.* 1983 Mar 04; 32 (8): 101-3.
  17. *Ibid.*
  18. CDC. A cluster of Kaposi's sarcoma and *Pneumocystis* pneumonia among homosexual male residents of Los Angeles and Orange Counties, California. *MMWR.* 1982 Jun 18; 31 (23): 305-7.

19. Auerbach. Cluster of cases of AIDS. 1984.
20. Jaffe. Epidemiologic results. 1983; Rogers. Laboratory results. 1983.

Chapter 5

1. Jaffe. Epidemiologic results. 1983; Rogers. Laboratory results. 1983.
2. Essex M, et al. Antibodies to cell membrane antigens associated with human T-cell leukemia virus in patients with AIDS. *Science*. 1983; 220 (4599): 859–62.
3. Gelmann EP, et al. Proviral DNA of a retrovirus, human T-cell leukemia virus, in two patients with AIDS. *Science*. 1983; 220 (4599): 862–65; Gallo RC, et al. Isolation of human T-cell leukemia virus in acquired immune deficiency syndrome. *Science*. 1983; 220 (4599): 865–67.
4. Barre-Sinoussi F, et al. Isolation of a T-lymphotropic retrovirus from a patient at risk for AIDS. *Science*. 1983; 220 (4599): 868–71.
5. Feorino PM, et al. Lymphadenopathy associated virus infection of a blood donor-recipient pair with AIDS. *Science*. 1984; 225 (4657): 69–72.
6. Popovic M, et al. Detection, isolation, and continuous production of cytopathic retroviruses (HTLV-III) from patients with AIDS and pre-AIDS. *Science*. 1984; 224 (4648): 497–500; Gallo RC, et al. Frequent detection and isolation of cytopathic retroviruses (HTLV-III) from patients with AIDS and at risk for AIDS. *Science*. 1984; 224 (4648): 500–03; Schupbach J, et al. Serological analysis of a subgroup of human T-lymphotropic retroviruses (HTLV-III) associated with AIDS. *Science*. 1984; 224 (4648): 503–5; Sarngadharan MG, et al. Antibodies reactive with human T-lymphotropic retroviruses (HTLV-III) in the serum of patients with AIDS. *Science*. 1984; 224 (4648): 506–8.
7. Feorino. Blood donor-recipient pair. 1984.
8. Levy JA, et al. Isolation of lymphocytopathic retroviruses from San Francisco patients with AIDS. *Science*. 1984; 225 (4664): 840–42.
9. Petricciani JC. Licensed tests for antibody to human T-lymphotropic virus type III. Sensitivity and specificity. *Ann Intern Med*. 1985; 103 (5): 726–29.

10. Ibid.
11. Staff Report of the Subcommittee on Oversight and Investigations Committee on Energy and Commerce, U.S. House of Representatives. Institutional Response to the HIV blood test patent dispute and related matters. Accessed 10/20/2015.
12. Coffin J, et al. What to call the AIDS virus? *Nature*. 1986; 321 (6065): 10.
13. Chermann JC, Barre-Sinoussi F. Role of human immunodeficiency virus in the physiology of AIDS. *Antibiot Chemother*. 1987; 38: 13–20.
14. Gurgo C, et al. An overview of human T-lymphotropic retroviruses and the role of HTLV-III/LAV in AIDS. *Antibiot Chemother*. 1987; 38: 1–12.
15. Schupbach. Serologic analysis. 1984; Gilden RV et al. HTLV-III Legend Correction. *Science*. 1986; 232 (4748): 307.
16. Beardsley T. AIDS Research. French virus in the picture. *Nature*. 1986; 320: 563.
17. Popovic. Detection, isolation, and continuous production. 1984.

Chapter 6

1. Shilts. *And the Band Played On*. 160–161.
2. Ehrenkranz NJ, Rubini JR. *Pneumocystis carinii* pneumonia complicating hemophilia A. *J Florida MA*. 1983 (Feb); 70 (2): 116–82; CDC. Pneumocystis carinii pneumonia among persons with hemophilia A. *MMWR*. 1982; 31:365–367.
3. Ibid.
4. CDC. Update on AIDS among patients with Hemophilia A. *MMWR*. 1982 (Dec 10); 31(48): 644–652.
5. CDC *Pneumocystis carinii* pneumonia among persons with hemophilia A. 1982; CDC. Update on AIDS. 1982.
6. Ibid.
7. Evatt BL. The tragic history of AIDS in the hemophilia population, 1982–1984. *Journal of Thrombosis and Haemostasis*. 2006 (Sep 14); 4 (11): 1–21.
8. Peterman T, Allen J. Recipients of Blood and Blood Products (Chapter 10, pages 179–193). In: *The Epidemiology of AIDS: Expression, occurrence, and control of Human Immunodeficiency Virus Type 1 infection*, Edited by Kaslow RA, Francis DP. Oxford University Press; 1989.

9. CDC. HIV infection and pregnancies in sexual partners of HIV-seropositive hemophiliac men—United States. *MMWR.* 1987 (Sept 11); 36 (35): 593–5.
10. Ragni MV, et al. HIV transmission to female sexual partners of HIV antibody-positive hemophiliacs. *Public Health Rep.* 1988 (Jan–Feb); 103 (1): 54–8.
11. CDC. Possible transfusion-associated AIDS—California. *MMWR.* 1982; 31:652–654; Ammann AJ, et al. AIDS in an infant: possible transmission by means of blood products. *Lancet.* 1983; i: 956–8.
12. CDC. Possible transfusion-associated AIDS. 1982; Curran JW, et al. AIDS associated with transfusions. *NEJM.* 1984; 310: 69–75.
13. *Ibid.*
14. *And the Band Played On.* HBO Films; 1993.
15. CDC. Current trends prevention of Acquired Immune Deficiency Syndrome (AIDS): Report of Inter-Agency Recommendations. *MMWR.* 1983 (Mar 4); 32 (8): 101–3.
16. *Ibid.*
17. *Ibid.*
18. Haverkos HW. Epidemiology of AIDS in Hemophiliacs and Blood Transfusion Recipients. *Antibiotics and Chemotherapy.* 1987; 38: 59–65.
19. *Ibid.*
20. Peterman TA, et al. Risk of human immunodeficiency virus (HIV) transmission from heterosexual adults with transfusion-associated infections. *JAMA.* 1988; 259:55–8.
21. Lawrence DN. Oral presentation. First International AIDS meeting. Atlanta, Georgia. April 1985.
22. Lui KJ, et al. A model-based approach for estimating the mean incubation period of transfusion-associated AIDS. Proceedings of the National Academy of Sciences USA. 1986; 83: 3051–3055.
23. Lui KJ, et al. A model-based estimate of the mean incubation period for AIDS in homosexual men. *Science.* 1988 Jun 3; 240 (4857): 1333–5.
24. Petricciani JC. Licensed tests for antibodies to human T-lymphotropic virus type III. Sensitivity and specificity. *Ann Intern Med.* 1985; 103 (5): 726–29.
25. Schorr JB, et al. Prevalence of HTLV-III antibody in American blood donors. *N Engl J Med.* 1985 (Aug 8); 313 (6): 384–5.
26. *Ibid.*
27. CDC. Revised Public Health Service definition of persons who should refrain from donating blood and plasma—United States. *MMWR.* 1985 (Sep 06); 34 (35): 547–8.
28. Miller PJ, et al. Potential liability for transfusion-associated AIDS. *JAMA.* 1985 (Jun 21); 253 (23): 3419–24; Matthews GW, Neslund VS. The initial impact of AIDS on public health law in the United States—1986. *JAMA.* 1987 (Jan 16); 257 (3): 344–52.
29. Riding A. A scandal over tainted blood widens in France. *New York Times.* Feb 13, 1994; Section 1; 16.
30. Data Source: CDC. HIV Surveillance Reports Archive. https://www.cdc.gov/hiv/library/reports/surveillance/cdc-hiv-serveillance.html. Accessed 3/17/2023.
31. Epstein JS, et al. Blood system changes since recognition of transfusion-associated AIDS. *Transfusion.* 2013 (Oct); 53: 2365–74.
32. Busch MP, et al. Prevention of transfusion-transmitted infections. *Blood.* 2019; 133: 1854–64 [PMID: 28953438]; FDA. Revised Recommendations for reducing the risk of HIV transmission by blood and blood products: Guidance for Industry. U.S. Department of Health and Human Services. April 2020, updated August 2020.
33. Klamroth R, et al. Pathogen inactivation and removal methods for plasma-derived clotting factor concentrates. *Transfusion.* 2014, 54: 1406–17.
34. Epstein. Blood system changes. 2013.

Chapter 7

1. Shilts. *And the Band Played On.* 168.
2. CDC. Current trends Acquired Immune Deficiency Syndrome (AIDS): Precautions for Clinical and Laboratory Staffs. *MMWR.* 1982 (Nov 5); 31(43): 577–80.
3. *Ibid.*
4. CDC. Recommendations for prevention of HIV transmission in Health-care settings. *MMWR.* 1987 (Aug 21); 36 (SU02): 1–15.

5. CDC. *MMWR* 1982 (Nov 5).
6. *Ibid.*
7. CDC. Epidemiologic Notes and Reports. An Evaluation of the Acquired Immunodeficiency Syndrome (AIDS) Reported in Health Care Personnel—United States. *MMWR.* 1983 (Jul 15); 32 (27): 358–60.
8. CDC. Acquired Immunodeficiency Syndrome (AIDS): Precautions for Health-Care Workers and Allied Professionals. *MMWR.* 1983 (Sep 2); 32 (34): 450–1.
9. CDC. Prospective evaluation of health-care-workers exposed via parenteral or mucous-membrane routes to blood and body fluids of patients with AIDS. *MMWR.* 1984 (Apr 6); 33 (13): 181–2; CDC. *MMWR.* 1983 (Sep 2); CDC. *MMWR.* 1983 (Jul 15); CDC. *MMWR.* 1983 (Sep 2); CDC. *MMWR.* 1984 (Apr 6).
10. CDC. *MMWR.* 1983 (Sep 2).
11. *Ibid.*
12. *Ibid.*
13. CDC. Recommendations for preventing possible transmission of human T-lymphotropic virus type III/lymphadenopathy-associated virus from tears. *MMWR.* 1985 (Aug 30); 34 (34): 533–4.
14. CDC. *MMWR.* 1984 (Apr 6).
15. CDC. Epidemiologic notes and reports update: Evaluation of HTLV-III/LAV infection in health-care personnel. *MMWR.* 1985 (Sep 27); 34 (38); 575–8.
16. *Ibid.*
17. *Ibid.*
18. CDC. Education and foster care of children infected with human T-lymphotropic virus type III/lymphadenopathy-associated virus. *MMWR.* 1985 (Aug 30); 34 (34): 717–21.
19. *Ibid.*
20. CDC. Recommendations for preventing transmission of infection for human T-lymphotropic virus type III /lymphadenopathy-associated virus in the workplace. *MMWR.* 1985 (Nov 15); 34 (45): 681–6, 691–5.
21. *Ibid.*
22. CDC. Apparent transmission of human T-lymphotropic virus type III/ lymphadenopathy-associated virus from a child to a mother providing health care. *MMWR.* 1986 (Feb 07); 35 (5): 76–9.
23. *Ibid.*
24. McCray E. The Cooperative Needlestick Surveillance Group. *N Engl J Med.* 1986 Apr 24; 314 (17):1127–32.
25. *Ibid.*
26. *Ibid.*
27. CDC. Epidemiologic notes and reports update: Human immunodeficiency virus infections in health-care workers exposed to blood of infected patients. *MMWR.* 1987 (May 22); 36 (19): 285–289.
28. CDC. Possible transmission of HIV to a patient during an invasive dental procedure. *MMWR.* 1990 (Jul 27); 39 (20): 489–93.
29. *Ibid.*; Myers G. Molecular investigation of HIV transmission. *Ann Intern Med.* 1994 (Dec 1); 121 (11): 889–90.
30. CDC. Recommendations for prevention of HIV transmission in Healthcare settings. *MMWR.* 1987 (Aug 21); 36 (SU02): 1–15.
31. Kuhar DT, et al. Updated U.S. Public Health Service guidelines for the management of occupational exposures to HIV and recommendations for postexposure prophylaxis. *Infect Control Hosp Epidemiol.* 2013 Sept: 34 (9): 875–92 [PMID: 24042369].

Chapter 8

1. Shilts. *And the Band Played On.* 135.
2. Moskowitz LB, et al. Unusual causes of death in Haitians residing in Miami. High prevalence of opportunistic infections. *JAMA.* 1983; 250: 1187–1191.
3. Memorandum from Harry Haverkos to Task Force Core Group. "Re: Anecdotes of sexual encounters in Haiti." 2 August 1982.
4. Pape JW, et al. Characteristics of AIDS in Haiti. *NEJM.* 1983; 309: 945–950.
5. Vierra J, et al. AIDS in Haitians: Opportunistic infections in previously healthy Haitian immigrants. *N Engl J Med.* 1983; 308: 125–129.
6. Hennigar GR, et al. PCP in an adult. Report of a case. *American Journal of Clinical Pathology.* 1961; 35: 353–364.
7. CDC. Unexplained immunodeficiency and opportunistic infections in infants—New York, New Jersey, California. *MMWR.* 1982; 31: 665–667.
8. Oleske J, et al. Immune deficiency syndrome in children. *JAMA.* 1983 May 6; 249 (17): 2345–2349.

9. CDC. Current trends update: AIDS—USA. *MMWR*. 1984; 32: 688–691 (Pediatric AIDS definition).
10. Scott GB, et al. AIDS in infants. *N Engl J Med*. 1984; 310: 76–81.
11. The Collaborative Study Group of AIDS in Haitian-Americans. Risk Factors for AIDS among Haitians residing in the United States. Evidence of heterosexual transmission. *JAMA*. 1987; 257 (5): 635–39.
12. *Ibid*.
13. Pape JW, et al. AIDS in Haiti. *Ann Intern Med*. 1985; 103: 564–578.
14. *Ibid*.
15. CDC. Current trends update: AIDS—United States. *MMWR*. (May 10, 1985) S4: 245–9.
16. Nordheimer J. Poverty-scarred town now stricken by AIDS. *New York Times*. May 2, 1985; Castro KG, et al. Transmission of HIV in Belle Glade, Florida: Lessons for other communities in the United States. *Science*. 1988; 239 (4836): 193–197.
17. Castro. Transmission of HIV. 1988.
18. CDC. Update: Acquired Immunodeficiency Syndrome (AIDS)—Worldwide. *MMWR*. (May 13, 1988) 37(18): 286–288, 293–295; Piot P, and Quinn TC. Response to the AIDS pandemic—A global health model. *N Engl J Med*. 2013; 368: 2210–2218.
19. Piot. Response to the AIDS pandemic. 2013.
20. *Ibid*.; CDC. Current trends update. May 10, 1985.
21. Piot. Response to the AIDS pandemic. 2013.
22. Haverkos HW, et al. Relative rates of AIDS among racial/ethnic groups by exposure categories. *J Natl Med Assoc*. 1999 Jan; 91 (1): 17–24.
23. Pape JW and Johnson, Jr. WD. HIV-1 infection and AIDS in Haiti, Chapter 12, in: Kaslow RA and Francis DP (editors). *The Epidemiology of AIDS: Expression, Occurrence, and Control of HIV-1 Infection*. Oxford University Press; 1989. 221–230.

Chapter 9

1. Giraldo G, Beth E (editors). Epidemic of AIDS and Kaposi's sarcoma. *Antibiotics and Chemotherapy*. 1984; 32: vii.
2. Clumeck N et al. AIDS in African patients. *N Engl J Med*. 1984; 310:492–7.
3. McCormick JB, Fisher-Hoch S. *Virus Hunters of the CDC: Level 4*. Barnes & Noble Books; 1996.
4. Piot P. *No Time to Lose: A Life in Pursuit of Deadly Viruses*. W.W. Norton & Company; 2012.
5. Piot P et al. AIDS in a heterosexual population in Zaire. *Lancet*. 1984; 2:65–69.
6. Cohen J. The Rise and Fall of Projet SIDA. *Science*. 1997 (Nov 28); 278 (5343): 1565–1568.
7. Mann J, et al. Poster M-43, 1st International AIDS meeting. Atlanta; April 1985; Quinn TC, et al. AIDS in Africa: an epidemiologic paradigm. *Science*. 1986; 234:855–863.
8. *Ibid*.; Quinn TC, Mann JM. HIV infection and AIDS in Africa (chapter 11). In: Kaslow RA and Francis DP (editors). *The Epidemiology of AIDS. Expression, Occurrence, and Control of HIV-1 Infection*. Oxford University Press; 1989. 194–220.
9. Van de Perre P et al. AIDS in Rwanda. *Lancet*. 1984; 2:62–65; Melbye M et al. Evidence for heterosexual transmission and clinical manifestations of HIV infection and related conditions in Lusaka, Zambia. *Lancet*. 1986; 2:1113–1115; Kreiss JK et al. AIDS virus infection in Nairobi prostitutes: Spread of this epidemic to East Africa. *N Engl J Med*. 1986; 314:414–18.
10. Piot. *No Time to Lose*. 2012; Cohen. *Rise and Fall*. 1997.
11. WHO. *Weekly Epidemiological Record*. 1983 Dec 2; 83: 369–71.
12. *Ibid*.
13. WHO. *Weekly Epidemiological Record*. 1986 Mar 7; 10: 70–73.
14. *Ibid*.; McCormick. *Virus Hunters*. 1996.
15. WHO. *Weekly Epidemiological Record*. 1986 Mar 7; 10: 70–73.
16. WHO. *Weekly Epidemiological Record*. 1986 Nov 21; 47: 361–3.
17. *Ibid*.
18. Chin J, Mann JM. The global pattern and prevalence of AIDS and HIV infection. *AIDS*. 1988; 2 (suppl 1): S247–S252; Quinn. AIDS in Africa. 1986.
19. Figure 3 in Chin J, Mann JM. The global pattern.
20. Chin J, Mann JM. The global pattern.
21. *Ibid*.
22. Chin J. Global estimates of HIV

infections and AIDS cases: 1991. *AIDS.* 1991, 5 (suppl 2): S57–S61.
23. Modified table in Chin J. Global estimates.
24. Chin J. *The AIDS Pandemic: The Collision of Epidemiology with Political Correctness.* Radcliffe Publishing; 2007.
25. Quinn. AIDS in Africa. 1986; Quinn. HIV-1 infection. 1989.
26. Bygbjerg IC. AIDS in a Danish surgeon (Zaire, 1976). *Lancet.* 1983 Apr 23; i: 925.
27. Quinn. HIV-1 infection. 1989.
28. Nahmias AJ, et al. Evidence for human infection with an HTLV-III/LAV-like virus in Central Africa, 1959. *Lancet.* 1986; 1:1279–80.
29. McCormick. *Virus Hunters.* 1996; 21. Nzilambi et al. The prevalence of infection with HIV over a 10-year period in rural Zaire. *NEJM.* 1988 Feb 4; 318:276–9.
30. Nzilambi et al. The prevalence of infection.
31. Modified table 2 in Nzilambi et al. The prevalence of infection.
32. Nzilambi et al. The prevalence of infection.
33. Kanki PJ, Barin F, M'Boup S, et al. New human T-lymphotropic retrovirus related to simian T-lymphotropic virus type III (STLV–IIIagm). *Science.* 1986 (Apr 11); 232: 238–43; Clavel F, Mansinho K, Chamaret S, et al. Human immunodeficiency virus type 2 infection associated with AIDS in West Africa. *N Engl J Med.* 1987; 316 (19): 1180–5.
34. *Ibid.*
35. Hemelaar J, et al. Global and regional molecular epidemiology of HIV-1, 1990–2015: a systematic review, global survey, and trend analysis. *Lancet Infect Dis.* 2019; 19: 143–55 Open access; Vallari A, et al. Confirmation of putative HIV-1 group P in Cameroon. *J Virol.* 2011 (Feb 1), 85 (3): https://doi.org/10.1128/jvi.02005-10.
36. Hemelaar. Global and regional molecular epidemiology. 2019.
37. Gao F, et al. Origin of HIV-1 in the chimpanzee, Pan troglodytes. *Nature.* 1999; 397: 436–41; Kalich ML et al. Recombinant viruses and early global HIV-1 epidemic. *Emerging Infectious Diseases.* 2004; 109(7):1227–34.
38. Plotkin SA. CHAT oral polio vaccine was not the source of HIV type 1 Group M for humans. *Clin Infect Dis.* 2001 (Apr 1); 32: 1068–84.
39. Hooper E. *The River: A Journey to the Source of HIV and AIDS.* Little Brown; 1999.
40. *Ibid.*; The Editors. "Origin of AIDS" Update. *Rolling Stone.* 1993 Dec 9: 39.
41. Plotkin. CHAT oral polio vaccine. 2001; Koprowski H. AIDS and the polio vaccine. *Science.* 1992; 257 (5073): 1024–1027.
42. Gryseels S, et al. A near full-length HIV-1 genome from 1966 recovered from formalin-fixed paraffin-embedded tissue. *PNAS.* 2020 May 19; 117 (22): 1222–9.
43. U.S. Department of Health, Education, and Welfare, Public Health Service, National Institutes of Health. National Primate Plan. Prepared by Interagency Primate Steering Committee, Publication No. (NIH) 80–1520; 1978 Oct: 1–98.

Chapter 10

1. Tolstoy L. *War and Peace*, 1869 Book XIII, Chapter 1 (Page 795. Translated by Louise & Aylmer Maude.
2. Jaffe. Epidemiologic results. 1983.
3. Haverkos. Disease manifestation. 1985.
4. *Ibid.*
5. *Ibid.*
6. *Ibid.*
7. *Ibid.*
8. *Ibid.*
9. *Ibid.*
10. *Ibid.*
11. *Ibid.*
12. Berg P. Use of "poppers" linked to Kaposi's sarcoma. *Washington Post.* 1985 April 24.
13. Moss AR, et al. Risk factors for AIDS and HIV seropositivity in homosexual men. *Am J Epidemiol.* 1987 Jun; 125 (6): 1035–47.
14. Haverkos. Disease manifestation. 1985.
15. Moss. Risk factors for AIDS and HIV. 1987.
16. Haverkos. Disease manifestation. 1985; Haverkos HW, et al. Nitrite inhalants: History, epidemiology, and possible links to AIDS. *Environ Health Perspect.* 1994; 102 (10) 858–61.
17. Montagnier L, Blanchard A. Myco-

plasmas as cofactors in infection due to the human immunodeficiency virus. *Clin Infect Dis.* 1993 Aug; 17 Suppl 1: S309–15.
 18. Duesberg P. Retroviruses as carcinogens and pathogens: Expectations and reality. *Cancer Research.* 1987 Mar 1; 47 (5): 1199–220; Duesberg P. *Inventing the AIDS Virus.* Regnery Publishing; 1996.
 19. Cohen J. AIDS research. Keystone's blunt message: "It's the virus, stupid." *Science.* 1993; 260: 292–3.

Chapter 11

 1. Harden VA. *AIDS at 30: A History.* Potomac Books; 2012. 125.
 2. PCP Therapy Project Group, Coordinator: Haverkos HW. Assessment of therapy for *Pneumocystis carinii* pneumonia. *Am J Med.* 1984; 76:501–508.
 3. *Ibid.*
 4. *Ibid.*
 5. *Ibid.*
 6. *Ibid.*
 7. Fauci AS (moderator). AIDS conference June 23, 1983: Epidemiology, clinical, immunologic, and therapeutic considerations. *Ann Intern Med.* 1984; 100: 92–106.
 8. *Ibid.*
 9. *Ibid.*; Lane HC et al. Partial reconstitution in a patient with AIDS. *N Engl J Med.* 1984 Oct 25; 311 (17): 1099–1103.
 10. Fauci AS (moderator). AIDS conference November 26, 1984: An update. *Ann Intern Med.* 1985; 102: 800–13; Lane HC, et al. Use of interleukin-2 therapy in patients with AIDS. *J Biol Response Mod.* 1984; 3: 512–16; INSIGHT-ESPRIT Study Group. Interleukin-2 therapy in patients with HIV infection. *NEJM.* 2009; 361:1548–59.
 11. Fauci. AIDS conference. 1983 and 1984; Volberding PA, et al. Recombinant interferon alpha in the treatment of AIDS-related Kaposi's sarcoma. *Seminars in Oncology.* 1985; 12(Suppl 5); 2–6.

Chapter 12

 1. Shilts. *And the Band Played On.* 93.
 2. TE Study Group, Coordinator: Haverkos HW. Assessment of therapy for *Toxoplasma* encephalitis. *Am J Med.* 1987 May; 82: 907–14.
 3. Sell KW, et al. Cyclosporine immunosuppression as the possible cause of AIDS. *N Engl J Med.* 1983 Oct 27; 309 (17): 1065.
 4. Kurian GT. *Government: A Historical Guide to the U.S. Government.* Oxford University Press; 1998. 408–414.
 5. *Ibid.*
 6. *Ibid.*

Chapter 13

 1. From an interview with Dr. Richard Krause at the NIH. November 17, 1988. Posted on the NIH website, "In their Own Words."
 2. "Update on the Status of Sodomy Laws," American Civil Liberties Union, Accessed February 16, 2023.
 3. Kinsey AC, et al. *Sexual Behavior in the Human Male.* W.B. Saunders; 1948.
 4. *Ibid.*
 5. Carter D. *Stonewall: The Riots that Sparked the Gay Revolution.* St. Martin's Press, 2004.
 6. *Ibid.*
 7. Cured. Independent Lens. WETA, Public Broadcasting Service, Season 23, Episode 1, released October 11, 2021; Lazarus A. Medical leadership and the strange case of "Dr. H. Anonymous." *The Pharos.* Winter 2019: 40–44.
 8. Jaffe HW, et al. National case-control study of Kaposi's sarcoma and *Pneumocystis carinii* pneumonia in homosexual men: Part 1. Epidemiologic results. *Ann Intern Med.* 1983; 99 (92): 145–51.
 9. Bland EF, and Jones TD. Rheumatic fever and rheumatic heart disease: A twenty-year report on 1000 followed since childhood. *Circulation.* 1951 Dec; 4: 836–43.
 10. Kaslow RA, et al. The Multicenter AIDS Cohort Study (MACS): Rationale, organization, and selected characteristics of the participants. *Am J Epidemiol.* 1987; 126 (2) :310–8.
 11. Winkelstein W, Jr., et al. Sexual practices and risk of infection by HIV. The San Francisco Men's Health Study. *JAMA,* 1987; 257:321–325.
 12. *Ibid.*; Kaslow. MACS. 1987.
 13. *Ibid.*
 14. Petricciani JC. Licensed tests for antibody to human T-lymphotropic virus type III: sensitivity and specificity. *Ann Intern Med.* 1985; 103: 726–9.

15. Bayer R, et al. HIV antibody screening. An ethical framework for evaluating proposed programs. *JAMA*. 1986; 256 (13):1768–74.
16. Shilts. *And the Band Played On*. 540–542.
17. CDC. Human T-lymphotropic virus type III/lymphadenopathy-associated virus antibody testing at alternate sites. *MMWR*. 1986 May 2; 35 (17): 284–7.
18. CDC. Current Trends. Additional recommendations to reduce sexual and drug abuse-related transmission of Human T-Lymphotropic virus type III/Lymphadenopathy-associated virus. *MMWR*. 1986 Mar 14; 35 (10): 152–5.
19. *Ibid*.
20. *Ibid*.
21. Shilts. *And the Band Played On*.
22. Gostin LO. *The AIDS Pandemic: Complacency, Injustice and Unfulfilled Expectations*. University of North Carolina Press; 2004; Matthews and Newlund. The initial impact of AIDS on public health law in the U.S.—1986. *JAMA*. 1987; 257: 344–52.
23. Kramer L. *The Tragedy of Today's Gays*. Jeremy P. Tarcher/Penguin; 2005.
24. Bayer. HIV antibody screening. 1986.
25. *Ibid*.
26. *Ibid*.
27. Kingsley LA, et al. Risk factors for seroconversion to human immunodeficiency virus among male homosexuals. Results from the Multicenter AIDS Cohort Study. *Lancet*. 1987; i (8529): 345–9.
28. *Ibid*.
29. Jaffe. National case-control study. 1983.
30. Kingsley. Risk factors. 1987.
31. Winkelstein. Sexual practices. 1987; Winkelstein W Jr., et al. The San Francisco Men's Health Study: III. Reduction in HIV transmission among homosexual/bisexual men, 1982–1986. *Am J Public Health*. 1987; 76 (9): 685–89.
32. Jaffe. National case-control study. 1983.
33. *Ibid*.; Kinsley. Risk factors. 1987; Winkelstein. Sexual practices. 1987; Winkelstein. San Francisco. 1987.
34. Samuel MC, et al. Factors associated with human immunodeficiency virus seroconversion in homosexual men in three San Francisco cohort studies, 1984–1989.

Journal of AIDS. 6 (3): 303–12; Ostrow DG, et al. A case-control study of human immunodeficiency virus type 1 seroconversion and risk-related behaviors in the Chicago Multicenter/CCS cohort, 1984–1992. *Am J Epidemiol*. 1995; 142: 875–83; Chu SY, et al. Epidemiology of reported cases of AIDS in lesbians, United States 1980–89. *Am J Public Health*. 1990; 80 (11): 1380–1.
35. Kingsley. Risk factors. 1987.
36. Ostrow DG, et al. Disclosure of HIV antibody status: Behavioral and mental health correlates. *AIDS Education and Prevention*. 1989; 1 (1): 1–11.
37. Abid SM, et al. Predictors of relapse in sexual practices among homosexual men. *AIDS Education and Prevention*. 1991; 3 (4): 293–304.
38. Pantaleo G, et al. The immunopathogenesis of HIV infection. *N Engl J Med*. 1993 Feb 4; 328 (5): 327–35.
39. Lui KJ, et al. A model-based approach for estimating the mean incubation period of transfusion-associated AIDS. *Proceedings of the National Academy of Sciences USA*. 1986; 83:3051–3055; Lui KJ, et al. A model-based estimate of the mean incubation period for AIDS in homosexual men. *Science*. 1988 Jun 3; 240 (4857): 1333–5.
40. *Ibid*.

Chapter 14

1. Campbell DJ. Venereal Diseases in the Armed Forces overseas. *Br J Venereal Dis*. 1946; 22: 158–64.
2. Redfield RR, et al. Frequent transmission of HTLV-III among spouses of patients with AIDS-related complex and AIDS. *JAMA*. 1985 Mar 15; 253 (11): 1571–3.
3. Haverkos HW, Edelman R. Female-to-male transmission of AIDS. *JAMA* (letter). 1985 Aug 23; 254 (8): 1036–7.
4. Redfield RR, et al. Heterosexually acquired HTLV-III/LAV disease (AIDS-related complex and AIDS). *JAMA*. 1985 Oct 18; 254: 561–3.
5. Polk BF. Female-to-male transmission of AIDS. *JAMA* (letter). 1985 Dec 13; 254 (22): 3177–8.
6. Tramont EC, et al. HTLV-III/LAV infections in the military. *Military Med*. 1987 (Feb); 152: 105–6.
7. Burke DS, et al. HIV infections

among civilian applicants for United States military service, October 1985 to March 1986: demographic factors associated with seropositivity. *N Engl J Med.* 1987: 317: 131–136.

8. McNeil JG, et al. Direct measurement of HIV seroconversion in a serially tested population of young adults in the U.S. Army, October 1985 to October 1987. *N Engl J Med.* 1989; 320: 1561–5.

9. Morgan WM, Curran JW. AIDS: Current and future trends. *Public Health Reports.* 1986; 101: 459–65.

10. Langmuir AD. AIDS projections are too high. In: *Pan American Health Organization, AIDS: Profile of an epidemic.* Scientific Publication No. 514; 1989 pp 179–185.

11. Masters WH, Johnson VE, et al. *Crisis: Heterosexual Behavior in the Age of AIDS.* Grove Press; 1988. 47–68.

12. Ibid.

13. Haverkos HW, Edelman R. The epidemiology of AIDS among heterosexuals. *JAMA.* 1988 Oct 07; 260 (13): 1922–9.

14. Ibid.

15. Handsfield HH. Heterosexual Transmission of HIV. *JAMA.* 1988 Oct 07; 260 (13):1943–4.

16. Edelman R, Haverkos HW. The suitability of HIV-positive individuals for marriage and pregnancy. *JAMA.* 1989; 261: 993.

17. Petersen LR, White CR. Premarital screening for antibodies to HIV type 1 in the United States. The Premarital Screening Study Group. *Am J Public Health.* 1990 Sep 1; 80 (9): 1087–90.

18. Ibid.

19. Quinn TC, et al. Viral load and heterosexual transmission of human immunodeficiency virus type 1. *N Engl J Med.* 2000 Mar 30; 342 (13): 921–2.

20. Piot P, Quinn TC. Global health: Response to the AIDS pandemic—a global health model. *N Engl J Med.* 2013 Jun 6; 368 (23): 2210–8.

Chapter 15

1. Shilts. *And the Band Played On.* 496.

2. Fauci AS, et al. The Acquired Immunodeficiency Syndrome: an update. *Ann Intern Med.* 1985 June; 102 (6): 800–13; Masur H. Prevention and treatment of Pneumocystis pneumonia. *N Engl J Med.* 1992 Dec 24; 327 (26): 1853–60.

3. Masur. Prevention and treatment. 1992.

4. Ibid.

5. The TE Study Group, Haverkos HW (Coordinator). Assessment of therapy for *Toxoplasma* encephalitis. *Am J Med.* 1987 May; 82 (5): 907–14.

6. Ibid.

7. Ibid.

8. Fauci AS. AIDS: an update. 1985; Porter SB, Sande MA. Toxoplasmosis of the central nervous system in the Acquired Immunodeficiency Syndrome. *N Engl J Med.* 1992 Dec 3; 327 (23): 1643–8.

9. Skowron G, Merigan TC. Chapter 17 Chemotherapy and Chemoprophylaxis. In: Kaslow RA, Francis DP. *The Epidemiology of AIDS: Expression, Occurrence, and Control of HIV-1 Infection.* Oxford University Press; 1989.

10. Rozenbaum W, et al. Antimoniotungstate (HPA 23) treatment of three patients with AIDS and one with prodrome. *Lancet.* 1985 Feb 23; 1 (8426): 450–1.

11. Dormont D, Maillet T, Di Maria H, et al. Second International Conference on AIDS. Paris; June 23–25, 1986.

12. Shilts. *And the Band Played On.* 1987.

13. Skowron. Chemotherapy and Chemoprophylaxis. 1989.

14. Mitsuya H, et al. Functional properties of antigen-specific T cells infected by Human T-Cell Leukemia-Lymphoma Virus (HTLV-I). *Science.* 1984; 225: 1484–86.

15. Mitsuya H, et al. Suramin protection of T cells in vitro against infectivity and cytopathic effect of HTLV-III/LAV. *Science.* 1984; 226: 172–4.

16. Skowron. Chemotherapy and Chemoprophylaxis. 1989; Fauci AS, Lane HC. *Annales de l'Institute Pasteur/Immunologie.* 1987; 138: 261.

17. Shilts. *And the Band Played On.* 1987.

18. Kweder SL, O'Neill RT, Beninger P. The New Drug Evaluation Process: FDA perspective. Chapter 3. In: Finklestein DM, Schoenfeld DA (editors). *AIDS Clinical Trials: Guidelines for Design and Analysis.* Wiley-Liss; 1995.

19. Ibid.

20. Broder S. Strategies for Experimental Therapy of the Retrovirus which causes AIDS. Chapter 30 In: Gluckman

JC, Vilmer E (editors); *Acquired Immunodeficiency Syndrome*. Elsevier; 1987; Yarchoan R, et al. Clinical pharmacology of 3'-azido2.'3'-dideoxythymidine (zidovudine) and related dideoxynucleotides. *N Engl J Med*. 1989 Sep 14: 321 (11): 726–38; Harden VA. *AIDS at 30: A History*. Potomac Books; 2012.
21. *Ibid*.
22. Fischl MA, Richman DD, Grieco MH, et al. The efficacy of azidothymidine (AZT) in the treatment of patients with AIDS and AIDS-related complex. A double-blind, placebo-controlled trial. *N Engl J Med*. 1987 Jul 23: 317 (4): 185–91.
23. *Ibid*.
24. Richman DD, Fischl MA, Grieco MH, et al. The toxicity of azidothymidine (AZT) in the treatment of patients with AIDS and AIDS-related complex: a double-blind, placebo-controlled trial. *N Engl J Med*. 1987 Jul 23; 317 (4): 192–7.
25. Wastila LJ, Lasagna L. The history of zidovudine (AZT). *Journal of Clinical Research and Pharmacoepidemiology*. 1990; 4: 25–37.
26. *Ibid*.
27. Fauci AS, et al. Ending the HIV epidemic: a plan for the United States. *JAMA*. 2019; 321 (9): 844–5.
28. Pitasi MA, et al. HIV testing in 50 local jurisdictions accounting for the majority of new HIV diagnoses and seven states with disproportionate occurrence of HIV in rural areas, 2016–2017. *MMWR*. 2019 Jun 28; 68 (25): 561–7.
29. Parran T. Syphilis: a public health problem. *Science*. 1938; 87(2251): 147–52.
30. CDC, Association of Public Health Laboratories. Laboratory testing for the diagnosis of HIV infection: updated recommendations. http://stacks.cdc.gov/view/cdc/23447. Published June 27, 2014, updated January 2019.

Chapter 16

1. Rothman KJ, Greenland S. *Modern Epidemiology*, second edition. Lippincott-Raven; 1998, 8.
2. Polk F, et al. Predictors of AIDS developing in a cohort of seropositive homosexual men. *N Engl J Med*. 1987; 316: 62–66.
3. Haverkos HW, Dougherty JA (editors). *Health Hazards of Nitrite Inhalants: NIDA Research Monograph 83*. U.S. Government Printing Office; 1988.
4. Haverkos HW, Drotman DP. Measuring inhalant nitrite exposure in gay men: implications for elucidating the etiology of AIDS-related Kaposi's sarcoma. In: Duesberg PH (editor). *AIDS: Virus- or Drug-Induced?* Kluwer Academic Publishers; 1996: 151–8.
5. *Ibid*.
6. Polk. Predictors of AIDS. 1987.
7. *Ibid*.
8. *Ibid*.
9. Haverkos HW, et al. Nitrite inhalants: History, epidemiology, and possible links to AIDS. *Environ Health Perspect*. 1994; 102 (10): 858–61.
10. *Ibid*.; Polk. Predictors of AIDS. 1987.
11. Personal communication, David Ostrow, M.D., Chicago, 2005.
12. Haverkos HW. Viruses, chemicals and co-carcinogenesis. *Oncogene*. 2004; 23: 6492–99.
13. Polk. Predictors of AIDS. 1987; Haverkos. Nitrite inhalants. 1994.
14. Haverkos. Nitrite inhalants. 1994.
15. Polk. Predictors of AIDS. 1987.
16. Armenian HK, et al. Composite risk score for KS based on a case-control and longitudinal study in MACS population. *Am J Epidemiol*. 1993; 138: 256–65.
17. Lauritsen J. NIDA meeting calls for research into the poppers–Kaposi's sarcoma connection. In: Duesberg PH (editor). *AIDS: Virus- or Drug Induced?* Kluwer Academic Publishers; 1996: 325–330.
18. Haverkos HW, Drotman DP. NIDA technical review: nitrite inhalants. *Biomed & Pharmacother*. 1996; 50: 228–30.
19. Haverkos. Nitrite inhalants. 1994.
20. Chang Y, et al. Identification of herpesvirus-like DNA sequences in AIDS-associated KS. *Science*. 1994; 266: 1865–1869.
21. Brunton TL. On the use of nitrite of amyl in angina pectoris. *Lancet*. 1867; 2: 97.
22. Frye WB. T. Lauder Brunton and amyl nitrite: a Victorian vasodilator. *Circulation*. 1986; 74 (2): 222–9.
23. Kaposi M. Idiopathic multiple pigmented sarcoma of the skin. *CA Cancer J Clin*. 1982; 1982; 32 (6): 342–347. Translated from German and reprinted from *Archiv Fur Dermatologie Und Syphilis*. 1872; 4: 265–273.

24. *Ibid.*
25. Surveillance, Epidemiology, and End Results: Incidence and mortality data, 1973-1977. NCI Monograph 57, NIH Publication No 81-2330. National Cancer Institute; 1981.
26. Safai B, et al. Association of Kaposi's sarcoma with second primary malignancies: possible etiopathogenic implications. *Cancer.* 1980; 45: 1472–9.
27. Safai B, Good RA. Kaposi's sarcoma: a review and recent developments. *CA—A Journal for Clinicians.* 1981; 31: 2–12.
28. Friedman-Kien AE. *Color Atlas of AIDS.* W.B. Saunders; 1989.
29. Giraldo G, et al. Kaposi's sarcoma: a new model in the search for viruses associated with human malignancies. *J Natl Cancer Inst.* 1972; 49: 1497–1507.
30. Giraldo G, Beth E, and Huang ES. KS and its relationship to CMV. *Int J Cancer.* 1980; 26: 23–29.
31. Levy JA, Pan L-Z, Beth-Giraldo E, et al. Absence of antibodies to the human immunodeficiency virus in sera from Africa prior to 1975. *Proc Natl Acad Sci USA.* 1986 Oct; 83: 7935–37.
32. Chang Y, Cesarman E, Pessin MS, et al. Identification of herpesvirus-like DNA sequences in AIDS-associated Kaposi's sarcoma. *Science.* 1994; 265: 1865–9.
33. Pauk J, Huang ML, Brodie SJ, et al. Mucosal shedding of human herpes virus 8 in men. *N Engl J Med.* 2000; 343: 1369–1377.
34. Giraldo. Kaposi's sarcoma. 1972.
35. Ziegler JL. Endemic KS in Africa and local volcanic soils. *Lancet.* 1993; 342: 1348–51; Ziegler JL, Simonart T, Snoeck R. Kaposi's sarcoma, oncogenic viruses and iron. *J Clin Virol.* 2001 Feb; 20 (3): 127–30.
36. Myers BD, et al. Kaposi's sarcoma in kidney transplant recipients. *Arch Intern Med.* 1974; 133:307–11; Penn I. Kaposi's sarcoma in organ transplant recipients: report of 20 cases. *Transplantation.* 1979; 27: 8–11; Hoshaw RA, Schwartz RA. Kaposi's sarcoma after immunosuppressive therapy with prednisone. *Arch Dermatol.* 1980; 116: 1280–2.
37. Haverkos HW. Multifactorial etiology of Kaposi's sarcoma: a hypothesis. *J Biosci.* 2008 Dec; 33 (5): 643–51.
38. CDC. Kaposi's sarcoma and *Pneumocystis* pneumonia among homosexual men—New York City and California. *MMWR.* 1981; 30 (25): 305–8.
39. Jaffe. Epidemiologic results. 1983; Rogers. Laboratory results. 1983.
40. Barre-Sinoussi. Isolation of a T-lymphotropic retrovirus. 1983.
41. Haverkos. Disease manifestation. 1985.
42. Marquart KH, et al. Disseminated Kaposi's sarcoma that is not associated with AIDS in a bisexual man. *Arch Pathol Lab Med.* 1986; 110:346–7.
43. Friedman-Kien AE, et al. Kaposi's sarcoma in HIV-negative homosexual men. *Lancet.* 1990; 335: 168–9.
44. Cesarman E, et al. Kaposi sarcoma: a primer. *Nat Rev Dis Primers.* 2019; 5 (1): 9.
45. Modified from Table 1 in Openshaw MR, et al. Taxonomic reclassification of Kaposi sarcoma identifies disease entities with distinct immunopathogenesis. *Journal of Translational Medicine.* 2023; 21: 283. https://doi.org/10.1186/s12967-023-04130-6.
46. Modified from Table 1 in Ruocco E, et al. Kaposi's sarcoma: Etiology and pathogenesis, inducing factors, causal associations, and treatment: Facts and controversies. *Clinics in Dermatology.* 2013; 31: 413–22.
47. Openshaw. Taxonomic reclassification. 2023.
48. Modified from Openshaw. Taxonomic reclassification. 2023.
49. Openshaw. Taxonomic reclassification. 2023.

Chapter 17

1. Kuhn TS. *The Structure of Scientific Revolutions.* University of Chicago Press; 1962. 144–5.
2. Koch R. *Reichsgesundheitsamt Mitteilungen.* 1884. Translated in Lechvalier & Solortorovsky. *Three Centuries of Microbiology.* Dover Publications; 1974. 85–109.
3. Snow J. The Cholera near Golden Square. In: Buck C, Llopis A, Najera E, Terris M (Editors). *The Challenge of Epidemiology: Issues and Selected Readings.* Pan American Health Organization; 1988. 415–418; Snow J. On the mode of communication of cholera. In: *The Challenge of Epidemiology: Issues and Selected Readings.* 1988. 42–45.

4. Howard-Jones N. Robert Koch and the cholera vibrio: a centenary. *Br Med J.* 1984 Feb 4; 288: 379–81.
5. *Ibid.*
6. Feorino PM, Kalyanaraman VS, Haverkos HW, et al. Lymphadenopathy associated virus infection of a blood donor—recipient pair with AIDS. *Science.* 1984; 225 (4657): 69–72.
7. Hill AB. The Environment and Disease: Association or Causation? *Proc R Soc Med.* 1965 May: 58 (5): 295–300. PMID 142 83879.
8. Doll R, Hill AB. Smoking and carcinoma of the lung: Preliminary report. *Br Med J.* 1950 Sep 30; 2 (4682): 739–48. doi: 10.1136/bmj.2.4682.739; CDC Epidemiology Program Office: Case studies in applied epidemiology. Cigarette Smoking and Lung Cancer, No. 731–703, EIS Summer Course, 2003.
9. *Ibid.*
10. Doll. Smoking and carcinoma. 1950.
11. Doll R, Hill AB. Mortality in relation to smoking: Ten years' observations of British doctors. *Br Med J.* 1964; 1: 1399–1410.
12. *Ibid.*
13. *Ibid.*
14. CDC. Case studies. 2003.
15. Hill. The Environment and Disease. 1965.
16. U.S. Department of Health, Education, and Welfare. *Smoking and Health.* Public Health Service Publication No. 1103; 1964.
17. Hill. The Environment and Disease. 1965.
18. *Ibid.*
19. Rothman KJ. Causes. *Am J Epidemiol.* 1976 (Dec); 104 (6): 587–92.
20. Mahmood SS, Levy D, Vasan RS, Wang TJ. The Framingham Heart Study and the Epidemiology of Cardiovascular Diseases: A Historical Perspective. *Lancet.* 2014 (March 15; 383 (9921): 999–1008.
21. *Ibid.*
22. *Ibid.*
23. Dawber TR, et al. Epidemiologic Approaches to Heart Disease: The Framingham Study. *Am J Public Health.* 1951 (Mar); 41: 279–86; Dawber TR, et al. Coronary Heart Disease in the Framingham Study. *Am J Public Health.* 1957 (Apr); 47 (4 Pt 2): 4–24; Dawber TR, et al. An Approach to Longitudinal Studies in a Community: The Framingham Study. *Ann NY Acad Sci.* 1963; 107:539–556.
24. Dawber. Coronary Heart Disease. 1957.
25. *Ibid.*
26. Kannel WB. An overview of the risk factors for cardiovascular disease. In: *The Challenges of Epidemiology: Issues and Selected Reading.* Buck C, et al. (editors). Pan American Health Organization, Scientific Publication No. 505; 1988. 699–718.
27. Truett J, et al. A multivariate analysis of the risk of coronary heart disease in Framingham. *J Chron Dis.* 1967; 20: 511–524.
28. Modified table in Truett J, et al. A multivariate analysis.
29. Kannel. An overview. 1988.
30. Modified table in Kannel. An overview.
31. Truett. A multivariate analysis.
32. Ford ES, Ajani UA, Croft JB, et al. Explaining the decrease in U.S. deaths, 1980–2000. *N Engl J Med.* 2007; 356: 2388–98.
33. *Ibid.*
34. Rogers. Laboratory results. 1983.
35. Haverkos. Disease manifestation. 1985.
36. Varani S, Landini MP. Cytomegalovirus-induced immunopathology and its clinical consequences. *Herpesviridae.* 2011; 2: 9. Published online 2011 Apr 7. doi: 10.1186/2042-4280-2-6. PMID 2147 3750; Varani S et al. Human cytomegalovirus targets different subsets of antigen-presenting cells with pathological consequences for host immunity: implications for immunosuppression, chronic inflammation and autoimmunity. *Rev Med Virol.* 2009 May; 19 (3): 131–45.
37. Jaffe. Epidemiologic results. 1983.
38. *Ibid.*
39. Table two in chapter 10 of Haverkos. Disease manifestation. 1985.
40. *Ibid.*; Moss. Risk factors. 1987; Armenian. Composite risk. 1993; Haverkos. Measuring inhalant. 1996.
41. Haverkos. Measuring inhalant. 1996.
42. Frye WB. T. Lauder Brunton and amyl nitrite: a Victorian vasodilator. *Circulation.* 1986; 74 (2): 222–9.
43. Haverkos. Measuring inhalant. 1996.
44. Dax EM, et al. Amyl nitrite alters human in vitro immune function. *Immuno-*

pharmacol Immunotoxicol. 1991; 13: 577-87.
45. Haverkos. Nitrite inhalants. 1994.
46. Haverkos. Disease manifestation. 1985.
47. *Ibid.*
48. Barre-Sinoussi. Isolation of a T-lymphotropic retrovirus. 1983.
49. Chang. Identification of herpesvirus-like DNA sequences. 1994.
50. Moore PS, Chang Y. The conundrum of causality in tumor virology: the cases of KSHV and MCV. *Seminars in Cancer Biology.* 2014; 26: 4-12.

Chapter 18

1. Haverkos HW. Viruses, chemicals and co-carcinogenesis. *Oncogene.* 2004; 23: 6492-99.
2. Rigoni-Stern D. Statistical facts about cancers on which Dr. Rigoni-Stern based his contribution to the Surgeons' subgroup at the IV Congress of the Italian Scientists on September 23, 1842. Translated by Bianca De Stavola. *Statistics in Medicine.* 1987; 6:881-4.
3. zur Hausen H. Human genital cancer: synergism between two virus infections or synergism between a virus and initiating events? *Lancet.* 1982; 2:1370-2.
4. Winkelstein W Jr., et al. Correlations of incidence rates for selected cancers in the nine areas of the Third National Cancer Survey. *American Journal of Epidemiology.* 1977; 105:407-9.
5. Winkelstein W Jr. Smoking and cervical cancer—current status: a review. *American Journal of Epidemiology.* 1990; 131: 945-57.
6. Haverkos HW, et al. Cigarette smoking and cervical cancer; Part 1: a meta-analysis. *Biomedicine and Pharmacotherapy.* 2003; 57:67-77.
7. Steckley SL, et al. Cigarette smoking and cervical cancer: Part II: a geographic variability study. *Biomedicine and Pharmacotherapy.* 2003; 57:78-83.
8. Working Group on the Evaluation of Carcinogenic Risks to Humans [IARC]. Tobacco smoke and involuntary smoking. IARC Monograph on Evaluation of Carcinogenic Risks to Humans. 2004; 83:1-1438; Haverkos HW, et al. Co-carcinogenesis: Human papillomaviruses, coal tar derivatives, and squamous cell cervical cancer. *Frontiers in Microbiology.* 2017; 8.2253.
9. *Ibid.*
10. International Collaboration of Epidemiologic Studies of Cervical Cancer (ICESCC). Comparison of risk factors for invasive squamous cell carcinoma and adenocarcinoma of the cervix: Collaborative reanalysis of individual data on 8,097 women with squamous cell carcinoma and 1,374 women with adenocarcinoma from 12 epidemiologic studies. *Int J Cancer.* 2007; 120: 885-91.
11. *Ibid.*
12. *Ibid.*; International Collaboration of Epidemiologic Studies of Cervical Cancer (ICESCC). Carcinoma of the cervix and tobacco smoking collaborative reanalysis of individual data on 13,541 women with carcinoma of the cervix and 23,017 women without carcinoma of the cervix from 23 epidemiologic studies. *Int J Cancer.* 2006; 118: 1481-95.
13. Ferrara A, et al. Co-factors related to the causal relationship between HPV and invasive cervical cancer in Honduras. *Int J Epidemiol.* 2000; 29:817-25.
14. Bennett C, et al. Commentary: Human papillomavirus and tar hypothesis for squamous cell cervical cancer. *Journal of Biosciences.* 2010; 35: 331-7.
15. Smith FR. Etiologic factors in carcinoma of the cervix. *American Journal of Obstetrics and Gynecology.* 1931; 21:18-25.
16. Lombard HL, Potter EA. Epidemiologic aspects of cancer of the cervix. *Cancer.* 1950; 3: 960-8; Rotkin ID. Epidemiology of cancer of the cervix. 3. Sexual characteristics of a cervical cancer population. *American Journal of Public Health.* 1967; 57: 815-29.
17. Haverkos H, et al. The cause of invasive cervical cancer could be multifactorial. *Biomed Pharmacother.* 2000; 54:54-9.
18. *Ibid.*
19. Rous P, Kidd JG. The carcinogenic effect of a papilloma virus on the tarred skin of rabbits. I. Description of the phenomenon. *Journal of Experimental Medicine.* 1938; 67: 399-428; Rogers S, Rous P. Joint action of a chemical carcinogen and a neoplastic virus to induce cancer in rabbits: Results of exposing epidermal cells to a carcinogenic hydrocarbon at the time of infection with Shope papilloma virus.

Journal of Experimental Medicine. 1951; 93: 459–88.

20. Working Group on the Evaluation of Carcinogenic Risks to Humans [IARC] Human Papillomaviruses. IARC Monograph on the Evaluation of Carcinogenic Risk to Humans. 1995; 64:1–379.

21. *Ibid.*; International Collaboration of Epidemiologic Studies of Cervical Cancer (ICESCC). Comparison of risk factors for invasive squamous cell carcinoma and adenocarcinoma of the cervix. 2006; 885–91; zur Hausen H. Papillomaviruses in the causation of human cancers—a brief historical account. *Virology.* 2009; 384:260–5; Bzhala D, et al. International standardization and classification of human papillomavirus types. *Virology.* 2015; 476: 341–4.

22. Future II Study Group. Quadrivalent vaccine against human papillomavirus to prevent high-grade cervical lesions. *N Engl J Med.* 2007; 356: 1915–27.

23. (SEARCH) Writing Group for the SEARCH for Diabetes in Youth Study Group. 2007. Incidence of diabetes in youth in the United States. *JAMA.* 2007; 297: 2716–24.

24. Adams SF. The seasonal variation in the onset of acute diabetes. *Arch Intern Med.* 1926; 37: 861–4.

25. Helfand, RF, et al. Serologic evidence of an association between enteroviruses and the onset of type 1 diabetes mellitus. *J. Infect. Dis.* 1995; 172: 1206–11; Oberste MS, Pallansch MA. Establishing evidence for enterovirus infection in chronic diseases. *Annals of the New York Academy of Sciences.* 2003; 1005: 23–31; Yeung WG, et al. Enterovirus infection and type 1 diabetes mellitus: systematic review meta-analysis of observational molecular studies. *British Medical Journal.* 2011; 342: 35.

26. Yoon JW, et al. Isolation of a virus from the pancreas of a child with diabetic ketoacidosis (virus induced diabetes mellitus). *N Engl J Med.* 1979; 300: 1173–9.

27. Concannon P, et al. Genetics of type 1A diabetes. *N Engl J Med.* 2009; 360: 1646–54; Concannon P, et al. Type 1 diabetes: evidence for susceptibility loci from four genome-wide linkage scans in 1,435 multiplex families. *Diabetes.* 2005; 54: 29995–3001.

28. Hypponen E, et al. Intake of vitamin D and risk of type 1 diabetes: a birth-cohort study. *Lancet.* 2001; 358: 1500–3.

29. Dahlquist, GG, et al. Dietary factors and the risk of developing insulin dependent diabetes in childhood. *British Medical Journal.* 1990; 300: 1302–6; Dahlquist GG, et al. The Swedish Childhood Diabetes Study—a multivariate analysis of risk determinants for diabetes in different age groups. *Diabetologia.* 1991; 34: 757–62.

30. Kalits I, Podar T. Incidence and prevalence of type 1 (insulin-dependent) diabetes in Estonia in 1988. *Diabetologia.* 1990; 33: 346–9; LaPorte RE, et al. Differences between blacks and whites in the epidemiology of insulin-dependent diabetes mellitus in Allegheny County, Pennsylvania. *American Journal of Epidemiology.* 1986; 123: 592–603.

31. Jankowsky C, et al. Viruses and vitamin D in the etiology of type 1 diabetes mellitus and multiple sclerosis. *Virus Research.* 2012; 163: 424–30.

32. *Ibid.*; Haverkos HW, et al. Enteroviruses and type 1 diabetes mellitus. *Biomedicine and Pharmacotherapy.* 2003; 57: 379–85.

33. *Ibid.*

34. Modified from Haverkos HW. HIV is necessary but not sufficient for AIDS. *Journal of Biosciences.* 2003; 28: 365–6.

35. Loh S-W et al. Primary cutaneous apocrine carcinoma. *Annals of Dermatology.* 2016; 28: 699–700.

Epilogue

1. World Health Organization (WHO) website on AIDS. Accessed 10/29/2023.

2. Piot P, Quinn TC. Response to the AIDS pandemic—a global health model. *N Engl J Med.* 2013; 368 (23): 2210–18.

3. Moore. Conundrum of causality in tumor virology. 2014.

4. Musher DM, Abers MS, Corrales-Medina VF. Acute infection and myocardial infarction. *N Engl J Med.* 2019; 180: 171–6.

5. Haverkos. Viruses, chemicals and co-carcinogenesis. 2004.

6. Haverkos HW, et al. Co-carcinogenesis: Human papillomaviruses, coal tar derivatives, and squamous cell cervical cancer. *Front Microbiol.* 2017; 8: 2253; Jankosky. Viruses and vitamin D. 2012;

Millegan J, Haverkos HW. What causes schizophrenia? *Research*. 2014 Nov 10; 1: 1172. doi.org/10.13070/rs.en.1.1172.

Appendix A

1. Gregg M. *Field Epidemiology*, third edition. Oxford University Press, 2008. 87.

Appendix B

1. Gregg M. *Field Epidemiology*, third edition. Oxford University Press, 2008. 87.

Bibliography

Altman L.K. *Who Goes First? The Story of Self-Experimentation in Medicine*, Random House, New York, 1987.
Amdur M.O., et al. *Casarett and Doull's Toxicology: Basic Science of Poisons* (4th edition), Pergamon Press, New York, 1991.
American Academy of Pediatrics. *Substance Abuse: A Guide for Health Professionals*, American Academy of Pediatrics, Elk Grove Village, Illinois, 1988.
American College of Physicians. "Medical Knowledge Self-Assessment Program 17: Infectious Diseases," ACP, 2015.
American Psychiatric Association. *Diagnostic and Statistical Manual of Mental Disorders* (4th edition) [DSM-IV], APA, Washington, D.C., 1994.
Ammann A.J. *Women, HIV, and the Church: In Search of Refuge*, Cascade Books, Eugene, Oregon, 2012.
Arguin P.M., et al. "Health Information of International Travel 2005–2006," U.S. Department of Health and Human Services, Elsevier Mosby, 2005.
Aschengrau A., and Seage G.R., III. *Essentials of Epidemiology in Public Health* (2nd edition), Jones and Bartlett Publishers, Sudbury, Massachusetts, 2008.
Barnett T., and W. Whiteside. *AIDS in the Twenty-First Century: Disease and Globalization*, Palgrave Macmillan, New York, 2002.
Bartlett J.G. *Pocket Book of Infectious Disease Therapy*, Williams & Wilkins, Baltimore, 1997.
Bartlett J.G., Redfield R.R., and Pham P.A. *Medical Management of HIV Infection*, Knowledge Source Solutions, Durham, NC, 2013.
Battjes R.J., and Pickens R.W. "Needle Sharing Among Intravenous Drug Abusers: National and International Perspectives," NIDS Research Monograph 80, U.S. Department of Health and Human Services, 1988.
Bayer R., and Oppenheimer G.M. *AIDS Doctors: Voices from the Epidemic*, Oxford University Press, Oxford, 2000.
Carter D. *Stonewall: The Riots that Sparked the Gay Revolution*, St. Martin's Griffin, New York, 2004.
Chin J. *The AIDS Pandemic: The Collision of Epidemiology with Political Correctness*, Radcliffe Publishing, Oxford, 2007.
Ciraulo D.A., and Shader R.I. *Clinical Manual of Chemical Dependence*, American Psychiatric Press, Inc., Washington, D.C., 1991.
Colton T. *Statistics in Medicine*, Little, Brown and Company, Boston, 1974.
Cornish D. *1980: The Emergence of HIV*, BookBaby, 2018.
Crewdson J. *Science Fictions: A Scientific Mystery, a Massive Cover-Up, and the Dark Legacy of Robert Gallo*, Little, Brown and Company, Boston, 2002.
Crichton M. *The Andromeda Strain*, Vintage, New York, 1969.
Culshaw R.V. *The Real AIDS Epidemic: How the Tragic HIV Mistake Threatens Us All* (2nd edition). Skyhorse Publishing, New York, 2023.
Darwin C. *The Voyage of the Beagle*, P.F. Collier, New York, 1937.

Bibliography

De Cock K.M., Jaffe H.W., and Curran J.W. *Dispatches from the AIDS Pandemic: A Public Health Story*, Oxford University Press, Oxford, 2023.

Duesberg P.H. *AIDS: Virus- or Drug-Induced? Contemporary Issues in Genetics and Evolution*, Volume 5, Kluwer Academic Publishers, Dordrecht, Netherlands, 1996.

Duesberg P.H. *Inventing the AIDS Virus*, Regnery Publishing, Washington, D.C., 1996.

Eng T.R., and Butler W.T. *The Hidden Epidemic: Confronting Sexually Transmitted Diseases* (summary), National Academy Press, Washington, D.C., 1997.

Evans A.S., and Kaslow R.A. *Viral Infections of Humans: Epidemiology and Control* (4th edition), Plenum Medical Book Company, New York, 1997.

Fauci A.S. et al. *Harrison's Principles of Internal Medicine* (17th edition), McGraw-Hill Medical, New York, 2008.

Finkelstein D.M., and Schoenfeld D.A. *AIDS Clinical Trials: Guidelines for Design and Analysis*, Wiley-Liss, New York, 1995.

Fumento M. *The Myth of Heterosexual AIDS: How a Tragedy Has Been Distorted by the Media and Partisan Politics*, Basic Books, New York, 1990.

Gallo R. *Virus Hunting: AIDS, Cancer and the Human Retrovirus: A Story of Scientific Discovery*, Basic Books, New York, 1991.

Garrett L. *The Coming Plague: Newly Emerging Diseases in a World Out of Balance*, Farrar, Straus and Giroux, New York, 1994.

Gilbert D.N. et al. *The Sanford Guide to Antimicrobial Therapy* (28th edition), Antimicrobial Therapy, Hyde Park, Vermont, 1998.

Giraldo G. et al. *AIDS and Associated Cancers in Africa*, Karger, Basel, 1988.

Giraldo G. et al. *Antibiotics and Chemotherapy*, Volume 38. "Recent Advances in AIDS and Kaposi's Sarcoma," Karger, Basel, 1987.

Giraldo G. et al. *Antibiotics and Chemotherapy*, Volume 48. "Development and Applications of Vaccines and Gene Therapy in AIDS," Karger, Basel, 1996.

Gregg M. *Field Epidemiology* (3rd edition), Oxford University Press, Oxford, 2008.

Groopman J. *The Measure of Our Days: A Spiritual Exploration of Illness*, Penguin Books, New York, 1997.

Gullotta T.P. et al. *Adolescent Sexuality*, Sage Publications, Newbury Park, California, 1993.

Gyanes R.P. *Germ Theory: Medical Pioneers in Infectious Diseases*, ASM Press, Washington, D.C., 2011.

Harden V.A. *AIDS at 30: A History*, Potomac Books, Washington, D.C., 2012.

Haverkos H.W. *On the Front Lines of the AIDS Pandemic*, Lambert Academic Publishing, Saarbrücken, Germany, 2012.

Haverkos H.W., and Dougherty J.A. "Health Hazards of Nitrite Inhalants: NIDA Research Monograph 83," U.S. Department of Health and Human Services, Public Health Service, Washington, D.C., 1988.

Hoeprich P.D. *Infectious Diseases: A Modern Treatise of Infectious Processes* (2nd edition), Harper & Row, Hagerstown, MD, 1977.

Hooper E. *The River: A Journey to the Source of HIV and AIDS*, Little, Brown and Company, Boston, 1999.

Hulley S.B., and Cummings S.R. *Designing Clinical Research*, Williams & Wilkins, Baltimore, 1988.

Institute of Medicine. *Confronting AIDS: Directions for Public Health, Health Care, and Research*, National Academy Press, Washington, D.C., 1986.

Institute of Medicine. *Scaling Up Treatment for the Global AIDS Pandemic: Challenges and Opportunities*, National Academies Press, Washington, D.C., 2005.

Joseph S.C. *Dragon Within the Gates: The Once and Future AIDS Epidemic*, Carroll & Graf Publishers, Inc., New York, 1992.

Kalichman S. *Denying AIDS: Conspiracy Theories, Pseudoscience, and Human Tragedy*, Springer, New York, 2009.

Kaslow R.A., and Francis D.P. *The Epidemiology of AIDS: Expression, Occurrence, and Control of Human Immunodeficiency Virus Type 1 Infection*, Oxford University Press, Oxford, 1989.

Bibliography

Kearney B. et al. *Project Inform: The HIV Drug Book*, Pocket Books, New York, 1995.
Kennedy R.F., Jr. *The Real Anthony Fauci: Bill Gates, Big Pharma, and the Global War on Democracy and Public Health*, Skyhorse Publishing, New York, 2021.
Kinsey A.C. et al. *Sexual Behavior in the Human Female*, W.B. Saunders Company, Philadelphia, 1953.
Kinsey A.C. et al. *Sexual Behavior in the Human Male*, W.B. Saunders Company, Philadelphia, 1948.
Klaassen C.D., and Watkins J.B., III. *Casarett and Doull's Essentials of Toxicology*, McGraw-Hill, New York, 2003.
Knobler S. et al. Institute of Medicine. "Considerations for Viral Disease Eradication: Lessons Learned and Future Strategies," National Academy Press, Washington, D.C., 2002.
Kontaratos N. *Dissecting a Discovery: The Real Story of How the Race to Uncover the Causes of AIDS Turned Scientists Against Disease, Politics Against Science, Nation Against Nation*, Xlibris, Bloomington, IN, 2006.
Kramer L. *Faggots*, Random House, New York, 1978.
Kramer L. *The Normal Heart*, Samuel French, London, 1985.
Krause R.M. *Emerging Infections*, Academic Press, San Diego, 1998.
Krause R.M. *The Restless Tide: The Persistent Challenge of the Microbial World*, National Foundation for Infectious Diseases, 1981.
Kucer A. et al. *The Use of Antibiotics: A Clinical Review of Antibacterial, Antifungal and Antiviral Drugs* (5th edition), Butterworth-Heinemann, Oxford, 1997.
Kulstad R., ed. The American Association for the Advancement of Science. AIDS 1988: AAAS symposia papers, AAAS Publication No. 88-19, AAAS, Washington D.C., 1988.
Kurian G.T., ed. *A Historical Guide to the U.S. Government*, Oxford University Press, Oxford, 1998.
Lauritsen J. *The AIDS War: Propaganda, Profiteering and Genocide from the Medical-Industrial Complex*, Asklepios, New York, 1993.
Leibowitch J. *A Strange Virus of Unknown Origin*, Ballantine Books, New York, 1985.
Ma P., and Armstrong D. *The Acquired Immune Deficiency Syndrome and Infections of Homosexual Men*, Yorke Medical Books, USA, 1984.
Mandell G.L. et al. *Principles and Practice of Infectious Diseases* (5th edition), Churchill Livingstone, Philadelphia, 2000.
Masters W.H. et al. *Crisis: Heterosexual Behavior in the Age of AIDS*, Grove Press, New York, 1988.
McCormick J.B., and Fisher-Hoch S. *Virus Hunters of the CDC: Level 4*, Barnes & Noble Books, New York, 1996.
Michael G.T. et al. *Sex in America: A Definitive Survey*, Little, Brown and Company, Boston, 1994.
Miller H.G. et al. National Research Council. *AIDS: The Second Decade*, National Academy Press, Washington, D.C., 1990.
Montagnier L. *Virus: The Co-Discoverer of HIV Tracks Its Rampage and Charts the Future*, W.W. Norton & Company, Inc., London, 2000.
Mukkerjee S. *The Emperor of All Maladies: A Biography of Cancer*, Scribner's, New York, 2010.
Mullan F. *Plagues and Politics: The Story of the United States Public Health Service*, Basic Books, New York, 1989.
Myerson B.E. et al. *Ready to Go: The History and Contributions of U.S. Public Health Advisors*, American Social Health Association, Research Triangle Park, NC, 2008.
Nelson K.E. et al. *Infectious Disease Epidemiology: Theory and Practice*, Jones and Bartlett, Sudbury, MA, 2004.
Pan American Health Organization. "AIDS: Profile of an Epidemic (Scientific Publication No. 514)," Pan American Health Organization, Washington, D.C., 1989.
Pan American Health Organization. "The Challenge of Epidemiology: Issues and Selected Readings (Scientific Publication No. 505)," Pan American Health Organization, Washington, D.C., 1988.
Pan American Health Organization. "The Challenge of Epidemiology: Issues and selected

readings (Scientific Publication No. 514)," Pan American Health Organization, Washington, D.C., 1989.

Pendergrast M. *Inside the Outbreaks: The Elite Medical Detectives of the Epidemic Intelligence Service.* Mariner Books, Boston, 2010.

Pepin J. *The Origins of AIDS*, Cambridge University Press, Cambridge, 2011.

Peters C.J. *Virus Hunter: Thirty Years of Battling Hot Viruses Around the World*, Anchor Books, New York, 1997.

Petrow S. et al. *Ending the HIV Epidemic: Community Strategies in Disease Prevention and Health Promotion*, Network Publications, Santa Cruz, CA, 1990.

Piot P., and Andre F. *Hepatitis B: A Sexually Transmitted Disease in Heterosexuals*, Excerpta Medica, New York, 1990.

Preston R. *The Hot Zone: A Terrifying True Story*, Random House, New York, 1994.

Ratner M.S. *Crack Pipe as Pimp: An Ethnographic Investigation of Sex-for-Crack Exchanges*, Lexington Books, New York, 1993.

Remington P.L. et al. *Chronic Disease Epidemiology and Control* (3rd edition), American Public Health Association, 2010.

Robertson P.B., and Greenspan J.S. *Oral Manifestations of AIDS: Diagnosis and Management of HIV-Associated Infections*, PSG Publishing Company, Littleton, MA, 1988.

Rondanelli E.G. *AIDS Clinical and Laboratory Atlas*, Edizioni Medico-Scientifiche, Pavia, Italy, 1989.

Root-Bernstein R.C. *Rethinking AIDS: The Tragic Cost of Premature Consensus*, Free Press, 1993.

Rothman K.J., and Greenland S. *Modern Epidemiology* (2nd edition), Lippincott-Raven, Philadelphia, 1998.

Roueche B. *Eleven Blue Men, and Other Narratives of Medical Detection*, Berkley Medallion, New York, 1955.

Roueche B. *The Medical Detectives*, Pocket Books, New York, 1982.

Rozenbaum W. *"La vie est une maladie sexuellment transmissible constamment mortelle, Le Grand Livre du Mois,"* Le Club, 1999.

Schellekens H., and Horzinek M.C. *Animal Models in AIDS*, Elsevier, Amsterdam, 1990.

Shilts R. *And the Band Played On: Politics, People, and the AIDS Epidemic*, St. Martin's Press, New York, 1987.

Shilts R. *Conduct Unbecoming: Gays and Lesbians in the U.S. Military*, St. Martin's Press, New York, 1993.

Smith B.L. *American Science Policy Since World War II*, Brookings Institution, Washington, D.C., 1990.

Szentivanyi A., and Friedman H. *Viruses, Immunity, and Immunodeficiency*, Plenum Press, New York, 1986.

Tolstoy L. *War and Peace*, Translated by Louise & Aylmer Maude, Wordsworth Classics, Hertfordshire, 1993.

Turner C.F., Miller H.G., and Moses L.E. National Research Council. *AIDS: Sexual Behavior and Intravenous Drug Abuse*, National Academy Press, Washington, D.C., 1989.

Verghese A. *My Own Country: A Doctor's Story*, Vintage Books, New York, 1994.

Index

AIDS Clinical Trials Group (ACTG) 3, 178
Auerbach, David 25, 32, 57, 123
AZT (azidothymidine, zidovudine) 3, 157, 173, 180–183, 188, 189

Barre-Sinoussi, Francois 70
Bayer, Ronald 158
Bregman, Dennis 123
Broder, Sam 177, 180–181
Brunton, T. Lauder 27, 129, 193, 218

Chang, Yuan 192
Chermann, Jean Claude 10, 62, 69, 176
Chin, James 115
Choi, Keewhan 51, 52
cryoprecipitate 40, 73
Curran, James "Jim" 8, 10, 21–22, 25–27, 31, 33–34, 38, 44–45, 54, 60–62, 75–76, 87, 97–98, 101–102, 104, 108, 110, 127, 131, 192
cytomegalovirus (CMV) 3, 11–14, 24, 27, 35, 44–45, 50, 61–62, 102, 108, 112, 125–126, 134–135, 138, 142–143, 162, 173, 176, 195–196, 216, 244

Darrow, William "Bill" 30–32, 57
Drotman, Peter 36, 38, 122–123
Duesberg, Peter 130, 191

Edelman, Robert "Bob" 136–137, 139–142, 149, 164, 169–170, 174, 178, 183–184
Epidemic Intelligence Service (EIS) 2–3, 8, 18, 20, 97–98, 167
Epstein, Jay 67, 70
Essex, Max 59–60, 119
Evatt, Bruce 71, 75–76

Fauci, Anthony "Tony" 129, 135, 143–144, 161, 178, 181–182
Feorino, Paul 60–61, 63–65
Francis, Donald "Don" 60–61, 77

Gallo, Robert "Bob" 59, 61, 64–70, 81, 129, 135, 138, 142–144, 151, 164, 177, 186, 191
gay marriage 155
Giraldo, Gaetano 24, 27, 61–62, 68–69, 108, 125, 195–196
Gottlieb, Michael 26–27, 40, 51, 63–64, 69, 177, 205
Guinan, Mary 37–38, 41, 123

Haverkos, Lynne 62, 111, 137, 228
Health Hazards of Nitrite Inhalants 186–187
hemophilia 33, 39–40, 42, 45–46, 56–58, 62, 68, 71–74, 76–78, 80–84, 101, 103, 123, 126, 169, 219
hepatitis B virus 3, 18, 72, 75–76, 79, 83–84, 86, 96, 105, 124
herpes simplex virus, type 1 (HSV-1) 4, 53, 192, 194–196, 199, 201–202, 220, 231, 235
Ho, Monto 12–13
HPA-23 173, 176–178, 188
human herpesvirus type 8 (HHV-8) 4, 53, 192, 194–196, 199, 201–202, 220, 231, 235
human immunodeficiency virus 67, 119, 197, 227

Institut Pasteur, Paris, France 62, 67, 69–70, 174, 176
interferon 8, 13–16, 99, 135–138, 176

Jaffe, Harold 26, 30–31, 44, 47, 49, 51–52, 122–123, 125, 127, 149, 151, 159–160, 191–192, 215
Jordan, William "Bill" 141–142, 163
Juranek, Dennis 21, 34, 37, 122, 132

Kaposi, Moricz 24, 193
Kaslow, Richard 137, 141, 149–151
Kinsey, Alfred 146–148
Koch, Robert 7, 63, 65, 144, 185, 202–205, 207, 222–223, 227, 235
Kramer, Larry 131, 138, 157

275

Index

Krause, Richard "Dick" 98–100, 109, 137–138, 140–141, 143, 146, 149–150, 157, 162

LaMontagne, John 178, 184
Langmuir, Alexander 20, 167–168
latency period 71, 76, 78–79, 81, 119, 161–162, 183
Lawrence, Dale 1–2, 71–72, 74, 76, 78–79, 81
Lui, Kong-Jung "KJ" 79

Mann, Jonathan 11–112, 115–116
Masur, Henry 34, 134–136, 140
Millstein, Richard 191
Mitsuya, Hiroaki "Mitch" or "Ron" 177, 180–181
Montagnier, Luc 68–70, 119, 130, 186
Moss, Andrew 128

Needlestick Study 89, 93
Ngali, Bosenga 111
nitrite inhalants 11, 27, 29, 35, 51, 52, 55, 122–130, 140–141, 162, 186–188, 190–193, 197–201, 216–220, 231
Nobel Prize in Physiology or Medicine 7, 70
Nzilambi, Eugene 111

Oleske, James 44
opportunistic infection 4, 8, 14, 16, 19, 22–23, 33, 35–36, 40–44, 46, 53, 72, 97, 100–102, 108, 110–112, 114, 123, 126, 128, 131, 134, 136–138, 140, 142–143, 161, 173, 176, 180, 198, 205, 216, 218, 220, 234, 238

Pape, Jean 99–100, 104, 107
Parasitic Diseases Drug Service 131
pentamidine 13, 22, 71, 131–135, 137, 174

Pickens, Roy 183, 222–223
Pickworth, Wallace "Wally" 224
Pinsky, Paul 10, 123
Piot, Peter 109–110
Polk, Frank 164–165, 186, 191
Projet SIDA 110–112, 115, 149

Quinn, Thomas 98, 109–110, 113, 171

Redfield, Robert 163–166, 182
Ribner, Bruce 7–8, 18
Rogers, Martha 31, 45
Rothman, Kenneth 7, 185, 202–203, 210–211, 215, 220, 235
Rozenbaum, Willy 176–177

Saah, Al 98, 137, 141
Sencer, David 57, 156
Shands, Kathy 22, 24–25
Stonewall Inn 146, 148
suramin 177–178

Thomas, Polly 25, 39, 45
Tramont, Edmund "Ed" 163, 165–167, 222

universal precautions 85, 95–96

White, Ryan 90–91, 94
Wilson, Hank 187–188, 191–192
Winkelstein, Warren 150–151, 160, 223–224
World Health Organization 1, 5, 62, 105, 108, 113, 117, 225, 227, 234

Yarchoan, Bob 177, 180–181

zur Hausen, Harald 70, 223

www.ingramcontent.com/pod-product-compliance
Ingram Content Group UK Ltd.
Pitfield, Milton Keynes, MK11 3LW, UK
UKHW041930140426
5217IPUK00014B/393